Maurice C. Haddad (Ed.), Mohamed E. Abd El Bagi, Jean C. Tamraz (Co-eds.)

Imaging of Parasitic Diseases

Maurice C. Haddad (Editor)
Mohamed E. Abd El Bagi, Jean C. Tamraz (Co-editors)

Imaging of Parasitic Diseases

Foreword by Albert L. Baert

With 426 Figures, 37 in Colour and 28 Tables and Boxes

Springer

Maurice C. Haddad, MD, FRCR
Department of Diagnostic Radiology
American University of Beirut Medical Center
P.O. Box 11-0236
Beirut
Lebanon

Mohamed E. Abd El Bagi, FFRRCSI, FRCR
Radiology and Imaging Department 920W
Riyadh Military Hospital
P.O. Box 7897
Riyadh 11159
Kingdom of Saudi Arabia

Jean C. Tamraz, MD, PhD
CHU Hotel-Dieu de France
P.O. Box 16-6830
Beirut
Lebanon

Library of Congress Control Number: 2007933310

ISBN 978-3-540-49353-2 Springer Berlin Heidelberg New York

Springer is a part of Springer Science+Business Media
springer.com

Editor: Dr. Ute Heilmann, Heidelberg, Germany
Desk Editor: Wilma McHugh, Heidelberg, Germany
Reproduction, typesetting and production: LE-TEX Jelonek, Schmidt & Vöckler GbR, Leipzig, Germany
Cover design: Frido Steinen-Broo, EStudio, Calamar, Spain

Printed on acid-free paper 24/3180/YL 5 4 3 2 1 0

Dedication

This book is dedicated to our parents, families, teachers, and residents.

M.C. Haddad
M.E. Abd El Bagi
J.C. Tamraz

I dedicate this book to my great teachers Professor Rafic Melhem (†), Professor Ghassan Rizk (†), and Dr. Chahine Abou Sleiman from Lebanon, and to Professor Kenneth Evans and Professor Geraint Roberts from the UK.

To my wife Roula, my son Rodrigue, and my daughter Tamara.

M.C. Haddad

To the soul of my mother, who wished me maximal success; to my father, the symbol of integrity; to my wife for everlasting support; and to my children, who are my beacons of hope.

M.E. Abd El Bagi

To my wife Claire, and my daughters Caroline and Eve.

J.C. Tamraz

Foreword

This volume offers a comprehensive overview of modern radiological imaging in patients with parasitic diseases. Its contents systematically cover all body organs. Each topic is introduced by concise but essential information about the pathogens, epidemiology, mode of transmission, pathology, clinical symptoms and laboratory diagnosis to be followed by a complete description of imaging features including classical X-ray as well as the modern cross-sectional techniques such as US, CT and MRI. Numerous excellent illustrations are available as well as tables summarizing key features and relevant clinical data for differential diagnosis.

The editor, Maurice C. Haddad, and the co-editors, Jean C. Tamraz and Mohamed E. Abd El Bagi, are assisted by a group of internationally well known experts in the field of radiological imaging of infectious diseases, particularly parasitic infections. I would like to congratulate the editors of this superb work which is a most welcome and much needed update of our knowledge on radiological imaging of parasitic diseases. It will fill a specific gap in the medical literature.

I am convinced that it will be of great interest for radiologists worldwide. Indeed, due to our actual lifestyle, frequent travelling as well as migration of the population, parasitic diseases are no longer primarily confined to some geographical areas of the world.

This work is highly recommended not only to radiologists but also to other clinicians involved in the management of patients with infectious diseases.

Albert L. Baert

Preface

The idea of publishing a book came into my mind (M.C.H.) when a few years ago I submitted a manuscript entitled "Imaging of Parasitic Diseases of the Hepatobiliary System" for publication in the major prestigious radiology journals. The manuscript was rejected, but an anonymous reviewer commented that the manuscript would be more suitable for publication as a chapter in a book. I took up the challenge and began the search for co-editors and authors to write other chapters. At this point, I would like to thank the reviewer for giving me the idea and throwing down the challenge.

The aim of this book is to introduce the concept of "Imaging of Infection," which includes bacterial, viral, fungal, and parasitic infections. The concept of "Tropical Radiology" is no longer valid; the term is actually a misnomer that has been propagated by generations of the medical profession for many years. This volume is limited to the description of the imaging findings of parasitic diseases only. Parasitic diseases are not confined only to the tropical and subtropical areas; indeed, they are increasing worldwide because of travel, immunosuppression, and other behavioral and living deficiencies, especially poor hygiene and sanitation. Some of these diseases are prevalent or clustered in poor or developing countries, but the majority are encountered worldwide, even in industrialized and developed countries.

In the radiologic bibliography, there is a shortage of books on the subject of "Imaging of Infection." This book is intended to partly rectify this shortfall and is aimed at radiologists all over the world.

Maurice C. Haddad
Mohamed E. Abd El Bagi
Jean C. Tamraz

Acknowledgements

It is obvious that this volume could not have been put together without the significant contributions of several friends and colleagues who provided material and images for illustration, citing Dr. Nabil Khoury, Prof. Halim Saad, Prof. Fadi Mourad, Prof. Ala' Sharara, Dr. Ghina Birjawi, Dr. Nadim Kanj, Dr. Claire Outin-Tamraz, Dr. Salam Koussa, Prof. Nuha Nuwayri-Salti, Prof. Mukbil Hourani, Dr. Zaher Chakhachiro, Dr. Ayman Tawil, Dr. Bassam Sammak, and Dr. Nabil Ammouri from Lebanon; Dr. Said Huwayjeh and Dr. Fayez Sandouk from Syria; Dr. Mohammad Al-Karawi, Dr. A.E. Mohamed, Dr. A. Haleem, Dr. A. Saeed, Dr. Mohamad Al Thagafi, Dr. Mona Al Shahed, Dr. Mohammad Al Mutairi, Dr. A. Muntashri, Dr. F. El Zein, Dr. A. Al Onazi, Dr. F. Hamid, Dr. A. Shaaban, Dr. M. Babiker, Dr. Jawda Nabulsi, and Dr. Mohamed El Sheikh from Saudi Arabia; Dr. Antonio Menezes da Silva from Portugal; Dr. Leandro Tavares Lucato, Dr. Lidia Mayumi Nagae Pœtscher, and Dr. Dany Jasinowodolinski from Brazil; Prof. Elias Melhem, Prof. Philip Goodman, Prof. Gordon Gamsu, and Prof. Edward Patz from the United States; Dr. Sung-Jong Hong from Korea; Dr. Fortunato Juarez from Mexico, and Prof. Thomas Franquet from Spain.

The material has been collected over the past 20 years from major medical institutions in the Middle East and the USA.

Special thanks go to Mrs. Leila Mushantaf, Mrs. Lilian Rizk Nabhan, and Mrs. Rosario Miraflor Reyes for their secretarial assistance and typing of the manuscripts; to Mrs. Aida Farha, Reference Librarian at the Saab Medical Library of the American University of Beirut for her valuable help in the literature search; the staff of the Department of Medical Illustration at Riyadh Armed Forces Hospital; Mr. Hasan Nisr from the Department of Medical Photography at the American University of Beirut; and Mr. Ziad Sourani from the Department of Diagnostic Radiology at the American University of Beirut Medical Center.

The editors are deeply indebted to the authors for writing excellent chapters – without their dedication to academic excellence this book would not exist; and to our residents Dr. Mohammad Arabi, Dr. Gisèle Ishak, Dr. Shukri Loutfi, Dr. Mayssoun Mehanna, Dr. Charif Sidani, Dr. Lara Nassar for gathering information from medical records and helping in the preparation of the manuscript.

The editors express their sincere gratitude to the publisher Springer-Verlag, especially Dr. Ute Heilmann and her co-workers, Mrs. Wilma McHugh, Mrs. Anne Strohbach, and Ms. Paula Francis, for their unlimited help and assistance during the preparation and publication of this book.

Finally, the editors respectfully thank and extend their deep appreciation to Professor Albert Baert, Editor-in-Chief of the journal European Radiology, for kindly agreeing to write the foreword of this book.

Contents

List of Contributors

Mohamed E. Abd El Bagi, FFRRCSI, FRCR
Radiology and Imaging Department 920W
Riyadh Military Hospital
P.O. Box 7897
Riyadh 11159
Kingdom of Saudi Arabia

Ghassan N. Al Awar, MD
Division of Infectious and Tropical Diseases
Department of Internal Medicine
American University of Beirut Medical Center
P.O. Box 11-0236
Beirut
Lebanon

Jorge A. Carrillo, MD
Universidad Nacional de Colombia
Avenida 9 #138–45
Bogota
Colombia

Tarek A. El-Diasty, MD
Department of Radiology
Urology and Nephrology Center
Mansoura University
Mansoura
Egypt

Ahmad Farouk El-Sherbiny, MD
Department of Radiology
Urology and Nephrology Center
Mansoura University
Mansoura
Egypt

Maurice C. Haddad, MD, FRCR
Department of Diagnostic Radiology
American University of Beirut Medical Center
P.O. Box 11-0236
Beirut
Lebanon

Roula G. Hourani, MD
Department of Diagnostic Radiology
American University of Beirut Medical Center
P.O. Box 11-0236
Beirut
Lebanon

Santiago Martinez, MD
Duke University Medical Center
Box 3808
Durham, NC 27705
USA

Carlos S. Restrepo, MD
University of Texas Health Science Center at San Antonio
Mail Code 7800, 7703 Floyd Curl Drive
San Antonio, TX 78229
USA

Jean C. Tamraz, MD, PhD
CHU Hotel-Dieu de France
P.O. Box 16-6830
Beirut
Lebanon

Chapter

Introduction

1

Maurice C. Haddad

Contents

1.1 Definition of Parasitosis

Parasitosis or zoonosis is a term used to describe a disease in animals that may be accidentally transmitted to humans.

1.2 Classification of Parasites

Table 1.1 shows the classification of parasites.

1.3 Modes of Transmission

Humans acquire parasitic diseases by ingesting infested raw or undercooked foods, or by drinking contaminated water or fluids, or by skin bites and cutaneous penetration (Table 1.1).

1.4 Clinical Aspects

The symptomatology of parasitic diseases depends on the site of infection or organ involvement; the symptoms are often nonspecific.

For parasitic diseases that affect the central nervous system the clinical manifestations are often nonspecific and depend on the type and location of the lesions; however, the frequently encountered symptoms are fever, headache, seizure, and neurologic deficit.

For parasitic diseases of the lungs the chief complaints are frequently fever, coughing, chest pain, and hemoptysis. Zoonoses that are associated with pulmonary abnormalities on a chest radiograph and blood eosinophilia include: toxocariasis, ascariasis, strongyloidiasis, schistosomiasis, filariasis, ankylostomiasis, and paragonimiasis, the so-called Loeffler's syndrome, or eosinophilic pneumonia.

For parasitic diseases of the liver, spleen, and biliary tree, the frequently encountered signs are hepatosplenomegaly, cholangitis, jaundice, and abnormal liver function tests. Parasitic diseases that are associated with fever and hepatosplenomegaly with or without lymph node enlargement include visceral leishmaniasis, acquired disseminated toxoplasmosis, malaria, toxocariasis, schistosomiasis (Katayama syndrome), and trypanosomiasis.

Gastrointestinal tract involvement is characterized by abdominal pain, diarrhea, weight loss, and anemia. Parasitic diseases associated with diarrhea include protozoan diseases without evidence of blood hypereosinophilia such as amebiasis, giardiasis, *Cryptosporidium* and *Microsporidium* species in immunocompromised patients, and helminthic diseases such as ascariasis, enterobiasis, taeniasis, hookworms, strongyloidiasis, and schistosomiasis with evidence of blood hypereosinophilia (Bourée and Bisaro 2007).

Parasitic diseases associated with peripheral blood eosinophilia include most of the helminthic infections such as schistosomiasis, strongyloidiasis, toxocariasis, trichinosis, filariasis, echinococcosis, cysticercosis, dicrocoeliasis, fascioliasis, gnathostomiasis, *A. suum*, pentastomiasis, ankylostomiasis, anisakiasis, capillariasis, dracunculiasis, loiasis, taeniasis, trichuriasis, and onchocerciasis. The eosinophils act as parasite killers. Parasitic diseases associated with anemia include: malaria, visceral leishmaniasis, giardiasis, hookworms (*Ancylostoma duodenale* and *Necator americanus*), trichuriasis, diphyllobothriasis, babesiosis, and balantidiasis.

Table 1.1 Classification of parasites, modes of transmission, and treatment

Species	Modes of transmission					Treatment
	Meat	Fish	Water	Vegetables and soil	Skin	
A. PROTOZOA (unicellular organisms)						
Common						
Plasmodium (P. malariae, P. vivax, P. ovale, P. falciparum)					+	Quinine
Entamoeba histolytica			+			MNZ
Toxoplasma gondii	+		+			Pyrimethamine Sulfamonomethoxine
Trypanosoma cruzi					+	Nifurtimox Benznidazole
Leishmania (L. donovani, L. tropica, L. infantum)					+	Miltefosine Amphotericin B
Giardia lamblia			+			MNZ, nitazoxanide
Cryptosporidium parvum			+			Nitazoxanide
Rare						
Babesia microti	+					Atovaquone Azithromycin
Balantidium coli	+		+			Tinidazole/ Metronidazole Pimaricin/oxyteracine
B. METAZOA (multicellular organisms)						
HELMINTHS (WORMS)						
NEMATODES (ROUND WORMS)						
Common						
Ascaris lumbricoides			+			PP, ABZ, levamizole
Toxocara (T. cati, T. canis)				+		ABZ, DEC
Strongyloides stercoralis					+	TCBZ, IVM
Rare						
Ascaris suum	+					ABZ
Gnathostoma spinigerum		+				ABZ, TCBZ
Wuchereria bancrofti					+	IVM
Enterobius vermicularis			+	+		ABZ, PP
Ancylostoma duodenale					+	PP, TCBZ, MBZ
Trichuris trichiura			+	+		ABZ, MBZ

Table 1.1 *(continued)* Classification of parasites, modes of transmission, and treatment

Species	Modes of transmission					Treatment
	Meat	Fish	Water	Vegetables and soil	Skin	
Anisakis marina		+				Symptomatic treatment, TCBZ
Capillaria (*C. philippinensis, C. hepatica*)		+				ABZ
Necator americanus					+	PP, ABZ
Angiostrongylus (*A. costaricensis, A. cantonensis*)		+		+		Symptomatic treatment TCBZ, PP, ABZ
Dirofilaria (*D. immitis, D. repens*)					+	DEC
Bayliascaris procyonis			+			ABZ
Onchocerca volvulus					+	IVM, DEC
Loa loa					+	DEC
Dracunculus medinensis				+		MNZ, TCBZ
Trichinella spiralis	+					TCBZ, DEC, MBZ
Dioctophyma renale		+	+			Conservative treatment. Surgery
CESTODES (TAPE WORMS)						PZQ
Common						
Taenia (*T. solium, T. saginata, T. multiceps*)	+		+			ABZ, PZQ
Echinococcus (*E. granulosus, E. multilocularis, E. vogeli, E. oligarthrus*)			+	+		ABZ, PZQ
Rare						
Hymenolepis nana				+		Niclosamide, PZQ
Spirometra (*S. mansoni, S. erinacei*)		+	+			PZQ
Diphyllobothrium latum		+				Niclosamide, PZQ
TREMATODES (FLUKES)						
Common						
Schistosoma (*S. mansoni, S. hematobium, S. japonicum, S. mekongi*)					+	PZQ
Clonorchis sinensis		+				PZQ
Opisthorchis viverrini		+				PZQ
Fasciola hepatica				+		TCBZ, bithionol
Rare						
Dicrocoelium dendriticum	+					PZQ, mirazid
Paragonimus westermani	+	+				PZQ, bithionol
Heterophyes heterophyes		+		+	+	PZQ
Echinostoma (*E. ilocanum, E. lindoense*)		+		+	+	Niclosamide, PZQ

Table 1.1 *(continued)* Classification of parasites, modes of transmission, and treatment

Species	Modes of transmission					Treatment
	Meat	Fish	Water	Vegetables and soil	Skin	
Fasciolopsis buski		+		+	+	Niclosamide, PZQ
Metagonimus yokogawai		+		+	+	PZQ
ARTHROPODS						
Armillifer armillatus	+					IVM
Linguatula serrata	+					PZQ
Fannia canicularis	+	+		+		Disodium octaborate tetrahydrate

MNZ metronidazole, *TBZ* thiabendazole, *IVM* ivermectin, *PZQ* praziquantel, *PP* pyrantel pamoate, *TCBZ* triclabendazole, *ABZ* albendazole, *DEC* diethylcarbamazine, *MBZ* mebendazole

Table 1.2 Parasites with radiologically visible calcifications

Site of infection	Zoonosis	Imaging appearance of calcifications
Brain	Cysticercosis Toxoplasmosis Echinococcosis Paragonimiasis Sparganosis	Oval with lucent center Round Egg-shell, punctate Round Small punctate
Muscle	Cysticercosis Pentastomiasis Paragonimiasis	Oval with lucent center Comma shape Round
Urinary system	Schistosomiasis Echinococcosis	Linear Egg-shell, punctate
Subcutaneous tissues	Dracunculiasis Loiasis Onchocerciasis	Irregular coiled Thread-like coil Filamentous
Peritoneum	Pentastomiasis	Comma shape
Liver	Echinococcosis (unilocular) Echinococcosis (alveolar) Schistosomiasis (*S. japonicum*) Pentastomiasis Paragonimiasis	Egg-shell Punctate, cotton ball Linear Comma shape Round
Lungs	Paragonimiasis Cysticercosis Pentastomiasis	Round Oval with lucent center Comma shape
Colon	Schistosomiasis	Pericolonic conglomerate
Spleen	Echinococcosis Pentastomiasis	Egg-shell, punctate Comma shape

Parasitic diseases associated with cutaneous or subcutaneous lesions or nodules include: gnathostomiasis (creeping eruption), schistosomiasis (swimmer's itch or cercarial dermatitis), onchocerciasis (sowda), cutaneous leishmaniasis (Oriental sore), trypanosomiasis (trypanosomal chancre), hookworms (cutaneous larva migrans), sparganosis, dracunculiasis, loiasis (Calabar swellings), dirofilariasis (*D. repens*), strongyloidiasis, cysticercosis and dioctophymiasis (subcutaneous), cutaneous myiasis, cutaneous amebiasis, and epizoonoses caused by ectoparasites such as scabies and lice.

Parasitoses associated with radiologically demonstrable calcifications are listed in Table 1.2 (Thomas 1986).

1.5 Diagnosis

A high index of clinical suspicion is essential, as diagnosis of parasitic infection requires special sampling techniques and laboratory procedures. Definitive diagnosis is usually achieved by detecting the parasite in the patient's tissues or body fluids by histological examination or culture, or by polymerase chain reaction amplification of the parasite-specific antigen sequence. Antibody detection using serological techniques is also possible in a few parasitic infections. Certain lesions have characteristic radiological appearances, hence the value of imaging, particularly in the cerebral syndromes (Barsoum 2006).

1.6 Prevention and Treatment

There is yet no effective vaccine against human parasitic diseases. The best method of eradication/control or prevention of the parasites is breaking their lifecycles. Good hygiene and sanitation with sufficient cooking or freezing of meat or fish, thorough cleaning and disinfection of vegetables before consumption, and drinking bottled purified water are also very efficient preventive measures. Parasitic diseases are often treatable and curable diseases. Some of the useful antiparasitic drugs are listed in Table 1.1 (Nakamura-Uchiyama et al. 2003). Treatment is usually straightforward using either broad spectrum or specific drugs, yet some species are drug-resistant.

References

Barsoum RS (2006) Parasitic infections in transplant recipients. Nat Clin Pract Nephrol 2(9):490–503

Bourée P, Bisaro F (2007) Parasitic diarrhea. Presse Med 36 (4 Pt 2):706–716

Nakamura-Uchiyama F, Hiromatsu K, Ishiwata K, Sakamoto Y, Nawa Y (2003) The current status of parasitic diseases in Japan. Intern Med 42(3):222–236

Thomas AMK (1986) Radiological manifestations of parasitic disease. Br J Hosp Med 35(5):503–511

Chapter

2 Imaging of Parasitic Diseases of the Central Nervous System

Roula G. Hourani, Jean C. Tamraz

Contents

2.1 Introduction

Infections of the central nervous system (CNS), especially parasitic infections, have increased in the last decade secondary to the acquired immunodeficiency syndrome (AIDS) epidemic, immunosuppressive therapy used in treatment of cancer, and in organ transplantation. CNS infection is a life-threatening disease; the prognosis depends on early detection and the correct diagnosis of the infection, because once an intracranial infestation is established, the pathogens may produce a severe inflammatory response and serious brain damage. Although laboratory analysis of CSF and CNS biopsy is the gold standard in the identification of the pathogenic agent, neuroimaging plays a crucial role in the early and specific diagnosis of the disease. It is useful not only in the differentiation of CNS infections, relying on the visualization of typical lesion patterns and based on the anatomical compartment involved, but also in the follow-up of treatment response. Magnetic resonance imaging (MRI) is more sensitive than computed tomography (CT) scanning in the detection of focal or diffuse parenchymal lesions and vasculitic complications. Furthermore, better detection and characterization of infectious brain lesions are possible today using the advanced MRI techniques, such as diffusion-weighted imaging (DWI), perfusion-weighted imaging, and proton MR spectroscopy imaging (^{1}H-MRSI), which sometimes produce specific imaging patterns.

This chapter summarizes the epidemiology, pathology, clinical presentation, laboratory analysis, and the imaging findings of the most important parasitic diseases that affect the CNS, excluding the maxillofacial region. For those readers interested in the latter subject an excellent review in the French language and without illustrative examples by Piette (1989) is available in the medical literature. CNS parasitoses include: the group of protozoa (amebiasis, toxoplasmosis, malaria and trypanosomiasis); the group of helminth roundworms (toxacariasis, baylisascariasis, gnathostomiasis, angiostrongyliasis and trichinosis), the group of helminth tapeworms (echinococcosis, cysticercosis, coenurosis, and sparganosis), and finally the group of helminth flukes (schistosomiasis, paragonimiasis).

2.2 Protozoa

2.2.1 Amebiasis

2.2.1.1 Parasite

Amebiasis is a widespread parasitic disease caused by the protozoans *Entamoeba histolytica*, *Naegleria fowleri*, *Acanthamoeba astronyxis*, and *Balamuthia mandrillaris* (Deol at al. 2000), which are found in the mud or fresh water of lakes. It probably colonizes 10–20% of the colons of the world's population, but only a small number of patients become symptomatic (Palmer and Reeder 2001).

2.2.1.2 Mode of Contamination

The infection can occur at any age, in healthy and immunocompromised patients. Usually, humans acquire amebiasis by ingesting cysts of *E. histolytica* in contaminated food or drinking water, from swimming in the contaminated water of lakes or inhaling dust or soil with amebic cysts.

2.2.1.3 Epidemiology

It is commonest in poor developing countries of the tropics: Asia, India, East, and South Africa, and portions of Central and South America (Argentina, Brazil, Mexico, Peru, and Venezuela).

2.2.1.4 Pathology

Cerebral amebiasis is rare; it occurs in less than 1% of patients with dysenteric amebiasis. However, it is the second commonest cause of death from parasites and accounts for 4.2–8.5% of deaths due to amebiasis. *E. histolytica* or *Balamuthia* arrives in the brain by hematogenous spread from the colon through the hepatic, pulmonary or vertebral veins or ascends directly along the nasal mucosa, olfactory nerves, or after skin trauma, mainly in the case of *Balamuthia mandrillaris*, to the brain leading to vasculitis of cerebral vessels and hemorrhagic necrosis (Galarza et al. 2002; White et al. 2004). It causes meningoencephalitis with single or multiple supratentorial lesions, varying in size from microscopic to 5 cm in diameter.

2.2.1.5 Clinical Presentation

The clinical symptoms depend on the type of amebic infection:

1. In primary amebic meningoencephalitis, there is rapid progression to coma and death.
2. Granulomatous amebic encephalitis is a slow, progressive disease characterized by headache, fever, seizures, signs of increased intracranial pressure, hemiplegia, and coma; one hallmark of the disease is that many patients present with typical skin lesions for a long period before the neurological symptoms appear.

2.2.1.6 Diagnosis and Laboratory Tests

Since the imaging features of amebic abscesses are nonspecific, they should be considered in the differential diagnosis of any intracranial abscess in endemic areas, especially if it is associated with chronic granulomatous skin disorder. Diagnosis is made on culture, serology or immunofluorescence on biopsy specimens. The culture of the pus is sterile most of the time because the parasite exists in the wall of the abscess.

2.2.1.7 Imaging Findings

Amebic encephalitis involves the cerebral hemispheres, mainly the frontal lobes and basal ganglia. CT features include diffuse brain edema, hypodense brain abscess; contrast administration shows single or multiple focal, punctate, nodular or ring-enhancing masses. On MRI, T1-weighted images (WI) demonstrate a centrally hypointense mass with surrounding edema and heterogeneous or ring enhancement after intravenous injection of gadolinium. T2-WI show a central hyperintense lesion with possible hemorrhage within it, with a hypointense rim, presumably from granulation tissue, and surrounded by hyperintense edema. MRI is superior to CT in demonstrating small brain lesions. These findings are nonspecific for amebic encephalitis and cannot be differentiated from brain abscesses of any other etiology (De Villiers and Durra 1998).

2.2.1.8 Treatment

After the diagnosis has been confirmed by serologic tests, treatment by metronidazole, ketoconazole and other appropriate antiamebic medication should be started. Pentamidine, azithromycin, and some phenothiazines are novel antiamebic medications at the experimental stage (Schuster and Visvesvara 1998). In rare cases, brain biopsy is made to work out the diagnosis and the excision of the brain lesion may be curative if the process is still localized; however, in most cases amebic encephalitis presents as diffuse encephalitis with multiple brain lesions limiting the treatment by surgical excision (Deol et al. 2000; Ofori-Kwakye et al. 1986).

2.2.2 Toxoplasmosis

2.2.2.1 Parasite

Toxoplasmosis is a parasitic infection due to the protozoan *Toxoplasma gondii.*

2.2.2.2 Mode of Contamination

Humans are infected by ingestion of food or water containing oocysts shed by cats or by eating or handling undercooked or raw meat (mainly pork and lamb) containing tissue cysts. From the small intestine, dissemination to all organs occurs: brain, eye, heart, skeletal muscle, placenta, and fetus. Maternal infection acquired for the first time during gestation or a few months before gestation results in congenital transmission to the fetus.

2.2.2.3 Epidemiology

It is an infection with worldwide prevalence, and is more frequent in the tropics, warm and humid climates and areas where cats are numerous.

2.2.2.4 Pathology and Clinical Manifestations

Primary infection (including pregnant women) is asymptomatic in 90% of cases. In the remaining 10%, the clinical manifestations are nonspecific: cervical or occipital lymphadenopathy and myalgia. Rarely, patients may have myocarditis, hepatitis, pneumonitis, or encephalitis. Intrauterine infection of the fetus manifests as chorioretinitis, encephalomyelitis, hydrocephalus, and microcephaly. In immunocompetent patients, *Toxoplasma* produces chorioretinitis, infection of the CNS with formation of many foci of necrosis and vasculitis in the cortex, basal ganglia, periventricular white matter, and periaqueductal gray matter with secondary periventricular calcification that leads to the characteristic, yet not pathognomonic, radiological findings of the disease. Hydrocephalus may be present, related to obstruction of the cerebral aqueduct. In immunocompromised patients, especially AIDS patients; the brain is the site most commonly infected by *T. gondii* in 3–40% of AIDS patients, resulting in multiple brain abscesses, mainly in the basal ganglia (Luft et al. 1983; Luft and Remington 1992; Montoya and Liesenfeld 2004). Clinical manifestations of toxoplasmic encephalitis include mental status changes, seizures, focal motor or sensory abnormalities, and cerebellar signs.

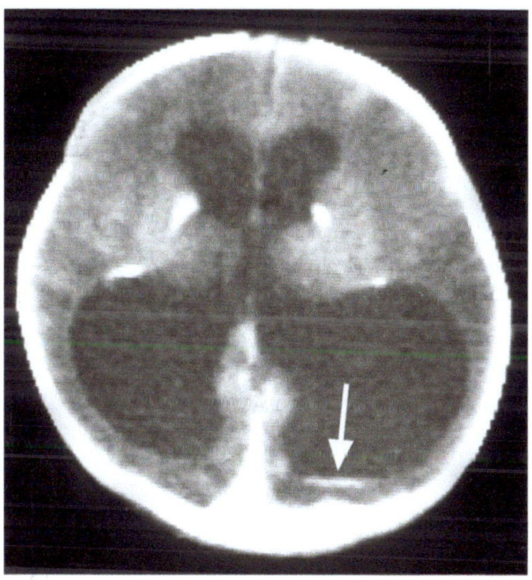

Fig. 2.1 Congenital toxoplasmosis. Axial non-enhanced CT scan of the brain shows periventricular calcifications and encephalomalacia, hydrocephalus, and intraventricular hemorrhage (*arrow*)

2.2.2.5 Diagnosis

Diagnosis can be established by direct detection of the parasite (cell culture or polymerase chain reaction [PCR] for *T. gondii* DNA) or by indirect serological techniques (Sabin-Feldman dye test, immunofluorescent antibody test, ELISA, etc.). Ophthalmologic and CSF examinations, and radiological studies are useful in the diagnosis of the congenital disease.

2.2.2.6 Imaging Findings

Congenital toxoplasmosis of the CNS manifests in the newborn as hydrocephalus, microcephaly, and scattered cerebral calcifications, mainly in the periventricular region, the basal ganglia, and the cortex (Fig. 2.1). In the adult form, CT demonstrates multiple hypo- or isodense lesions with surrounding edema and mass effect that show thin, smooth rim or solid nodular enhancement on post-contrast images. The lesions are located in the basal ganglia in 75% of cases, in the thalamus and cerebral hemispheres at the corticomedullary junction; they appear hypointense on T1-WI, hyperintense on T2 WI with evidence of ring enhancement on gadolinium-enhanced T1-WI, often with hypointense surrounding edema (Fig. 2.2). In problematic cases with atypical lesions, distinguishing toxoplasmosis from primary CNS lymphoma may be difficult and advanced MR modalities are useful in this regard. DWI shows no restriction of water diffusion in the center of the lesion, the apparent diffusion coefficient (ADC) is either equal to or greater than the normal white matter due to marked brain

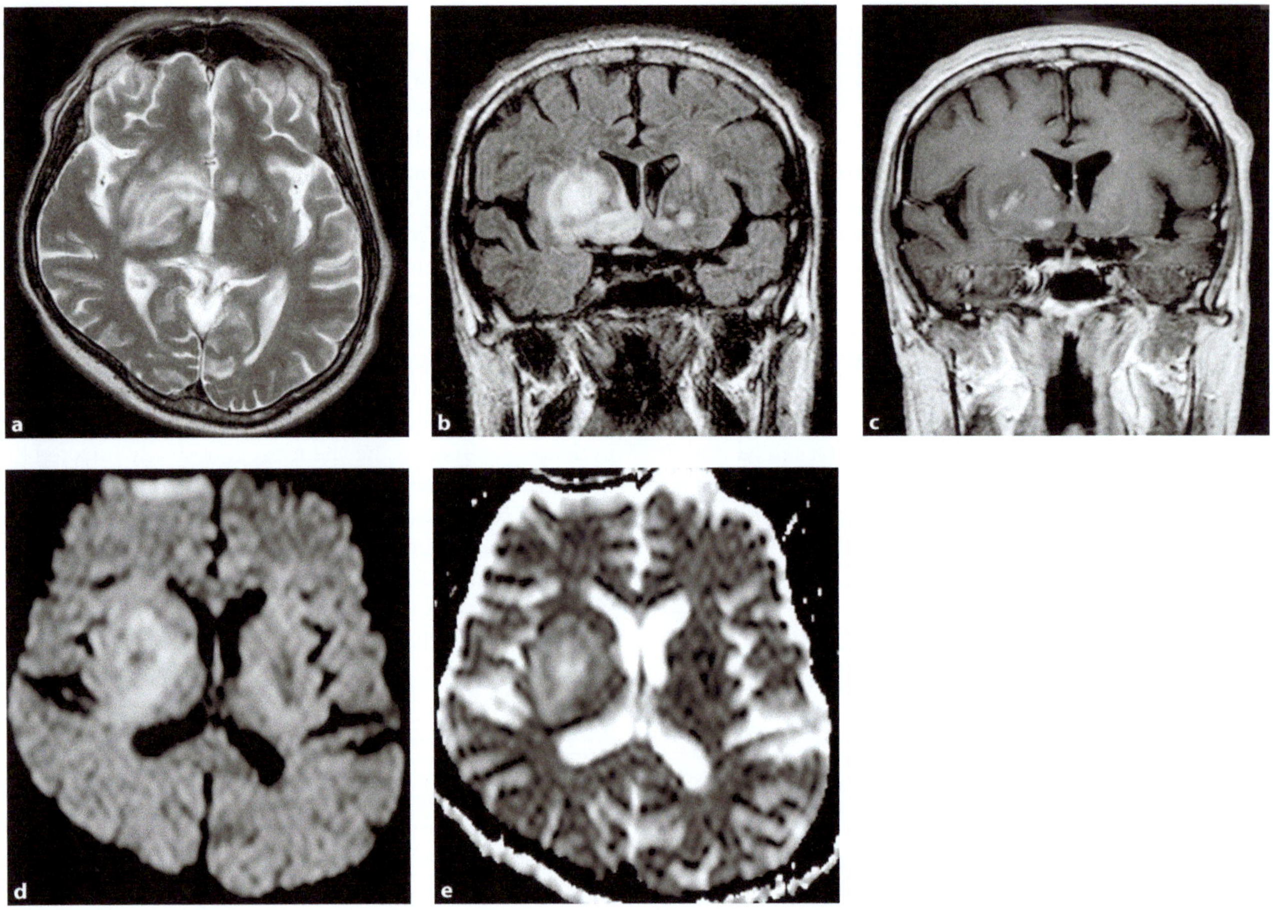

Fig. 2.2 An adult AIDS patient with toxoplasmosis. **a** Axial T2-weighted MR image. There is abnormal high signal in both basal ganglia. **b,c** Coronal FLAIR and T1-weighted gadolinium-enhanced MR images. The lesion in the right basal ganglia has irregular heterogeneous enhancement. **d** Diffusion-weighted image ($b = 1{,}000$ s/mm^2). The core of the lesion demonstrates unrestricted diffusion. **e** Apparent diffusion coefficient (ADC) map. The core of the lesion has an ADC that is increased relative to that of normal white matter

edema, in contrast to lymphoma and pyogenic abscess where the ADC is low (Fig. 2.2) (Chong-Han et al. 2003). Perfusion CT and MRI reveal decreased relative cerebral blood volume (rCBV) in *Toxoplasma* lesions and increased rCBV in lymphoma (Ernst et al. 1998). Proton MR spectroscopy is characterized by predominant lipid and lactate peaks and a decrease in all other metabolites, whereas lymphoma demonstrates a mild to moderate increase in lipid and lactate peaks, but a large increase in the choline peak. Thallium-201 brain SPECT shows marked uptake of isotope tracer in case of lymphoma, but not in *Toxoplasma* abscess (Kastrup et al. 2005). PET scan demonstrates hypometabolic lesions, in contrast to lymphoma, which looks hypermetabolic (Camacho et al. 2003). In immunocompromised patients, the differential diagnosis of toxoplasmic encephalitis includes: CNS lymphoma, progressive multifocal leukoencephalopathy (infection by JC polyomavirus virus), cytomegalovirus encephalitis and other opportunistic infections such as *Cryptococcus neoformans*, *Aspergillus*, *Mycobacterium tuberculosis*, *Nocardia* or pyogenic abscess.

2.2.2.7 Treatment

In immunocompetent hosts, the infection is self-limiting and does not require any treatment; however, if needed the combination of pyrimethamine, sulfadiazine, and folinic acid is considered the best treatment, whereas in pregnant woman with recent infection, medical treatment should be initiated as soon as possible and continued throughout pregnancy (Mandell et al. 2000; Torre et al. 1998).

2.2.3 Malaria

2.2.3.1 Parasite

Malaria is a disease secondary to human infection by one of the *Plasmodium: P. falciparum* or *P. vivax*, which are the most common, and less likely by *P. malariae* or *P. ovale*. *P. falciparum* malaria is considered the most significant human parasitic infection involving the CNS.

2.2.3.2 Mode of Contamination and Epidemiology

Malaria infects one hundred million people and two million die every year, one million in Africa alone. Malaria has worldwide prevalence, is most common and serious in the tropics and subtropics, and transmission from person to person occurs by female *Anopheles* mosquitoes and rarely during blood transfusion.

2.2.3.3 Pathology

There are different hypotheses concerning the pathogenesis of the neurological symptoms of *P. falciparum*, the parasite remains confined in the intravascular space and does not enter the brain parenchyma. One of the hypotheses is that the parazited red blood cells (PRBC) packed in the cerebral capillaries lead to obstruction of the cerebral microvasculature and impair cerebral perfusion with subsequent edema in the brain. The "permeability" hypothesis suggests that PRBC adhere to capillary endothelium and cause functional changes in the blood–brain barrier. The "toxic" hypothesis proposed that binding the PRBC to the endothelium activates the production of neuroactive mediators, cytokines, and nitric oxide that alter the neuronal function and cause serious brain complications and swelling (Gitau and Newton 2005).

2.2.3.4 Neurological Manifestations

The neurological manifestations of *P. falciparum* occur in 2% of all malaria cases, but they are not specific. Cerebral malaria is a rapidly progressive, potentially fatal complication of *P. falciparum* infection with a high mortality rate 15–40% (Muehlethaler et al. 2005). It is a diffuse encephalopathy presenting as impaired consciousness and coma. Other neurologic features include headache, agitation psychosis, and seizures.

2.2.3.5 Diagnosis

The diagnosis is made by the identification of trophozoites in thick or thin Giemsa-stained blood smears or by the dip-stick test, which is specific and sensitive. *P. falciparum* antigen (HRP-2, aldolase) can be also detected by means of an immunochromatographic assay.

2.2.3.6 Imaging Features

Malaria has a predilection to the basal ganglia and the cortex. Non-enhanced CT may demonstrate four patterns depending on the severity of the disease and the outcome:

1. Normal brain in 30–50% of cases, and it is indicative of favorable outcome (Newton et al. 1994; Patankar et al. 2002).
2. Diffuse brain edema, cytotoxic and vasogenic in origin, seen in 67% of cases, and indicates a good prognosis.
3. Diffuse cerebral edema with focal infarct and possible secondary hemorrhage in the cortex, basal ganglia, thalamus, pons or cerebellum. These infarcts are rarely seen in cerebral malaria, more frequently in children, and are secondary to severe reduction in cerebral perfusion and hypoglycemia. Four to twenty-one percent of patients have neurological sequelae, such as hemiparesis, ataxia, cortical blindness, or generalized spasticity (Brewster et al. 1990; Molyneux 2000).
4. Diffuse brain edema with symmetrical hypodensity in the thalami and cerebellum related to infarctions in the territories of the thalamoperforating and cerebellar arteries; it is seen in deeply comatose patients and correlated with a poor prognosis (100% mortality rate) (Patankar et al. 2002).

The petechial hemorrhages in the cerebrum and cerebellum constantly seen in the autopsy are not visualized on CT. MRI shows cortical and subcortical infarcts that are hypointense on T1-WI, with some high signal foci representing petechial hemorrhage; T2-WI demonstrate hyperintensity in the cortex, white matter, the basal ganglia, and cerebellum (Fig. 2.3). T2* (gradient-echo) sequence is useful for the detection of petechial hemorrhages that appear as small foci of hyposignal intensity.

2.2.3.7 Treatment

Malaria must be suspected in all febrile patients returning from areas in which malaria is endemic; therefore, a good clinical and travel history is mandatory. The treatment includes appropriate antimalarial antibiotics, together with anticonvulsant drugs and supportive therapy (Molyneux 2000). Delays in the diagnosis and treatment increase the risk of mortality and morbidity.

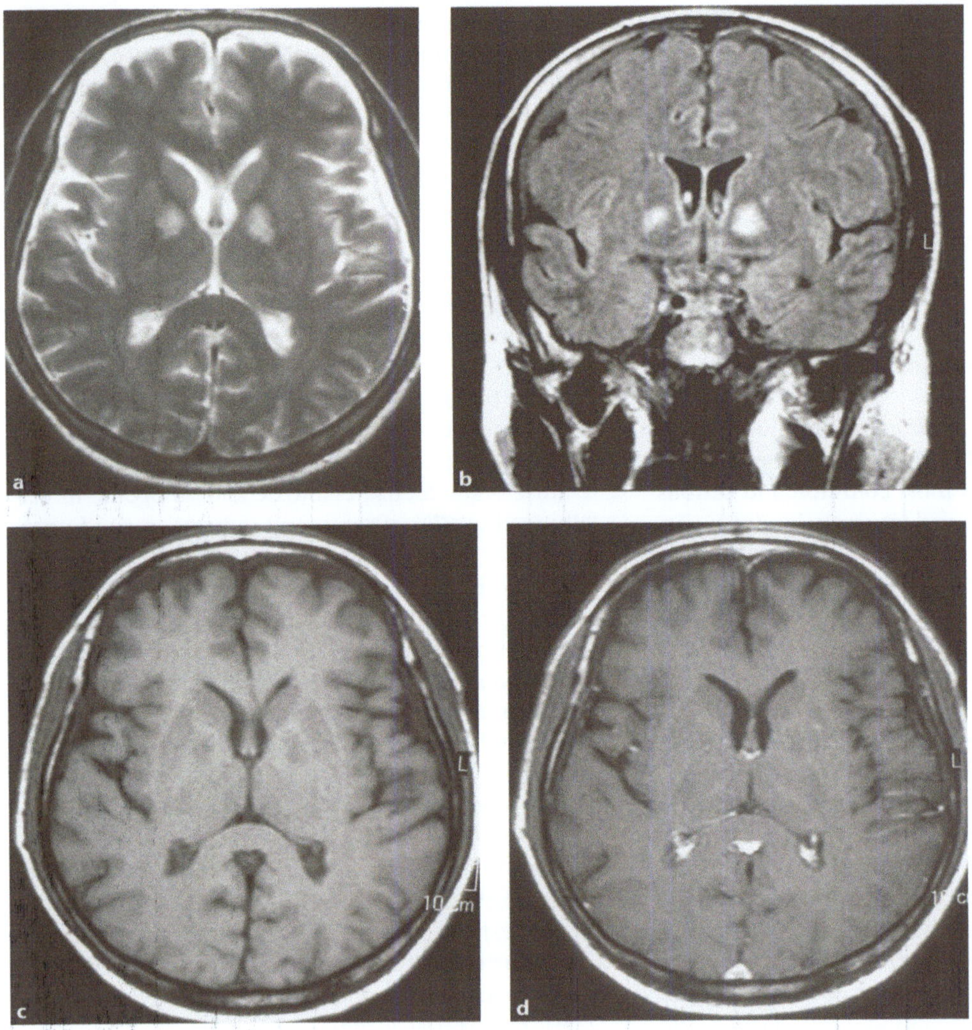

Fig. 2.3 Cerebral malaria. **a,b** Axial T2-weighted and coronal FLAIR MR images of the brain. There is abnormally high signal in the globi pallidi bilaterally. **c,d** Axial T1-weighted image pre- (**c**) and post-gadolinium enhancement (**d**). The lesions in the globi pallidi are hypointense with no evidence of abnormal enhancement

2.2.4 Trypanosomiasis

Trypanosomiasis results from infection by the parasite *Trypanosoma cruzi*. There are two types of trypanosomiasis: American trypanosomiasis (Chagas' disease) and African trypanosomiasis (sleeping sickness).

2.2.4.1 African Trypanosomiasis

2.2.4.1.1 Mode of Contamination

African trypanosomiasis is transmitted to humans by the tsetse fly.

2.2.4.1.2 Pathology

It invades the meninges, subarachnoid spaces, and Virchow-Robin spaces causing meningoencephalitis, brain edema, and congestion with secondary petechial hemorrhages.

2.2.4.1.3 Clinical Presentation

The clinical presentation includes behavioral changes, indifference, and daytime somnolence.

2.2.4.1.4 *Imaging Findings*

Brain CT scans demonstrate diffuse brain edema with scattered petechial hemorrhage (Osborn et al. 2004). A case of human African trypanosomiasis was reported by Sabbah et al. (1997), caused by *T. brucei rhodesiense*. After the febrile period of parasite dissemination, the patient had meningeal involvement, but a normal CT scan. Contrast-enhanced MRI showed thick enhancing meninges compatible with meningitis, but no abnormality in the brain parenchyma was initially detected. After two sessions of arsenical treatment, a severe drug-induced encephalopathy occurred, appearing as low-density lesions in the internal capsules on non-enhanced CT scans of the brain, and as high signal intensities in the posterior limbs of the internal capsules and middle cerebellar peduncles on T2-WI (Sabbah et al. 1997).

2.2.4.2 American Trypanosomiasis (Chagas' Disease)

2.2.4.2.1 *Mode of Contamination*

American trypanosomiasis is transmitted to humans by the reduviid bug (known as the "kissing" or "assassin" bug). The bugs live in cracks in the walls of rural houses made of mud. Man becomes infected when the infected insect bites the skin and the site becomes contaminated by the bug's feces. Transmission can also occur via blood transfusion and organ transplantation.

2.2.4.2.2 *Epidemiology*

In endemic areas, it affects poor people, and many of them contract the infection during childhood. Chagas' disease is confined to Central and South America from Texas to Argentina, particularly in Brazil, Argentina, Uruguay, and Chile.

2.2.4.2.3 *Pathology and Clinical Manifestations*

The insect bite causes severe edema, which is called "Romana's sign" when it is periorbital or "Chagoma" in other parts of the body (Deol et al. 2000). Acute infection causes fever, generalized illness, a swollen face, and conjunctivitis. In the chronic stage, the central nervous system may be involved after reactivation of the disease in immunosuppressed patients including AIDS patients where the disease could be very severe. *T. cruzi* most frequently affects the heart and gastrointestinal system with increased risk of cardioembolic stroke (9–36% of patients with Chagas' disease have cerebral infarction) (Carod-Artal et al. 2003); however, in patients with AIDS, cerebral infection is the most common form of reactivation, it causes perivascular inflammation with secondary fatal meningoencephalitis (mortality risk of 2–10%).

The meningoencephalitis syndrome includes fever, seizure, headache, focal neurological dysfunction, and signs of intracranial hypertension.

2.2.4.2.4 *Diagnosis*

The diagnosis is made by identifying the parasite and/or the antibodies to the parasite in the host's blood.

2.2.4.2.5 *Imaging Findings*

Computed tomography scanning demonstrates single or multiple ring-enhancing lesions, hypodense tumor-like lesions that enhance after contrast administration, and has also been described in AIDS patients (Palmer and Reeder 2001; Pagano et al. 1999; Yoo et al. 2004). The lesions have a nonspecific appearance and are located in the white matter, corpus callosum, deep and subcortical white matter, and the cerebellum. On MRI, they appear hypointense on T1-WI, hyperintense on T2-WI with evidence of ring enhancement on T1 post-gadolinium (Fig. 2.4). On diffusion-weighted images the lesions may demonstrate restricted diffusion (Fig. 2.4d) (Yoo et al. 2004; Lury and Castillo 2005). Hemorrhage within the lesions may be seen. Similar inflammatory lesions may occur in the spinal cord with the appearance of multiple enhancing intramedullary lesions.

Chagas' disease should be included in the differential diagnosis with lymphoma and toxoplasmosis in patients with AIDS presenting with brain lesions.

2.2.4.2.6 *Treatment*

There is no vaccine or preventive therapy for Chagas' disease. Treatment includes nifurtimox and benznidazole, both efficient when given in the acute stage of the infection. In the chronic stage, the medication is less effective (Lury and Castillo 2005).

2.3 Helminths Roundworms (Nematodes)

2.3.1 Toxocariasis

2.3.1.1 Parasite

Toxocariasis is a human helminthiasis parasitic infection with worldwide prevalence, caused by *Toxocara canis* or rarely *Toxocara cati*, the roundworms of dogs and cats respectively.

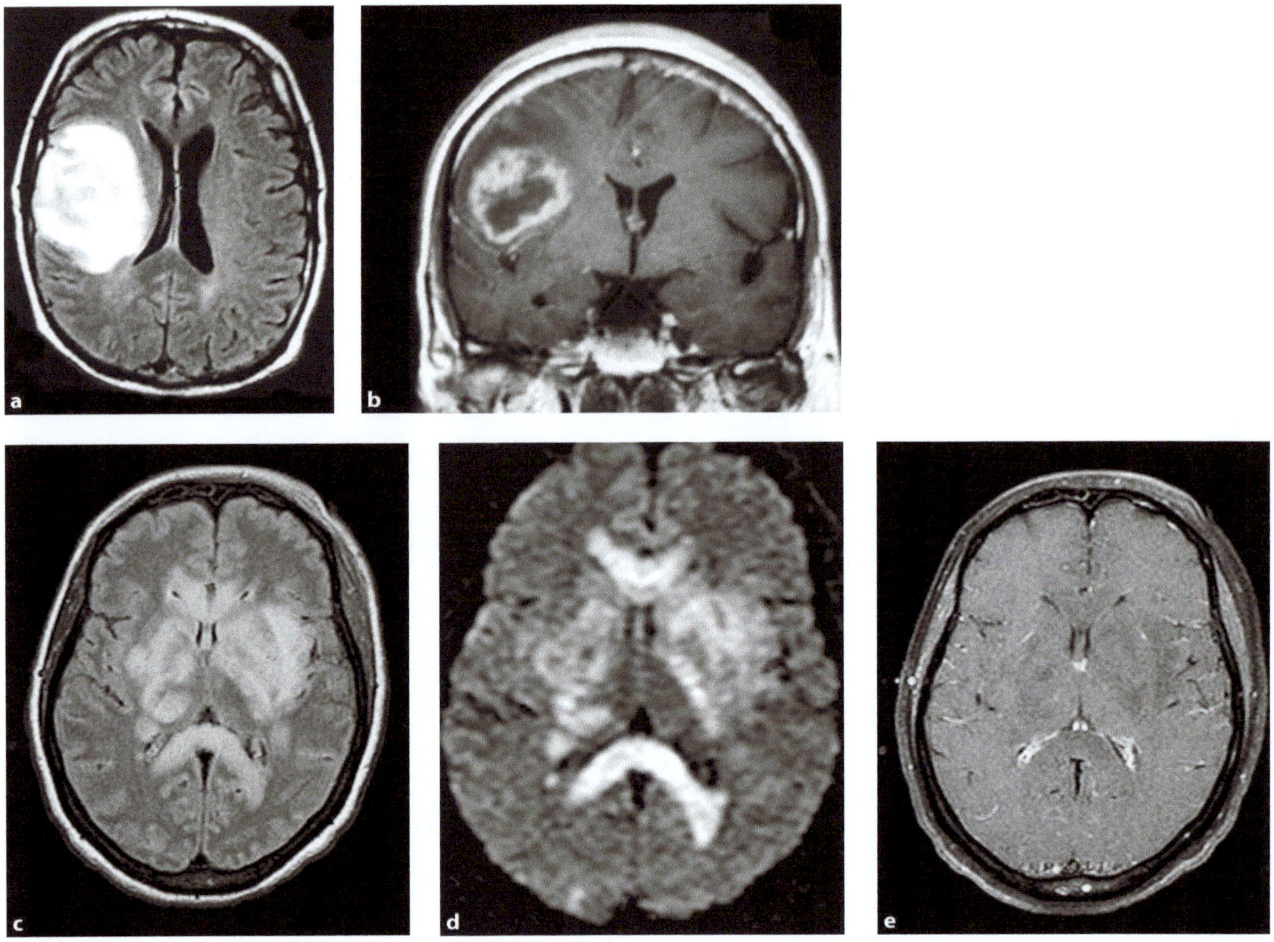

Fig. 2.4 Chagas' disease (American trypanosomiasis) **a,b** Chagas' disease reactivation in a 46-year-old man, status post-cardiac transplantation. Pseudotumoral presentation. **a** Axial FLAIR image shows a mass lesion in the right cerebral hemisphere, with peripheral edema. **b** Coronal T1 post-gadolinium image demonstrates the necrotic center with irregular enhancing border of this lesion. CSF study disclosed trypomastigote forms of *T. cruzi*. **c,d,e** Chagas' disease reactivation in a 33-year-old woman, HIV positive. Meningoencephalitic presentation. **c** Axial FLAIR image discloses multiple coalescent foci of hyperintensity, including basal ganglia, thalami, corpus callosum, and internal and external capsules. **d** Diffusion-weighted image shows restriction to water motion in these lesions, as hyperintensity. **e** Axial T1 post-gadolinium image demonstrates no significant enhancement (Courtesy of Drs Leandro Tavares Lucato and Lidia Mayumi Nagae Poetscher, Department of Radiology of the Clinics Hospital of the University of Sao Paolo, School of Medicine, Sao Paolo, Brazil)

2.3.1.2 Mode of Contamination

Humans are infected by oral ingestion of infected eggs of *T. canis* via regular contact with dogs and cats, consumption of noncooked vegetables or undercooked giblets. The higher risk of infection is in children, because of their play and hygiene habits.

2.3.1.3 Epidemiology

The seroprevalence for *Toxocara* is high in rural and some tropical areas, the West Indies, Nepal, Brazil, Columbia, the Netherlands, Thessaloniki, Greece, Cuba, and Germany (Bachli et al. 2004; Eberhardt et al. 2005; Xinou et al. 2003).

2.3.1.4 Pathology

There are three clinical forms of the disease depending on the number of larvae entering the brain and the severity of CNS inflammation: occult, ocular larva migrans, and visceral larva migrans. The latter form is a multisystemic disease involving the liver, heart, lungs, muscle, skin, eyes, and CNS. The clinical involvement of the CNS is rare and seen in all age groups (Xinou et al. 2003; Moreira-Silva et al. 2004).

2.3.1.5 Clinical Manifestations

Several clinical pictures have been reported, most importantly eosinophilic meningitis, encephalitis, meningoencephalitis, vasculitis, myelitis, radiculopathy, and rarely spinal cord compression by an epidural abscess.

The most common manifestations of cerebral toxocariasis are headache and isolated seizures, less likely ataxia and cognitive decline. *Toxocara* myelitis exhibits sensory and motor deficits.

2.3.1.6 Diagnosis and Laboratory Tests

The diagnosis is based on laboratory findings: CSF and/or blood eosinophilia, high titers of *T. canis* antibodies measured with enzyme linked immunosorbent assays (ELISA) or Western blot analysis. Positive serology with IgM anti-*Toxocara* in the serum and CSF (Eberhardt et al. 2005; Xinou et al. 2003).

2.3.1.7 Imaging Findings

Computed tomography and MR findings are nonspecific as neurotoxocariasis induces a granulomatous reaction similar to that seen with other parasitic CNS infections. They include multifocal, circumscribed lesions, hypoattenuating on CT scan, hypointense on T1-WI, and hyperintense on T2-WI, strongly and homogeneously enhancing after gadolinium. The distribution is cortical and subcortical involving the white matter of the centrum semi-ovale. Enhancement is thought to result from focal disruption of the blood–brain barrier and can occasionally be absent. Rarely, there is evidence of foci of microhemorrhages or cortical necrosis that appear hyperdense on CT scans and hyperintense on both T1- and T2-WI.

- The lesions may contain calcifications best depicted on non-enhanced CT scans. Cerebral toxocariasis presenting as a solitary mass lesion is very rare (Bachli et al. 2004; Eberhardt et al. 2005; Xinou et al. 2003; Vidal et al. 2003; Nelson et al. 1990).
- Focal meningeal enhancement may be seen adjacent to the inflammatory focus.
  Spinal cord lesions are hyperintense on T2-WI, and characteristically more extensive than predicted based on the clinical symptoms. Contrast-enhanced T1-WI show a characteristic nodular pattern of enhancement involving the peripheral aspect of the cord, sparing the central portions, and less extensive than the abnormal T2 signal (Fig. 2.5) (Jabbour et al. 2004; Kumar and Kimm 1994).
- The prognosis is very good with regression and healing of the lesion on follow-up MRI. Cortical laminar necrosis and hyperintense cortex on T1- and T2-WI have been described after treatment and remission (Xinou et al. 2003).
- Vasculitis rarely complicates *Toxocara* infection, resulting in multiple brain infarcts.

Neurotoxocariasis should be included in the differential diagnosis of CNS granulomatous infection with hypereosinophilia.

2.3.1.8 Treatment

Treatment is based on administration of antihelminthic drugs, primarily albendazole (Albenza, Zentel), mebendazole (Vermox), thiabendazole (Mintezol), and diethylcarbamazine (Hetrazan). Oral corticosteroids are frequently added to prevent autoimmune inflammatory reaction and progression of the edema (Bachli et al. 2004; Eberhardt et al. 2005).

2.3.2 Baylisascariasis

2.3.2.1 Parasite

It is a rare but fatal human neurological infection caused by the intestinal roundworm of raccoons, *Baylisascaris procyonis*.

2.3.2.2 Epidemiology

It is endemic in raccoons in most regions of the United States: in California, Illinois, Minnesota, Pennsylvania, and Missouri, and in Japan and Europe: Germany, Poland, etc.

2.3.2.3 Mode of Contamination

Humans are infected by the ingestion of infective eggs from the environment.

2.3.2.4 Pathology and Clinical Manifestations

Three types of human *B. procyonis* infection exist. The first is ocular larva migrans, in which the eyes are infected and which results in subacute neuroretinitis, permanent vision loss, and optic nerve impairment. The second is visceral larva migrans, resulting in abdominal pain and eosinophilia with a severe outcome. The third category is the neural larva migrans where the brain is

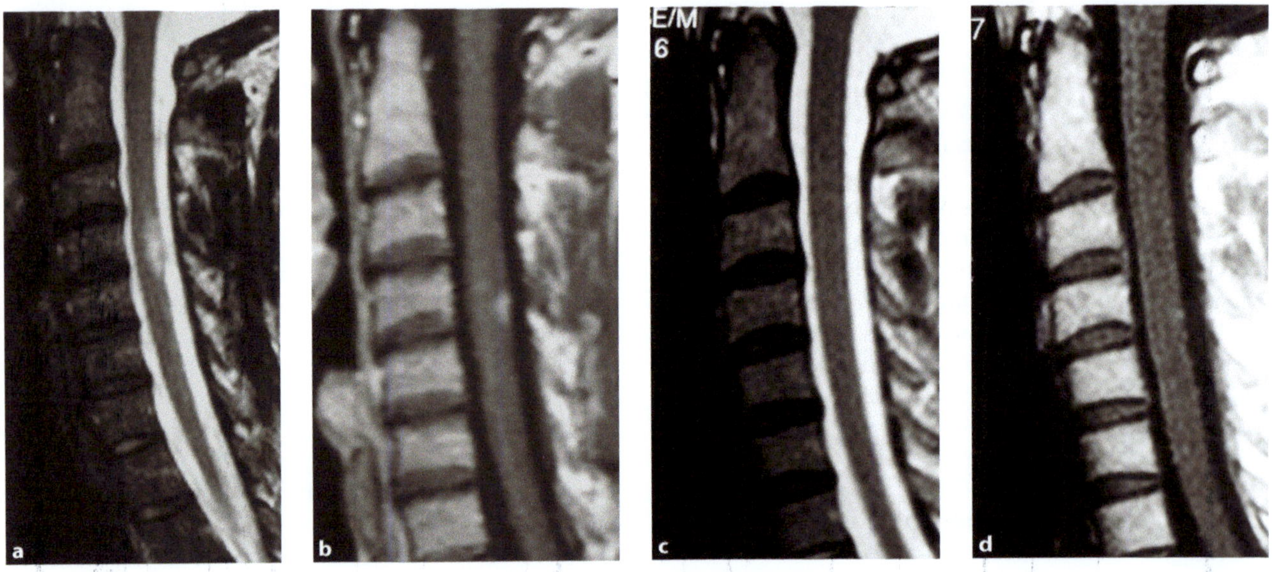

Fig. 2.5 Spinal cord toxocariasis in a 40-year-old man presenting with myelopathy. **a** Sagittal T2-WI of the cervical spine shows increased signal intensity of the posterior aspect of the spinal cord at the C4–C5 level associated with swelling of the cord at this level. **b** Sagittal T1-WI after contrast administration. The area of abnormality showed a focus of peripheral, nodular enhancement much smaller than the T2 abnormality. **c,d** Follow-up examinations following treatment with albendazole. There is complete resolution of the increased signal seen on T2-WI (**c**) and a significant decrease in the abnormal enhancement (**d**) (Courtesy of Dr Mukbil Hourani, Department of Diagnostic Radiology, American University of Beirut Medical Center, Beirut, Lebanon)

the primary site of larval migration causing severe damage to the brain, inflammatory reactions and often fatal CNS illness; 46% of neural infections have been fatal and 54% result in permanent neurologic sequelae like paralysis, developmental disability, and blindness.

2.3.2.5 Diagnosis and Laboratory Tests

Baylisascariasis should be considered in the differential diagnosis of children presenting with encephalitis and eosinophilia. The diagnosis is made by immunologic tests (ELISA, Western blot) and epidemiologic findings of possible exposure to raccoons; however, the definitive diagnosis is based on the identification of the larvae in brain biopsy specimens.

2.3.2.6 Imaging Findings

Brain MRI of patients with *B. procyonis* encephalitis show diffuse high signal intensity on T2-WI in the periventricular white matter, the corona radiata, and the brainstem, accompanied later by diffuse brain atrophy. There is no evidence of meningeal or parenchymal enhancement on post-contrast images (Rowley et al. 2000).

2.3.2.7 Treatment

Albendazole is the treatment of choice; however, since the diagnosis is difficult in most cases, and once the larvae have entered the CNS, they cause significant damage, and the treatment is usually ineffective. In this setting, efforts at prevention are critical and good hygiene, handwashing after outdoor activity, and soil decontamination by propane torch are recommended to prevent children from infection (Wise et al. 2005). Simultaneous administration of corticosteroids with albendazole can be used (Park et al. 2000).

Of particular interest to radiologists, levamisole (the L-isomer of tetramisole), an antihelminthic imidazothiazole drug that has been frequently used when taken in a single 150-mg dose to treat ascariasis, has been reported from China and Lebanon to induce a type of encephalopathy called antihelminthic imidazole-induced encephalopathy (AIIE). On imaging, CT scans revealed multiple hypodensities of the white matter while MRI demonstrated bilateral asymmetric multiple lesions of high signal intensity on T2-WI in the deep periventricular white matter, corona radiata, centrum semi-ovale, putamen, and internal capsules. The lesions showed ring enhancement on gadolinium-enhanced T1-WI. AIIE resembles the acute disseminated encephalitis (ADEM) and the differentiation from multiple sclerosis is primarily based on the monophasic clinical and radiological pattern of the disease. The treatment consists of steroids, and it carries a good prognosis (El Kallab et al. 2003).

2.3.3 Gnathostomiasis

Gnathostomiasis is a parasitic infection caused by *Gnathostoma spinigerum*, which is a parasite of cats and dogs endemic in Southeast Asia, Japan, and China. It causes eosinophilic myeloencephalitis with focal hemorrhage, involvement of the spinal cord, nerve root pain, and hemorrhagic CSF (Weller 1993).

2.3.4 Angiostrongyliasis Cantonensis

Angiostrongyliasis cantonensis is caused by the *Angiostrongylus cantonensis* infection. It is one of the most frequent causes of eosinophilic meningitis, more prevalent in Southeast Asia and the Pacific Islands. Brain CT scans show no focal lesions since the infection involves only the meninges (Rowley et al. 2000; Punyagupta et al. 1975).

2.3.5 Trichinosis/Trichinellosis

2.3.5.1 Parasite

Trichinosis, or trichinellosis, is caused by the nematode *Trichinella spiralis*.

2.3.5.2 Mode of Contamination

Humans are infected after ingestion of raw or undercooked pork or horse meat.

2.3.5.3 Epidemiology

The disease is prevalent worldwide, and is especially common among pork-consuming people.

2.3.5.4 Pathology

The larvae have a predilection for striated muscles. Neurological complications of trichinosis occur in 10–24% of cases (Ellrodt et al. 1987).

2.3.5.5 Clinical Manifestations

The clinical symptoms include meningitis, meningoencephalitis, paresis, aphasia, seizures, and symptoms of focal cerebral lesions with hemorrhage.

2.3.5.6 Diagnosis

The diagnosis is made by identifying anti-*Trichinella* antibodies in the CSF.

2.3.5.7 Imaging Findings

Computed tomography scanning demonstrates multiple brain hypodensities in the white matter representing lacunar infarcts, or focal granulomas with nodular enhancement seen on post-contrast images. Large infarcts in the territory of the middle cerebral artery, brain edema, hemorrhage, either punctate or large, could also be seen secondary to venous thrombosis (Fig. 2.6) (El Koussa et al. 1994).

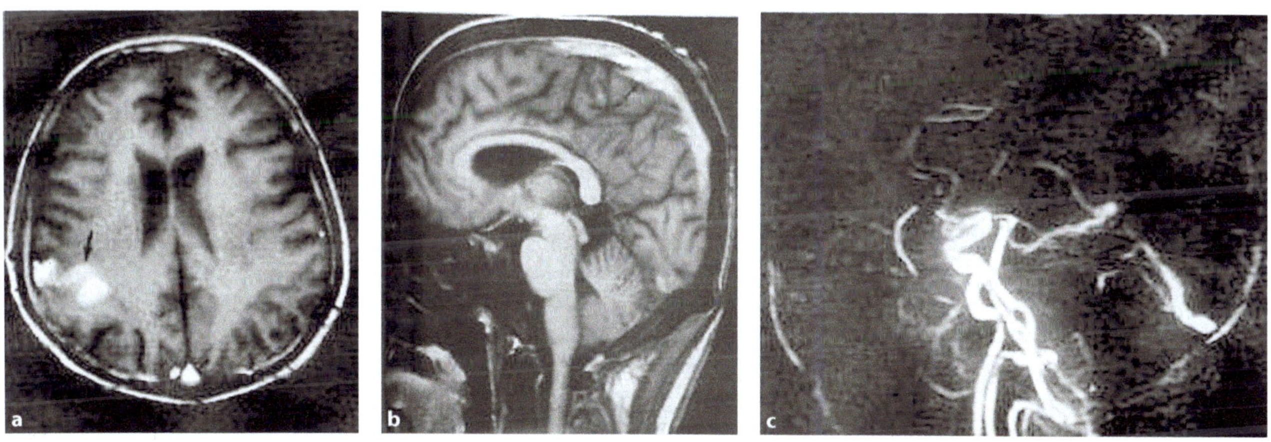

Fig. 2.6 Neurotrichinosis. **a,b** Axial and sagittal T1-weighted MR images of the brain showing hyperintense signal of the superior sagittal sinus compatible with sinus thrombosis, confirmed by MR venography in image **c**. Note also the presence of a hemorrhagic venous infarct *(arrow)* in the right parietal lobe involving the cortical and subcortical regions seen in image **a** (Courtesy of Dr. Salam El Koussa, Department of Medicine, Hotel Dieu de France-CHU, Beirut, Lebanon)

2.3.5.8 Treatment

The treatment of choice consists of mebendazole and flubendazole.

2.4 Helminths – Tapeworms (Cestodes)

2.4.1 Echinococcosis (Hydatid Disease)

2.4.1.1 Parasite

Neuroechinococcosis, or hydatid disease is caused by infection of the CNS by the larvae of the tapeworm: *Taenia echinococcus*. In humans, hydatid disease is produced by two types of echinococcus: *E. granulosus* most commonly and *E. multilocularis* (*alveolaris*) (Bukte et al. 2004).

2.4.1.2 Epidemiology

Together with neurocysticercosis, echinococcosis is the most frequent of the cerebral parasitic infections. It is usually endemic in sheep- and cattle-raising developing countries, particularly in the Middle East, Portugal, Spain, France, Italy, Greece, Croatia, Turkey, Australia, New Zealand, South America, and Africa. Given the human migration from endemic to non-endemic areas, hydatid disease has become a worldwide infection.

2.4.1.3 Mode of Contamination

Dogs, foxes or other carnivores are the primary hosts; sheep, cattle, and horses are the intermediate hosts. Humans may become infected through direct contact with infected dogs or through ingestion of food or drink contaminated by ova, i.e., parasite eggs shed from the stools of infected animals.

2.4.1.4 Pathology

The embryos penetrate the intestinal mucosa and reach the liver and lungs via the portal system and lymphatics. Infection occurs usually in the liver (50–77%) and lungs (8.5–43%), only the embryos bypassing the hepatic and pulmonary filters may involve any organ in the body through the systemic circulation, including brain involvement in approximately 2% of infected patients (Tuzun et al. 2002). Cerebral echinococcus represents 2% of intracranial masses in endemic areas and it is most common in children and young adults (50–70%) (Lunard et al. 1991; Haliloglu et al. 1997; El-Shamam et al. 2001). Cerebral echinococcus presents usually as a single cyst; multiple cysts are extremely rare, secondary to spontaneous, traumatic or surgical rupture of intracranial cysts or ruptured cysts elsewhere in the circulation, and embolization to the brain (Karadag et al. 2004; Al-Zain et al. 2002; Demir et al. 1991). They can occur anywhere in the brain; however, most cysts are supratentorial, in the territory of the middle cerebral artery, especially in the parietal lobe. Intraventricular localization, the spinal region (Fig. 2.7), posterior fossa, and the foramen magnum, is very rare (Boudawara et al. 1999).

The rate of growth of cerebral hydatid cysts is 1–5 cm per year (Guney et al. 2002; Altimors et al. 2000). The cerebral hydatid cyst thus grows slowly and remains asymptomatic until quite large; clinical manifestations are secondary to the mass effect related to the lesion location. The parasitic cyst has three layers: an inner germinal layer (endocyst) that produces scolices, daughter cysts and "hydatid sands," which are brood capsules for daughter cysts, an outer laminated acellular membrane layer (ectocyst), and an external fibrous capsule (pericyst) formed by the host tissue reaction containing inflammatory and giant cells. The pericyst contains blood vessels.

2.4.1.5 Clinical Manifestations

The most common presenting symptoms and signs are headache, vomiting, seizures, visual field disturbances, papilledema, hemiparesis, and ataxia (Bukte et al. 2004; Lunardi et al. 1991; Haliloglu et al. 1997; El-Shammam et al. 2001; Polat et al. 2003).

2.4.1.6 Diagnosis and Laboratory Tests

The diagnosis relies on positive serologic tests and imaging features. Serological tests, including indirect hemagglutination, latex agglutination, ELISA, and immunoelectrophoresis, are controversial in the diagnosis of hydatid disease, with common false-positive and -negative results (Karadag et al. 2004; Guney et al. 2002; Altinors et al. 2000; Polat et al. 2003; Ouboukhlik et al. 1994). The main role of the serological tests is in the follow-up of treated patients, where decreases in titers indicate resolution and response of the disease. Histopathologic diagnosis is the best diagnostic method, yet the aspiration of cysts is not recommended because of spillage and risk of anaphylaxis or secondary lesions (Bouckaert et al. 2000).

2.4.1.7 Imaging Findings

Computed tomography (CT) and magnetic resonance imaging (MRI) are both helpful in the diagnosis of neuroechinococcosis. Although CT is better at detecting cal-

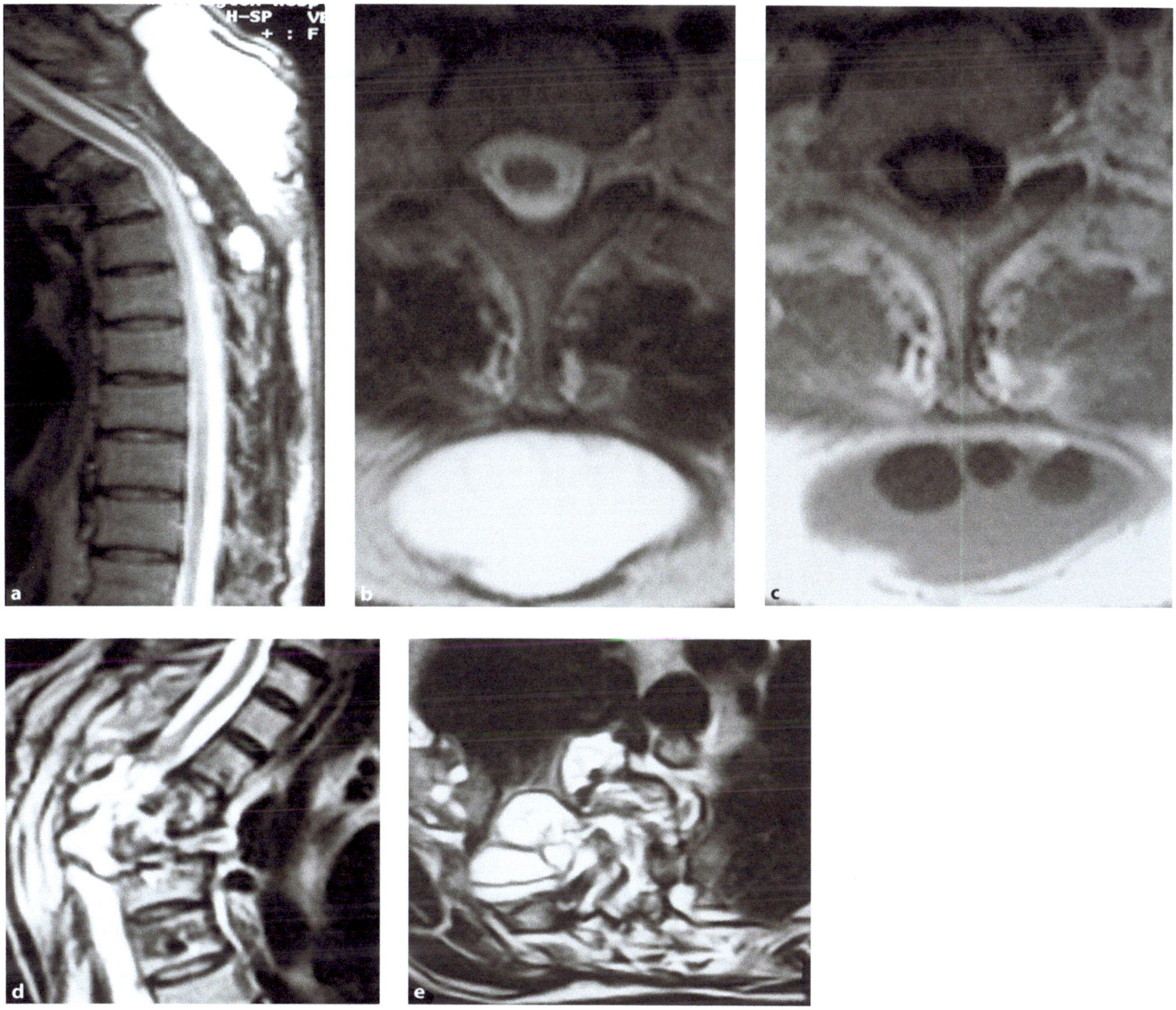

Fig. 2.7 Spinal hydatid disease. **a** Sagittal T2-weighted MR image of the thoracic spine showing hyperintense cystic lesions in the paravertebral space as well as in the posterior epidural space. **b,c**, Axial T2-WI and T1-WI demonstrate the cyst with a hyperintense signal on T2-WI compared with the CSF; the rim has hypointense signal intensity on T2. The presence of daughter cysts within it is a pathognomonic finding of hydatid cysts. **d,e** Sagittal and axial T2-weighted MR images of the thoracic spine in another patient known to have a spinal hydatid cyst. There is a multiloculated hyperintense cystic lesion with a hypointense rim in the spinal canal invading the spinal cord, the thoracic vertebral bodies, and extending to the paravertebral and prevertebral spaces

cification within the cyst wall or septa, MRI is more often used as diagnostic tool, provides better definition of the exact anatomic location of the lesion, and it is more sensitive in demonstrating multiple lesions.

E. granulosus (the most common form) (Fig. 2.8): on CT, the brain lesion presents as a spherical, well-defined, homogenous, smooth, thin-walled, cystic lesion isodense to the CSF with or without surrounding edema. The cyst wall is iso- or hyperdense relative to the brain parenchyma. Calcifications of the wall are rare, accounting for less than 1% of cases. After contrast, there is typically no enhancement. On MRI, the cyst is isointense to CSF on T1- and T2-WI, with a hypointense rim on T1- and T2-WI and no perilesional edema in untreated or uncomplicated cysts (Tuzun and Hekimoglu 1998). On fluid-attenuated inversion recovery (FLAIR) images, the fluid of the hydatid cyst is hyperintense. The gadolinium-enhanced T1-WI typically shows no enhancement; how-

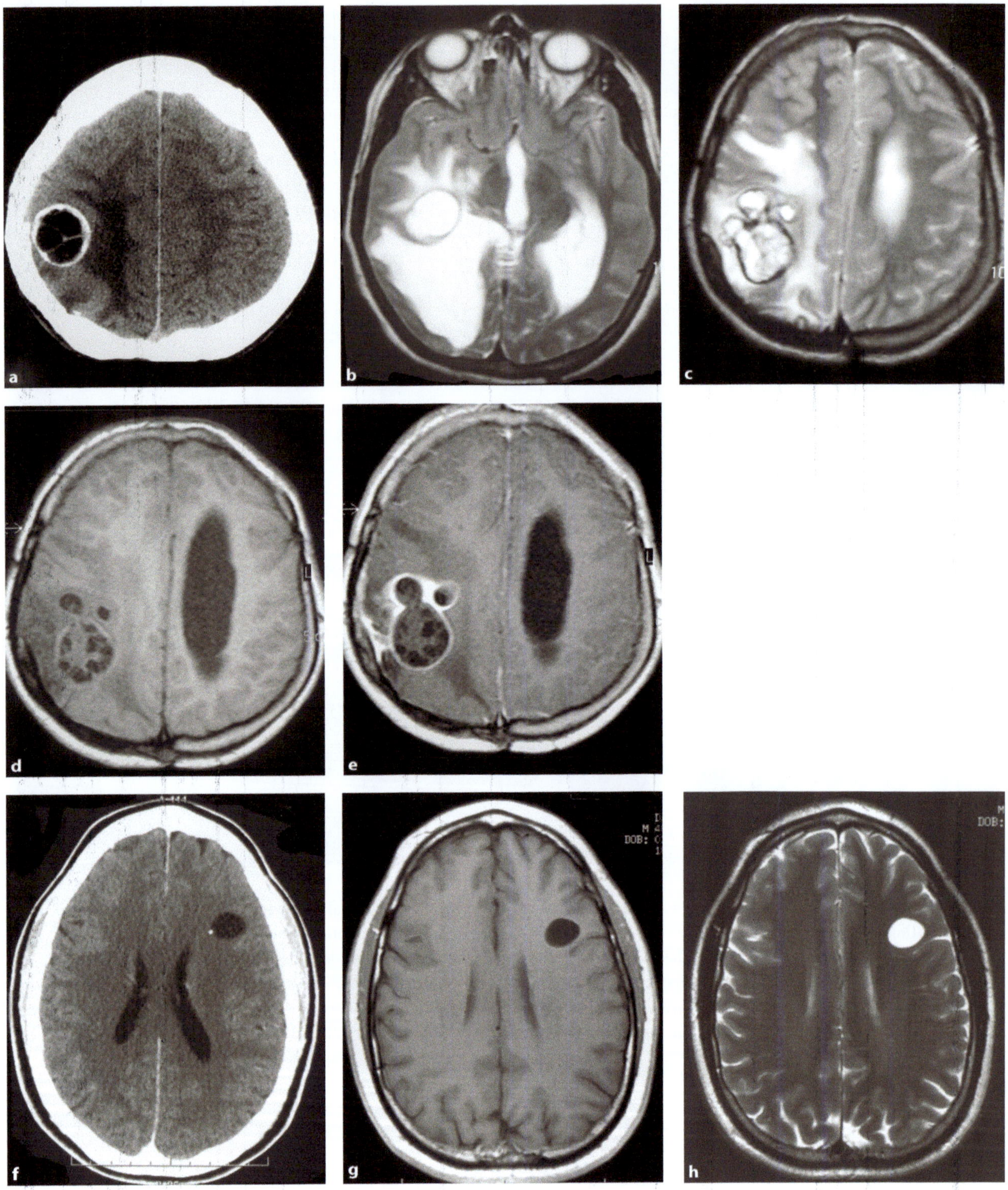

Fig. 2.8 Cerebral hydatid cysts. **a** Axial unenhanced CT scan shows a spherical, well-defined cystic lesion with a septated solid component and wall calcifications. **b,c** Axial T2-WI MR images of the same patient 2 years later demonstrate multiple large hyperintense simple and multiseptated cystic lesions in the right cerebral hemisphere showing a hypointense rim on T2-WI and surrounding edema. The largest lesion in the right frontal lobe shows a solid portion, multiple internal septae, and contains daughter cysts. There is rupture of its anterior wall with adjacent satellite exocystic daughter cysts. **d,e** Axial T1-WI pre- and post-contrast demonstrate rim of enhancement. **f–h** Contrast-enhanced CT scan, T1-WI, and T2-WI images of the brain showing a unilocular left cerebral hemisphere hydatid cyst with a peripheral punctate calcification better appreciated by CT than MRI. Note the lack of surrounding edema or mass effect of the hydatid cyst

ever, a fine rim of enhancement may be seen (Fig. 2.8e) (Osborn et al. 2004). The presence of detached germinal membrane, daughter cysts or "hydatid sands" within the cyst is pathognomonic of the disease; however, they are rarely present (Haliloglu et al. 1997; Patrikar et al. 1993). The hydatid sand is seen as a fluid–fluid level within the cyst, hyperdense on CT, and exhibiting hyposignal on T2-WI and FLAIR images.

In the case of *E. multilocularis* infection, CT and MRI demonstrate one or multiple well-defined mixed solid and multiloculated cystic lesions, containing calcifications in the solid portion, better assessed by means of CT, with peripheral surrounding edema. After contrast administration there is partial or total enhancement (Bensaid et al. 1994; Reittner et al. 1996). The lesions may show foci of low signal on T1- and T2-WI due to the presence of microcalcifications (Piotin et al. 1997).

2.4.1.8 Diagnosis

The differential diagnosis of cerebral hydatid cysts includes porencephalic cysts, arachnoid cysts, cystic tumors, and abscesses. Arachnoid cysts are extra-axial masses and they are not spherical, in contrast to hydatid cysts, and show a similar signal to CSF in all sequences. Mainly, arachnoid cysts suppress like CSF on FLAIR images, whereas hydatic cysts show a high signal within. The porencephalic cyst typically communicates with the ventricle and shows peripheral gliosis and encephalomalacia. A cystic neoplasm is characterized by the enhancement of a mural nodule or thick irregular margin with perilesional edema. A pyogenic abscess presents surrounding edema, intense rim enhancement, which is thinner on the ventricular margin, and restricted diffusion on the ADC map. Neurocysticercosis should be always included in the differential diagnosis of hydatid cysts. Differential diagnosis of cerebral echinococcosis alveolaris includes tumors, tuberculomas, and fungal infections. The correct diagnosis is facilitated by the identification of hepatic or pulmonary localization, laboratory findings, and presence in endemic geographical areas (Tuzun et al. 2002, Reittner et al. 1993; Piotin et al. 1997).

Proton magnetic resonance spectroscopy (^{1}HMRS) is a non-invasive, relatively new MR technique used to characterize the metabolic content of intracranial lesions. It has been recently used in the evaluation of hydatid cysts and demonstrates resonance of lactate, succinate, and acetate (Shukla-Dave et al. 2001; Kim et al. 1998).

2.4.1.9 Treatment

Neuroechinococcosis should be suspected in the presence of cystic brain lesions. Exact preoperative diagnosis is essential to avoid intraoperative cyst rupture and spillage of daughter cysts and scolices. Medical treatment alone is not effective; however, it is recommended in inoperable cases, when the cysts are too numerous, and to prevent a secondary echinococcosis. The aim of the surgery is intact removal of the cyst without causing any spillage because of the risk of anaphylactic reaction and recurrence. During surgery, silver nitrate (0.5%), hypertonic saline (20%), and other chemicals are often injected into the cysts to inactivate the scolices.

If the cyst ruptures, the cyst content should be aspirated with irrigation of the operative bed by hypertonic saline solution associated with albendazole treatment (Karadag et al. 2004; Guney et al. 2002). Surgery is the treatment of choice in patients with symptoms of intracranial hypertension (Talan-Hranilovic et al. 2002).

2.4.2 Neurocysticercosis

2.4.2.1 Parasite

Neurocysticercosis (NCC) is the most common parasitic disease of the central nervous system, secondary to infection by the larval form of the pork tapeworm *Taenia solium*.

2.4.2.2 Epidemiology

It is an infection with worldwide prevalence, mainly in areas with large immigrant populations: Central and South America, India, Africa, East Asia, China, and Eastern Europe (Hawk et al. 2005; White 2000; Garcia and Del Brutto 2000). It occurs at any age, more commonly in young and middle-aged adults.

2.4.2.3 Mode of Contamination

Taenia solium involves the pig as an intermediate host where the embryos of the parasites spread hematogenously and infect the muscles, eyes, and the CNS. The human is the definitive host; if he eats the infected pork meat undercooked or raw, he acquires cysticercosis; and as in the pig, the embryos traverse the intestinal mucosa and reach the muscles, eyes, CNS and subcutaneous soft tissues (Hawk et al. 2005; Garcia and Del Brutto 2000).

2.4.2.4 Pathology

Involvement of the CNS occurs in 60–90% of infected patients by hematogenous spread. The most common location is the convexity subarachnoid space, then the cisterns, brain parenchyma and the ventricular system, which is infected via the choroid plexus. The localization in the posterior fossa is possible, although rare according to the literature (Talan-Hranilovic et al. 2002; White 2000).

2.4.2.5 Clinical Manifestations

The clinical manifestations depend on the location, number, size, and stage of the parasite and the patient's immunologic reactivity. The main presentations are seizures and symptoms of increased intracranial pressure: headache, nausea and vomiting and focal neurological deficits depending on the location of the disease. Manifestations include also: meningitis, communicating or noncommunicating hydrocephalus, basal arachnoiditis, and angiitis of the intracranial vessels with subsequent infarcts (Hawk et al. 2005; Amar et al. 2000; Couldwell et al. 1995). Most of the time, cerebral infarcts associated with NCC result from vasculitis of small perforating arteries, and large territorial infarcts are rare (Couldwell et al. 1995). Since seizures occur in 50–80% of patients with NCC, it must be considered in the differential diagnosis of adult-onset epilepsy in endemic regions (White 2000; Medina et al. 1990).

2.4.2.6 Diagnosis and Laboratory Tests

The diagnosis is made by a combination of the clinical examination, and neuroradiological and serological studies. Immunologic tests like complement fixation tests and ELISA are sensitive in the case of viable subarachnoid parasites, but the sensitivity decreases in the case of intraparenchymal disease with no contact with the CSF and at the nodular calcified stage (Aditya et al. 2004).

2.4.2.7 Imaging Findings

Computed tomography and MRI are considered the best tools for diagnosing NCC. The imaging findings vary with the parasite's location, the developmental stage, and the host's response to the disease; even though lesions of different stages of development can be seen in the same patient. There are four pathologic stages of parenchymal cysticercosis (Escobar's stages): the vesicular stage (viable larva), the colloidal vesicular stage (degenerating larva), the granular nodular stage (healing), and the nodular calcified (healed) stage. MRI is the most sensitive imaging modality for the diagnosis of all stages of the disease, except the end-stage calcified disease, which is better detected by non-enhanced CT (Osborn et al. 2004).

At the vesicular stage the parasite is viable with no or minimal inflammation in the surrounding tissue. It presents as a small marginal nodule representing the embryo that projects into a small cyst with clear fluid. The parasite may remain at this stage for years. CT shows a smooth, thin-walled cyst lodging typically at the gray–white matter junction, isodense to the CSF and containing a hyperdense "dot" representing the protoscolex, with no or minimal surrounding edema and wall enhancement. MRI demonstrates a cystic lesion isointense to CSF in all MRI pulse sequences: T1-WI, T2-WI, and FLAIR, containing an eccentric scolex hyperintense to the CSF with no surrounding edema and no or mild rim enhancement after gadolinium administration (Fig. 2.9).

At the colloidal vesicular stage, after 5–7 years, the larva begins to degenerate as a result of the host's immune response. The scolex shows signs of hyaline degeneration and gradual shrinkage; the cyst wall thickens and the fluid becomes turbid and proteinaceous with the appearance of surrounding inflammation. CT shows hyperdense fluid in the cyst and ring enhancement on enhanced study; MRI shows the cyst with hyperintense content relative to the CSF in all pulse sequences: T1-WI, T2-WI, and FLAIR with mild or marked surrounding edema (Fig. 2.10). After contrast administration, the wall of the cyst enhances as well as the eccentric scolex.

At the granular nodular stage there is absorption of the cyst fluid and further thickening of the capsule, the scolex mineralizes; as a result CT and MRI show a retracted, thickened cyst with mild surrounding edema. The contrast enhancement shows homogenous enhancement (Fig. 2.11).

At the nodular calcified stage the dead larva is calcified and best identified on CT as multiple small calcified nodules with no surrounding edema (Fig. 2.12). MRI shows a small calcified lesion, better identified on T2* gradient echo sequences as a hypointense nodule with rare minimal enhancement on T1 after contrast.

On diffusion MR images, the cystic lesion is typically isointense to the CSF at the vesicular stage. There are few reports in the literature of ^{1}HMRS in NCC. In a case of a racemose cysticercal cyst ^{1}HMRS shows a predominant peak of pyruvate at 2.4 ppm, elevated lactate (1.3 ppm), alanine (1.6 ppm), acetate (2.2 ppm), succinate (2.4 ppm), and choline (3.2 ppm), and decreased N-acetyl aspartate (2.02 ppm) and creatine (3 ppm) (Chang et al. 1998; Jayakumar et al. 2004). Pyruvate is presumed to be the end-product of glycolysis; it is also present in hydatid cysts and is helpful in differentiating a cysticercal cyst from an epidermoid cyst, an arachnoid cyst, and a cystic glioma (Kohli et al. 1995; Gupta et al. 1995).

Imaging characteristics of other forms of cysticercosis include:

1. Intraventricular cysticercosis is seen in 10–20% of NCC. The fourth ventricle is the most common location, and it usually presents as a single cyst. The intraventricular cyst is not well seen on CT, one may just see hydrocephalus. However, the cyst could be better delineated after contrast opacification of the ventricular system through a lumbar puncture and intrathecal injection of contrast, or directly via an intraventricular ventriculoperitoneal shunt. On MRI, the cyst wall and content may be difficult to identify, however, when the cyst content becomes proteinaceous, T1, FLAIR and proton density sequences detect hyperintense cyst compared with the CSF. Gadolinium-enhanced T1-

weighted images show enhancement of the cyst wall as well as the scolex. The complications are ventriculitis, ependymitis and or hydrocephalus.

2. Subarachnoid and cisternal cysticercosis is an infestation of the subarachnoid space and may lead to the formation of a large multiloculated, grape-like, cystic lesion, typically without scolex, called the racemose form or a single cyst with an eccentric scolex. The most common location of the lesions is the sylvian fissure and basal cisterns; however, any sulcus or cistern could be involved. The content of the cysts appears isodense on CT, and isointense to CSF on MRI; the septae of racemose cysts could be seen on T1- and T2-WI with mild or no enhancement of the cyst wall on enhanced T1-WI. The potential complications are meningitis with subsequent hydrocephalus and vasculitis secondary to chronic basilar granulomatous meningitis. The major intracranial vessels might be occluded resulting in large territorial infarcts (4–12%) (Scharf 1988). CT and MR imaging features in subarachnoid NCC include hydrocephalus, abnormal enhancement of the leptomeninges at the level of the basal cisterns.
3. Spinal cysticercosis is rare, reported in 1–5% of NCC. Usually, it involves the subarachnoid space with formation of intradural cysts or arachnoiditis. The intradural cysts are identified on CT myelography as filling defects. On MRI, they demonstrate the same findings as cerebral subarachnoid cysticercosis. Involvement of the spinal cord is rare and intraspinal cysts show similar imaging characteristics to cerebral intraparenchymal cysts.
4. "Encephalitic cysticercosis" seen in children as diffuse multiple enhancing nodules with diffuse brain edema.

Neurocysticercosis and neuroechinococcosis should be considered in the differential diagnosis of cystic lesions of the brain, especially in developing countries.

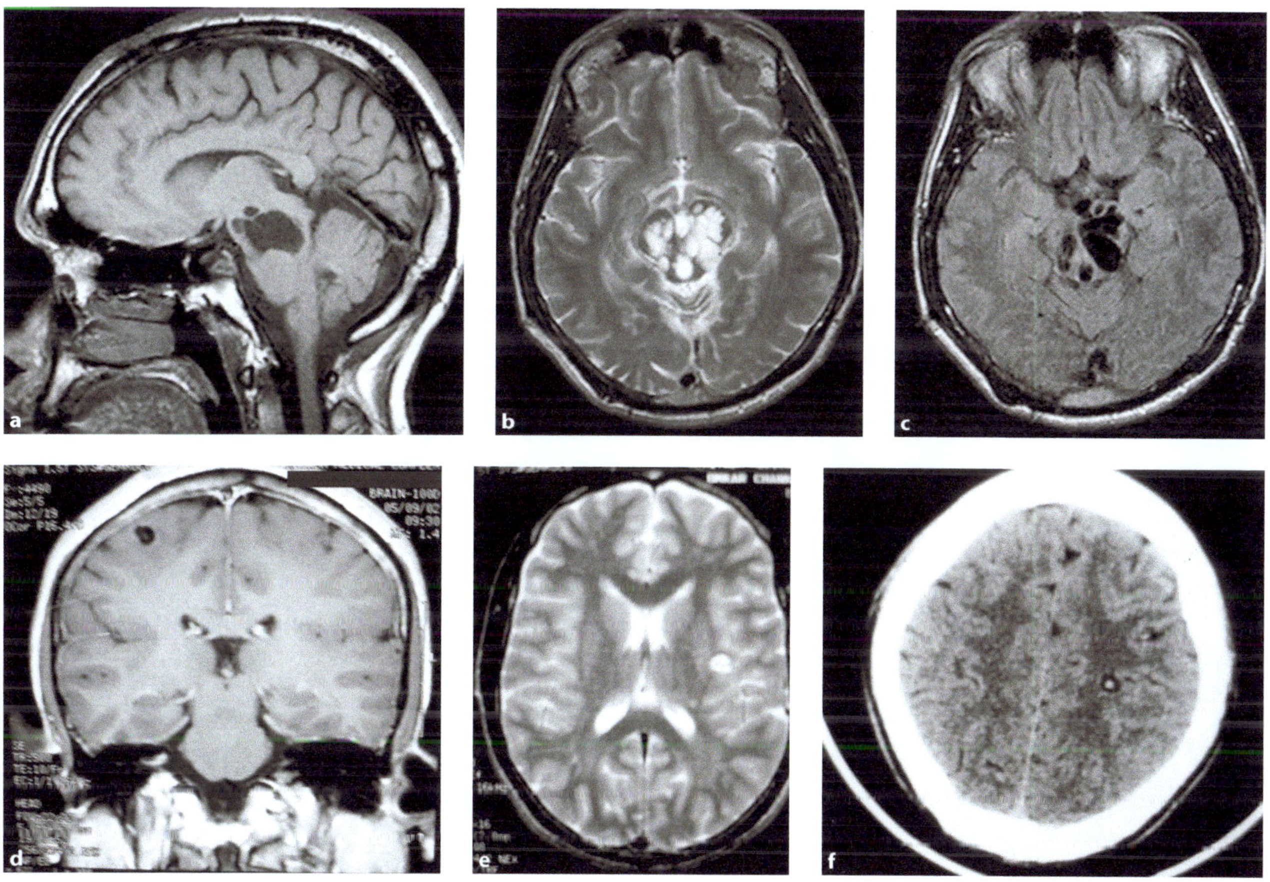

Fig. 2.9 Neurocysticercosis at the vesicular stage. **a** Sagittal T1-weighted, **b,c** axial T2-weighted, and FLAIR MR images of the brain demonstrate multiple cystic lesions in the tegmentum, containing fluid that is isointense to the CSF in all MRI pulse sequences with no evidence of surrounding edema. (Images **a–c** courtesy of Dr. Elias R. Melhem, Division of Neuroradiology, Hospital of University of Pennsylvania, Philadelphia, USA). **d** Coronal gadolinium-enhanced T1-WI, **e** axial T2-WI, and **f** non-enhanced CT scan of the brain showing typical changes of the cysticercus larva. Note the embryo projecting into the cyst on MRI in image **e**, and the hyperdense "dot" sign representing the protoscolex on the non-enhanced CT scan in image **f** (Images **d–f**, courtesy of Dr. F. El Zein, Department of Infectious Diseases, Riyadh Military Hospital, Riyadh, Saudi Arabia)

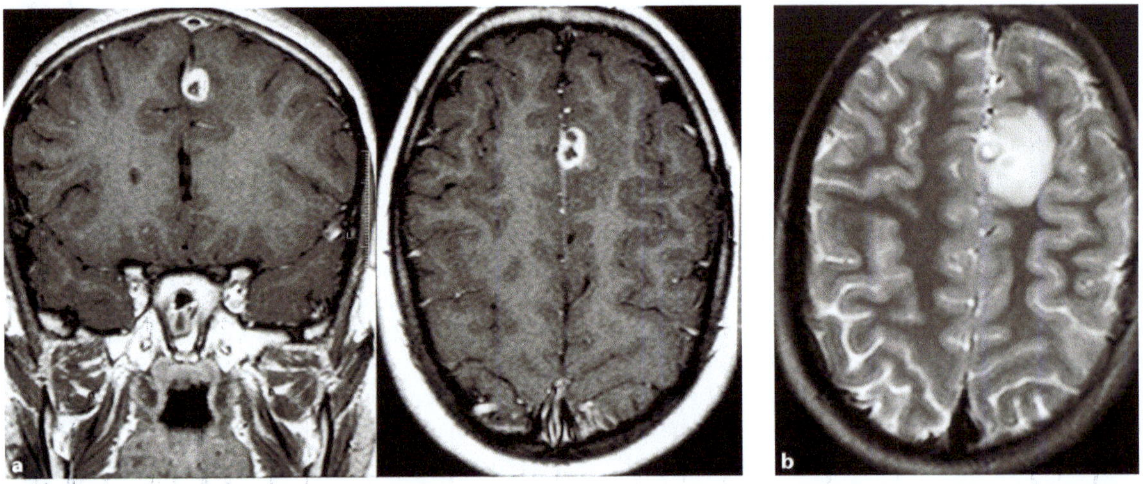

Fig. 2.10 Neurocysticercosis at the colloidal vesicular stage. **a,b** Coronal and axial T1-WI gadolinium-enhanced (**a**) and axial T2-WI (**b**) MR images showing a ring-enhancing lesion containing fluid, with surrounding brain edema, in the left cerebral hemisphere (Courtesy of Dr. Claire Outin-Tamraz, Department of Radiology, Trad Hospital, Beirut, Lebanon)

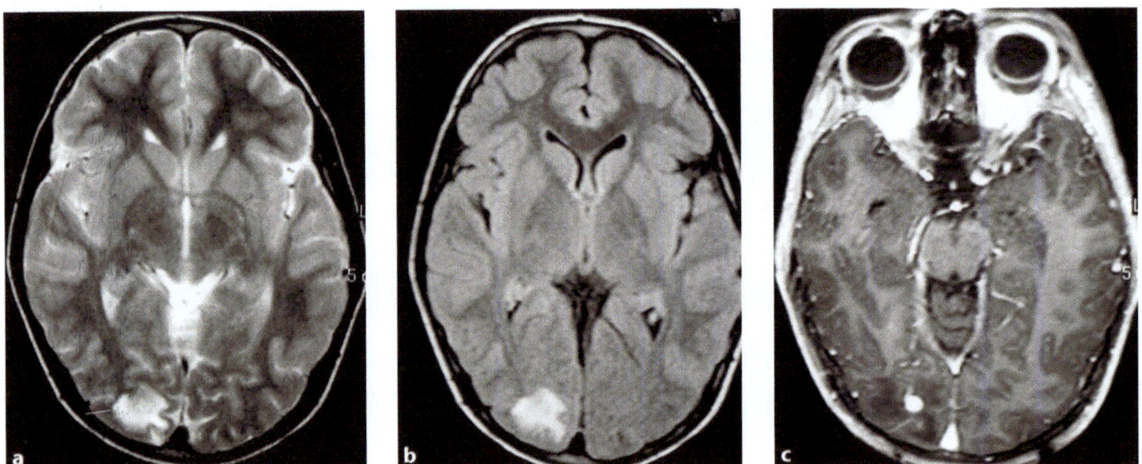

Fig. 2.11 Neurocysticercosis at the granular nodular stage. **a,b** Axial T2-WI and FLAIR images show a T2 hyperintense lesion in the right occipital lobe with mild surrounding edema. **c** Axial gadolinium-enhanced MRI demonstrates nodular homogenous enhancement corresponding to the retracted, thickened cyst

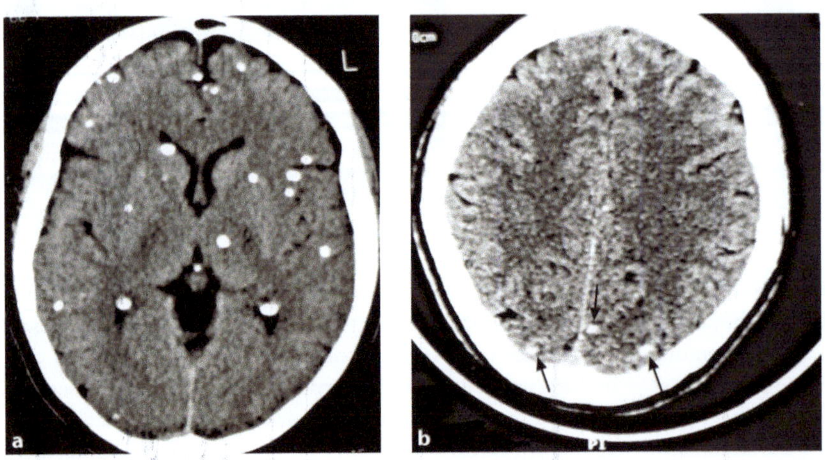

Fig. 2.12 Neurocysticercosis at the nodular calcified stage. **a,b** Axial non-enhanced CT scans of the brain show multiple, punctate, calcified parenchymal nodules (*arrows*) with no surrounding edema (Image **b**, courtesy of Dr. F. El Zein, Department of Infectious Diseases, Riyadh Military Hospital, Riyadh, Saudi Arabia)

A Cysticercosis Working Group in Peru has reported on the capability of magnetic resonance spectroscopy (MRS) in differentiating between cerebral tuberculosis and neurocysticercosis, thus avoiding brain biopsies or unnecessary antituberculous treatments. Tuberculomas show a high peak of lipids, more choline, and less N-acetylaspartate and creatine. The choline/creatine ratio was greater than 1 in all the tuberculomas, but in none of the cysticerci (Pretell et al. 2005).

2.4.2.8 Treatment

Treatment depends on the location of the cysts. Parenchymal cysticercosis is effectively treated by antihelminthic medication: albendazole and praziquantel. Surgical excision or drainage of parenchymal lesions may be required as a second option to relieve the mass effect or treat hydrocephalus or seizure (Wichert-Ana et al. 2004). Surgery is the treatment for patients with posterior fossa neurocysticercosis with symptoms of intracranial hypertension (Talan-Hranilovic et al. 2002). Antiepileptic drugs and steroids could also be used to treat seizures secondary to NCC and to decrease brain edema during medical therapy respectively. The efficacy of medical therapy is limited in intraventricular and cisternal cysticercosis. In these cases surgical treatment is recommended: CSF diversion to treat hydrocephalus or endoscopical resection of intraventricular lesions.

2.4.3 Sparganosis

2.4.3.1 Parasite

Sparganosis is a parasitic infection caused by the larvae of migrating tapeworms of the *Spirometra* genus.

2.4.3.2 Mode of Contamination

Humans become infected by drinking contaminated water, ingesting raw or undercooked snakes, frogs or fish, and by the use of a poultice of raw infected flesh applied to a wound, a common treatment in parts of Asia (Cummings et al. 2000).

2.4.3.3 Epidemiology

It is most prevalent in Japan, China, Taiwan, and Korea.

2.4.3.4 Pathology

The parasite has occasionally been reported to spread to the brain, ventricles or spinal canal, producing chronic and granulomatous inflammation. Cerebral sparganosis most frequently involves the frontal and parietal lobes, and rarely occurs in the posterior fossa or spinal canal. Most patients present with seizures, hemiparesis or chronic headache.

2.4.3.5 Diagnosis

Definitive diagnosis is made by identifying the sparganum or antisparganum IgG antibody. However, nowadays, MRI and CT brain imaging play a significant role in establishing the diagnosis (Moon et al. 1993).

2.4.3.6 Imaging Findings

Characteristic CT findings include the presence of hypodense areas in the cerebral white matter with adjacent cortical atrophy and ex-vacuo ventricular dilatation. There can be one or multiple small punctate foci of calcification, important diagnostic clues, which are not detected on MRI. Contrast enhancement shows linear, irregular or nodular enhancing lesions reflecting active granulomatous inflammation (Chang et al. 1992).

Magnetic resonance imaging is more sensitive than CT in imaging cerebral sparganosis. It shows better the localized cortical atrophy and the difference between normal and abnormal tissue. MRI features include:

1. Widespread white matter degeneration, hypointense on T1- and hyperintense on T2-WI with adjacent cortical atrophy and ipsilateral ventricular dilatation.
2. Small foci of petechial hemorrhage in the cortex and subcortical white matter exhibiting hyperintense signal on T1- and hypointense signal on T2-WI.
3. A mixed-signal intensity lesion showing a hypointense center and high signal in its periphery on T2-WI.
4. After gadolinium administration, the lesions demonstrate irregular, nodular or conglomerate ring or beaded pattern of contrast enhancement.
5. The lesions may change in location and shape on follow-up examinations, suggesting migration of the worm (Cummings et al. 2000; Moon et al. 1993).

The differential diagnosis includes cysticerosis, other granulomatous disease and metastasis; however, the presence of cortical atrophy and ipsilateral ventricular dilatation and the mobility of the lesions suggest sparganosis (Moon et al. 1993).

2.4.3.7 Treatment

The best treatment for cerebral sparganosis is removal of the worm and granuloma as no effective chemotherapy is available.

2.4.4 Coenurosis

Cerebral coenurosis is a rare parasitic infection caused by the larvae of the tapeworm *Taenia multiceps*. Human infections have been reported from Italy and Tanta in Egypt (Pau et al. 1987; Sabbatani et al. 2004; Antonios and Mina 2000). Cerebral coenurus cysts cause ventricular obstruction and increased intracranial pressure. On CT scans viable cysts appear as lucent lesions surrounded by a contrast-enhanced peripheral rim. On MRI, the cyst content is characterized by a CSF-like signal intensity pattern (Pau et al. 1987).

2.5 Helminths – Flukes (Trematodes)

2.5.1 Cerebral Schistosomiasis

2.5.1.1 Parasite

Schistosomiasis (bilharziasis) is a parasitic infection caused by trematode worms *Schistosoma*. There are five species of *Schistosoma* that infect humans: *mansoni*, *haematobium*, *japonicum*, *mekongi*, and *intercalatum*.

2.5.1.2 Epidemiology

This infection is endemic in South America, sub-Saharan Africa, the Middle East, and some Caribbean islands (Betting et al. 2005).

2.5.1.3 Mode of Contamination

Infection is acquired via direct contact with water contaminated by the larval form of the parasite known as cercariae. These larvae penetrate the human skin and reach the vascular system where they mature.

2.5.1.4 Pathology

The gastrointestinal, pulmonary, urinary, and CNS systems may be involved. Possible routes of spread to the brain or the spinal cord include embolization of eggs through the arterial system, venous shunts or retrograde migration of the worms via the valveless venous plexus of Batson (Betting et al. 2005; Ching et al. 1994). The central nervous system is rarely affected (2–4% of all patients are infected by *S. mansoni* (Preidler et al. 1996).

2.5.1.5 Clinical Manifestations

The clinical manifestations of cerebral schistosomiasis are attributable to an inflammatory reaction to the parasitic eggs. The most common neurological manifestation is transverse myelitis, usually caused by *S. mansoni*. Involvement of the brain presents with headache, seizures, and focal neurological deficits, most frequently resulting from infestation with *S. japonicum*.

2.5.1.6 Diagnosis

Confirmation of the diagnosis is difficult. Blood and CSF eosinophilia or antibody detection (CSF ELISA test) are variably positive. Kato-Katz thick smear examination of the stools can establish the presence of eggs in the stool. Definitive diagnosis requires the pathological demonstration of parasite eggs, i.e., ova in brain tissue obtained at biopsy (Mehta et al. 1997).

2.5.1.7 Imaging Findings

Computed tomography scan and MRI of the brain demonstrate single or multiple tumor-like lesions with surrounding vasogenic edema and mass effect. In the tumoral form, CT reveals a hyperdense or isodense space-occupying lesion with variable enhancement surrounded by edema without calcification or hemorrhage (Fig. 2.13a). Rarely, neuroschistosomiasis may present with intracerebral hematomas caused by necrosis of the vessel walls with secondary hemorrhage (Preidler et al. 1996). On MRI, the mass is heterogeneous, isointense to the gray matter on T1- and hyperintense on T2-WI, most commonly located in the cerebellum, less often in the thalamus, in the temporo-parietal, occipital, and frontal lobes (Fig. 2.13b,c). After contrast administration, MR may reveal either homogenous nodular enhancement of the mass (Ching et al. 1994), or punctate pattern of enhancement with multiple enhancing nodules, 1–2 mm, distributed throughout the mass, corresponding in pathology to aggregates of granulomas (Mehta et al. 1997), or an "arborized" appearance of central linear enhancement surrounded by multiple punctate nodules, clustered in the mass; this unique pattern is very suggestive of CNS schistosomiasis and was described in the brain as well as in the spinal cord (Fig. 2.13d,e) (Sanelli et al. 2001). Transverse myelitis is best demonstrated on MRI as focal enlargement of the cord with areas of hypersignal on T2-WI and heterogeneous contrast enhancement (Carod-Artal and Vargas 2004). The unique arborized pattern of enhancement may be present in the spinal cord lesions (Sanelli et al. 2001). The lower part of the cord and the conus are most commonly affected (Palmer and Reeder 2001).

2.5.1.8 Treatment

Treatment relies on the antiparasitic drugs oxamniquine and praziquantel associated with corticosteroids, with a favorable outcome (Betting et al. 2005). In the setting of acute paraplegia with intramedullary granulomas, surgical decompression may be warranted.

2.5.2 Cerebral Paragonimiasis

2.5.2.1 Parasite

Paragonimiasis is an infection with lung flukes of the genus *Paragonimus*, most frequently caused in humans by *P. westermani*.

2.5.2.2 Epidemiology

It is endemic in the Far East: Korea, China, Japan, Philippines, and Taiwan.

2.5.2.3 Mode of Contamination

The infection is acquired by eating raw or poorly cooked crabs, crayfish or shrimps infected with the metacercariae.

2.5.2.4 Pathology

The metacercariae penetrate the intestinal wall, enter the abdominal cavity, and thereafter migrate through the diaphragm to the lungs causing granulomatous infection. The most important extrapulmonary site for paragonimiasis is the brain. The reported frequency of cerebral involvement varies between 1 and 45%. The worms reach the brain by migration along the sheaths of the carotid arteries and jugular veins resulting in involvement of the temporal and occipital lobes most frequently (Choo et al. 2003).

2.5.2.5 Clinical Manifestations

Clinical manifestations of cerebral paragonimiasis include epilepsy, commonly of the Jacksonian type, headache, nausea, vomiting, hemiplegia, monoplegia, hemiparesis, and aphasia. Visual disturbances can rarely be seen secondary to a basal arachnoiditis. Subarachnoid hemorrhage has also been reported in association with cerebral paragonimiasis (Choo et al. 2003).

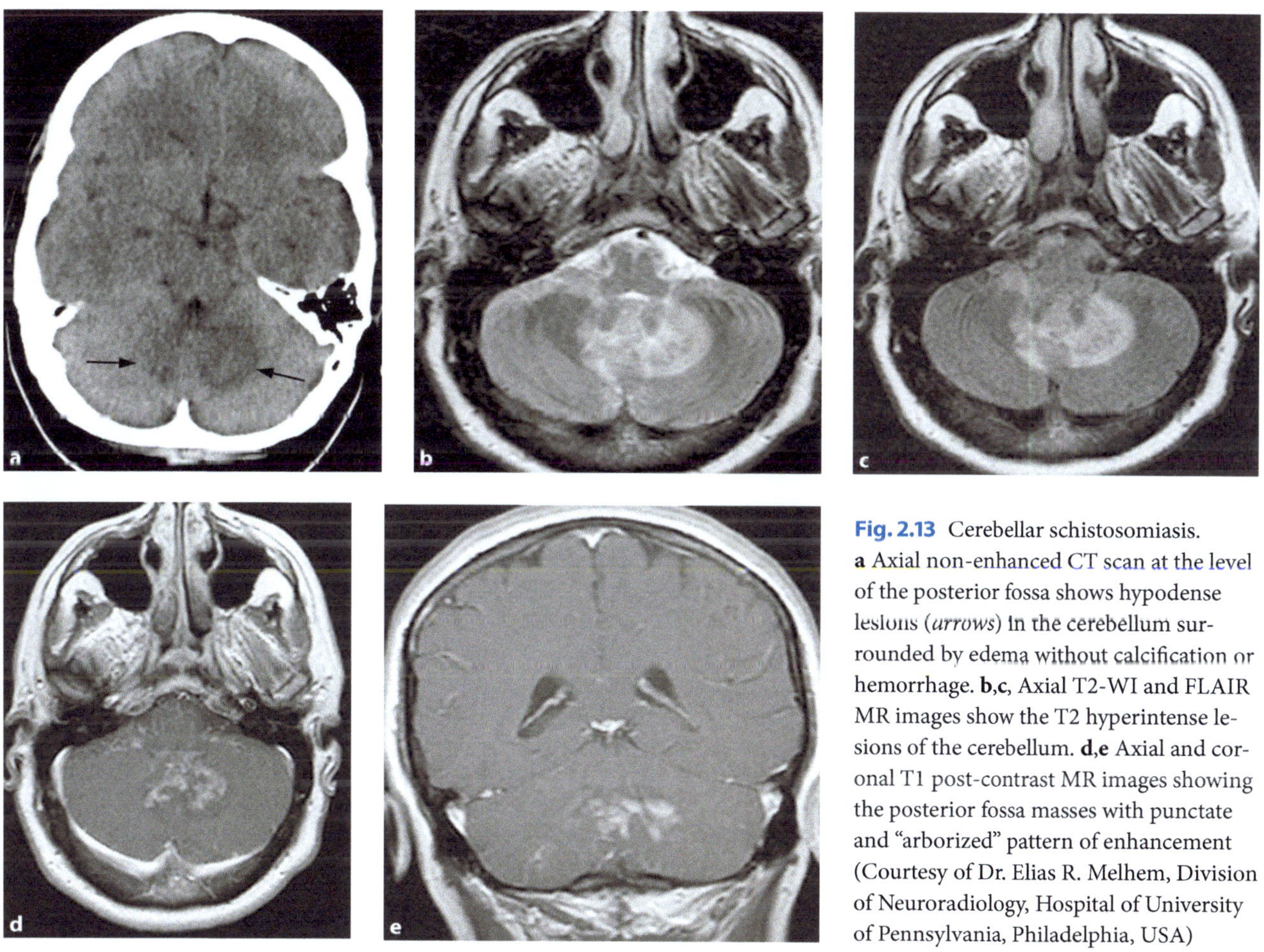

Fig. 2.13 Cerebellar schistosomiasis. **a** Axial non-enhanced CT scan at the level of the posterior fossa shows hypodense lesions (*arrows*) in the cerebellum surrounded by edema without calcification or hemorrhage. **b,c**, Axial T2-WI and FLAIR MR images show the T2 hyperintense lesions of the cerebellum. **d,e** Axial and coronal T1 post-contrast MR images showing the posterior fossa masses with punctate and "arborized" pattern of enhancement (Courtesy of Dr. Elias R. Melhem, Division of Neuroradiology, Hospital of University of Pennsylvania, Philadelphia, USA)

2.5.2.6 Diagnosis and Laboratory Tests

Several laboratory tests are useful in making the diagnosis and are variably positive. They include ELISAs for the serum and cerebrospinal fluid, IgG antibody for *Paragonimus westermani*, intradermal tests, and stool and sputum examinations (Kang et al. 2000).

2.5.2.7 Imaging Findings

The radiological findings are relatively typical. The CT and MRI findings consist of one or conglomerates of multiple ring-shaped enhancing lesions, representing abscesses surrounded by edema. The ring-like lesions resemble "grape clusters" usually involving one hemisphere (Choo et al. 2003). Each "ring" is round or oval, measuring 1–3 cm. Calcified lesions appear hyperdense on CT (Fig. 2.14a), they may be egg-shell, curvilinear or irregular, whereas on MRI, the calcified lesions show a rim of hyposignal intensity on T1- and T2-WI and a center that is iso- or hypointense on T1- and hyperintense on T2-WI. The wall of the ring-like lesions is isointense to the brain on T1-WI, iso- or hypointense on T2-WI, and enhanced on post-contrast T1-WI (Fig. 2.14b). Foci of hemorrhage may be observed. In the chronic stage, all the granulomas calcify, resulting in congregated multiple round or cystic calcified lesions called "soap bubbles."

2.5.2.8 Treatment

Treatment is based on the antiparasitic drug praziquantel, which can be curative (Kang et al. 2000).

2.6 Conclusion

Neurocysticercosis is the most common parasitic infection of the CNS in immunocompetent individuals. MRI is superior to CT scanning in the evaluation of most CNS parasitic infections, while CT has the capability of demonstrating calcified lesions to a better advantage than MRI. The use of the newer techniques of DWI, perfusion imaging, and MRS help in the differentiation of toxoplasmosis from lymphoma and neurocysticercosis from tuberculosis, thus avoiding brain biopsies. Diagnosis of brain parasitosis is based on imaging, laboratory analysis of CSF, serology tests, and brain lesion biopsy. Early diagnosis is of great importance, since brain parasitic infections are potentially treatable diseases.

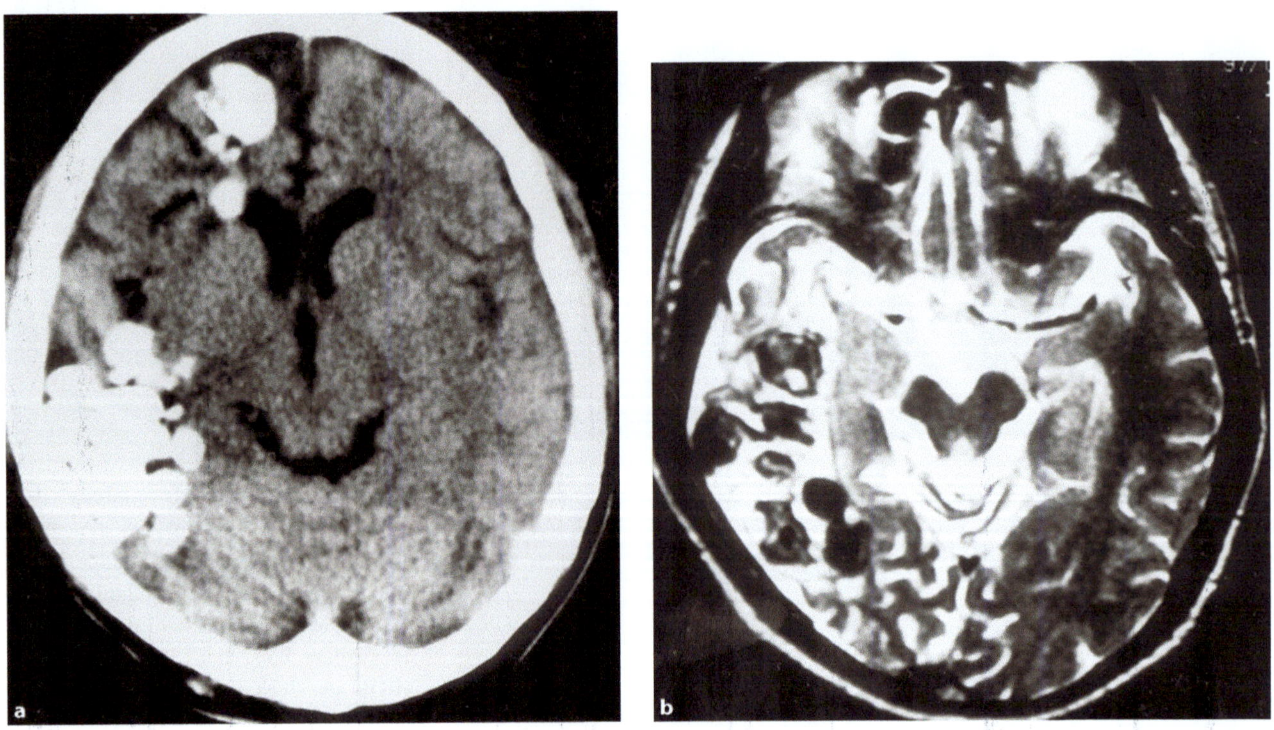

Fig. 2.14 Cerebral paragonimiasis. **a** Axial non-enhanced CT scan of the brain shows multiple calcified densities in the right frontal and temporal lobes. **b** Axial T2-weighted MR image shows congregated multiple round hypointense calcified lesions with inflammatory changes in the surrounding tissue (Courtesy of Dr Sung-Jong Hong, Department of Parasitology, Chung-Ang University, Faculty of Medicine, Seoul, Korea)

References

Aditya GS, Mahadevan A, Santosh V, Chickabasaviah YT, Ashwathnarayanarao CB, Krishna SS (2004) Cysticercal chronic basal arachnoiditis with infarcts, mimicking tuberculous pathology in endemic areas. Neuropathology 24:320–325

Altinors N, Bavbek M, Caner HH, Erdogan B (2000) Central nervous system hydatidosis in Turkey: a cooperative study and literature survey analysis of 458 cases. J Neurosurg 93:1–8

Al Zain TJ, Al-Witry SH, Khalili HM, Aboud SH, Al Zain FT Jr (2002) Multiple intracranial hydatidosis. Acta Neurochir (Wien) 144:1179–1185

Amar AP, Ghosh S, Apuzzo ML (2000) Treatment of central nervous system infections: a neurosurgical perspective. Neuroimaging Clin N Am 10:445–459

Antonios SN, Mina SN (2000) A case report of human coenurosis cerebralis in Tanta, Egypt. J Egypt Soc Parasitol 30(3):959–960

Bachli H, Minet JC, Gratzl O (2004) Cerebral toxocariasis: a possible cause of epileptic seizure in children. Childs Nerv Syst 20:468–472

Bensaid AH, Dietemann JL, de la Palavesa MM, et al. (1994) Intracranial alveolar echinococcosis: CT and MRI. Neuroradiology 36:289–291

Betting LE, Pirani C Jr, de Souza Queiroz L, Damasceno BP, Cendes F (2005) Seizures and cerebral schistosomiasis. Arch Neurol 62:1008–1010

Bouckaert MM, Raubenheimer EJ, Jacobs FJ (2000) Maxillofacial hydatid cysts. Oral Surg Oral Med Oral Pathol Oral Radiol Endod 89:338–342

Boudawara MZ, Jemel H, Ghorbel M, et al. (1999) [Hydatid cysts of the brain stem. Two cases]. Neurochirurgie 45:321–324

Brewster DR, Kwiatkowski D, White NJ (1990) Neurological sequelae of cerebral malaria in children. Lancet 336:1039–1043

Bukte Y, Kemaloglu S, Nazaroglu H, Ozkan U, Ceviz A, Simsek M (2004) Cerebral hydatid disease: CT and MR imaging findings. Swiss Med Wkly 134:459–467

Camacho DL, Smith JK, Castillo M (2003) Differentiation of toxoplasmosis and lymphoma in AIDS patients by using apparent diffusion coefficients. AJNR Am J Neuroradiol 24:633–637

Carod-Artal FJ, Vargas AP (2004) [Myelopathy due to Schistosoma mansoni. A description of two cases and review of the literature]. Rev Neurol 39:137–141

Carod-Artal FJ, Vargas AP, Melo M, Horan TA (2003) American trypanosomiasis (Chagas' disease): an unrecognised cause of stroke. J Neurol Neurosurg Psychiatry 74:516–518

Chang KH, Chi JG, Cho SY, Han MH, Han DH, Han MC (1992) Cerebral sparganosis: analysis of 34 cases with emphasis on CT features. Neuroradiology 34:1–8

Chang KH, Song IC, Kim SH, et al. (1998) In vivo single-voxel proton MR spectroscopy in intracranial cystic masses. AJNR Am J Neuroradiol 19:401–405

Ching HT, Clark AE, Hendrix VJ, Kobrine AI, Schwartz AM (1994) MR imaging appearance of intracerebral schistosomiasis. AJR Am J Roentgenol 162:693–694

Chong-Han CH, Cortez SC, Tung GA (2003) Diffusion-weighted MRI of cerebral toxoplasma abscess. AJR Am J Roentgenol 181:1711–1714

Choo JD, Suh BS, Lee HS, et al. (2003) Chronic cerebral paragonimiasis combined with aneurysmal subarachnoid hemorrhage. Am J Trop Med Hyg 69:466–469

Couldwell WT, Chandrasoma P, Apuzzo ML, Zee CS (1995) Third ventricular cysticercal cyst mimicking a colloid cyst: case report. Neurosurgery 37:1200–1203

Cummings TJ, Madden JF, Gray L, Friedman AH, McLendon RE (2000) Parasitic lesion of the insula suggesting cerebral sparganosis: case report. Neuroradiology 42:206–208

Demir K, Karsli AF, Kaya T, Devrimci E, Alkan K (1991) Cerebral hydatid cysts: CT findings. Neuroradiology 33:22–24

Deol I, Robledo L, Meza A, Visvesvara GS, Andrews RJ (2000) Encephalitis due to a free-living amoeba (Balamuthia mandrillaris): case report with literature review. Surg Neurol 53:611–616

De Villiers JP, Durra G (1998) Case report: amoebic abscess of the brain. Clin Radiol 53:307–309

Eberhardt O, Bialek R, Nagele T, Dichgans J (2005) Eosinophilic meningomyelitis in toxocariasis: case report and review of the literature. Clin Neurol Neurosurg 107:432–438

El Kallab K, El Khoury J, Elias E, Chelala A (2003) Encephalopathy induced by antihelminthic use of levamisole. A report of two patients. J Med Liban 51(4):221

El Koussa S, Chemaly R, Fabre-Bou Abboud V, Tamraz J, Haddad N (1994) Trichinosis and cerebral sinocavernous thrombosis. Rev Neurol (Paris) 150(6–7):464–466

Ellrodt A, Halfon P, Le Bras P, et al. (1987) Multifocal central nervous system lesions in three patients with trichinosis. Arch Neurol 44:432–434

El-Shamam O, Amer T, El-Atta MA (2001) Magnetic resonance imaging of simple and infected hydatid cysts of the brain. Magn Reson Imaging 19:965–974

Ernst TM, Chang L, Witt MD, et al. (1998) Cerebral toxoplasmosis and lymphoma in AIDS: perfusion MR imaging experience in 13 patients. Radiology 208:663–669

Galarza M, Cuccia V, Sosa FP, Monges JA (2002) Pediatric granulomatous cerebral amebiasis: a delayed diagnosis. Pediatr Neurol 26:153–156

Garcia HH, Del Brutto OH (2000) Taenia solium cysticercosis. Infect Dis Clin North Am 14:97–119

Gitau EN, Newton CR (2005) Review article: blood-brain barrier in falciparum malaria. Trop Med Int Health 10:285–292

Guney O, Ozturk K, Kocaogullar Y, Eser O, Acar O (2002) Submandibular and intracranial hydatid cyst in an adolescent. Laryngoscope 112:1857–1860

Gupta RK, Poptani H, Kohli A, Chhabra DK, Sharma B, Gujral RB (1995) In vivo localized proton magnetic resonance spectroscopy of intracranial tuberculomas. Indian J Med Res 101:19–24

Haliloglu M, Saatci I, Akhan O, Ozmen MN, Besim A (1997) Spectrum of imaging findings in pediatric hydatid disease. AJR Am J Roentgenol 169:1627–1631

Hawk MW, Shahlaie K, Kim KD, Theis JH (2005) Neurocysticercosis: a review. Surg Neurol 63:123–132; discussion 132

Jabbour R, Atweh, S, Kanj, S, Ishak G, Hourani, M (2004) MRI appearance of toxocara canis myelopathy. Am J Roentgenol 182:71

Jayakumar PN, Chandrashekar HS, Srikanth SG, Guruprasad AS, Devi BI, Shankar SK (2004) MRI and in vivo proton MR spectroscopy in a racemose cysticercal cyst of the brain. Neuroradiology 46:72–74

Kang SY, Kim TK, Kim TY, Ha YI, Choi SW, Hong SJ (2000) A case of chronic cerebral paragonimiasis westermani. Korean J Parasitol 38:167–171

Karadag O, Gurelik M, Ozum U, Goksel HM (2004) Primary multiple cerebral hydatid cysts with unusual features. Acta Neurochir (Wien) 146:73–77; discussion 77

Kastrup O, Wanke I, Maschke M (2005) Neuroimaging of infections. NeuroRx 2:324–332

Kim YJ, Chang KH, Song IC, et al. (1998) Brain abscess and necrotic or cystic brain tumor: discrimination with signal intensity on diffusion-weighted MR imaging. AJR Am J Roentgenol 171:1487–1490

Kohli A, Gupta RK, Poptani H, Roy R (1995) In vivo proton magnetic resonance spectroscopy in a case of intracranial hydatid cyst. Neurology 45:562–564

Kumar J, Kimm J (1994) MR in Toxocara canis myelopathy. AJNR Am J Neuroradiol 15:1918–1920

Luft BJ, Remington JS (1992) Toxoplasmic encephalitis in AIDS. Clin Infect Dis 15:211–222

Luft BJ, Conley F, Remington JS, et al. (1983) Outbreak of central-nervous-system toxoplasmosis in western Europe and North America. Lancet 1:781–784

Lunardi P, Missori P, Di Lorenzo N, Fortuna A (1991) Cerebral hydatidosis in childhood: a retrospective survey with emphasis on long-term follow-up. Neurosurgery 29:515–517; discussion 517–518

Lury KM, Castillo M (2005) Chagas' disease involving the brain and spinal cord: MRI findings. AJR Am J Roentgenol 185:550–552

Mandell G, Bennett J, Dolin R (2000) Principles and practice of infectious diseases. Churchill Livingstone, Philadelphia, pp 2858–2888

Medina MT, Rosas E, Rubio-Donnadieu F, Sotelo J (1990) Neurocysticercosis as the main cause of late-onset epilepsy in Mexico. Arch Intern Med 150:325–327

Mehta A, Teoh SK, Schaefer PW, Chew FS (1997) Cerebral schistosomiasis. AJR Am J Roentgenol 168:1322

Molyneux ME (2000) Impact of malaria on the brain and its prevention. Lancet 355:671–672

Montoya JG, Liesenfeld O (2004) Toxoplasmosis. Lancet 363:1965–1976

Moon WK, Chang KH, Cho SY, et al. (1993) Cerebral sparganosis: MR imaging versus CT features. Radiology 188:751–757

Moreira-Silva SF, Rodrigues MG, Pimenta JL, Gomes CP, Freire LH, Pereira FE (2004) Toxocariasis of the central nervous system: with report of two cases. Rev Soc Bras Med Trop 37:169–174

Muehlethaler K, Scheurer E, Zollinger U, Markwalder R, Nguyen XM (2005) Fulminant cerebral malaria in a Swiss patient. Infection 33:33–35

Nelson J, Frost JL, Schochet SS Jr (1990) Unsuspected cerebral Toxocara infection in a fire victim. Clin Neuropathol 9:106–108

Newton CR, Peshu N, Kendall B, et al. (1994) Brain swelling and ischaemia in Kenyans with cerebral malaria. Arch Dis Child 70:281–287

Ofori-Kwakye SK, Sidebottom DG, Herbert J, Fischer EG, Visvesvara GS (1986) Granulomatous brain tumor caused by Acanthamoeba. Case report. J Neurosurg 64:505–509

Osborn A, Blaser S, Salzman K (2004) Diagnostic imaging: brain, 1st edn. Saunders, Philadelphia, p 992

Ouboukhlik A, Choukri M, Elazhari A, Elkamar A, Boucetta M (1994) [Cerebral hydatid cyst. Apropos of 48 cases]. Neurochirurgie 40:242–246

Pagano MA, Segura MJ, Di Lorenzo GA, et al. (1999) Cerebral tumor-like American trypanosomiasis in acquired immunodeficiency syndrome. Ann Neurol 45:403–406

Palmer P, Reeder M (2001) The imaging of tropical diseases: with epidemiological, pathological and clinical correlation, 2nd edn. Springer, Heidelberg, p 1684

Park SY, Glaser C, Murray WJ, et al. (2000) Raccoon roundworm (Baylisascaris procyonis) encephalitis: case report and field investigation. Pediatrics 106:E56

Patankar TF, Karnad DR, Shetty PG, Desai AP, Prasad SR (2002) Adult cerebral malaria: prognostic importance of imaging findings and correlation with postmortem findings. Radiology 224:811–816

Patrikar DM, Mitra KR, Bhutada VR (1993) Cerebral hydatid disease. Australas Radiol 37:226–227

Pau A, Turtas S, Brambilla M, Leoni A, Rosa M, Viale GL (1987) Computed tomography and magnetic resonance imaging of cerebral coenurosis. Surg Neurol 27(6):548–552

Piette E (1989) General review of parasitoses involving the maxillo facial region. Acta Stomatol Belg 86:175–210

Piotin M, Cattin F, Kantelip B, Miralbes S, Godard J, Bonneville JF (1997) Disseminated intracerebral alveolar echinococcosis: CT and MRI. Neuroradiology 39:431–433

Polat P, Kantarci M, Alper F, Suma S, Koruyucu MB, Okur A (2003) Hydatid disease from head to toe. Radiographics 23:475–494; quiz 536–537

Preidler KW, Riepl T, Szolar D, Ranner G (1996) Cerebral schistosomiasis: MR and CT appearance. AJNR Am J Neuroradiol 17:1598–1600

Pretell EJ, Martinot C, Garcia HH, Alvarado M, Bustos JA, Martinot C, for the Cysticercosis Working Group in Peru (2005) Differential diagnosis between cerebral tuberculosis and neurocysticercosis by magnetic resonance spectroscopy. J Comput Assist Tomogr 29(1):112–114

Punyagupta S, Juttijudata P, Bunnag T (1975) Eosinophilic meningitis in Thailand. Clinical studies of 484 typical cases probably caused by Angiostrongylus cantonensis. Am J Trop Med Hyg 24:921–931

Reittner P, Szolar DH, Schmid M (1996) Case report. Systemic manifestation of Echinococcus alveolaris infection. J Comput Assist Tomogr 20:1030–1032

Rowley HA, Uht RM, Kazacos KR, et al. (2000) Radiologic-pathologic findings in raccoon roundworm (Baylisascaris procyonis) encephalitis. AJNR Am J Neuroradiol 21:415–420

Sabbah P, Brosset C, Imbert P, Bonardel G, Jeandel P, Briant JF (1997) Human African trypanosomiasis: MRI. Neuroradiology 39:708–710

Sabbatani S, Zucchelli M, Calbucci F, Roncaroli F, Chiodo F (2004) A case of cerebral coenurosis. Infez Med 12(3):205–210

Sanelli PC, Lev MH, Gonzalez RG, Schaefer PW (2001) Unique linear and nodular MR enhancement pattern in schistosomiasis of the central nervous system: report of three patients. AJR Am J Roentgenol 177:1471–1474

Scharf D (1988) Neurocysticercosis. Two hundred thirty-eight cases from a California hospital. Arch Neurol 45:777–780

Schuster FL, Visvesvara GS (1998) Efficacy of novel antimicrobials against clinical isolates of opportunistic amebas. J Eukaryot Microbiol 45:612–618

Shukla-Dave A, Gupta RK, Roy R, et al. (2001) Prospective evaluation of in vivo proton MR spectroscopy in differentiation of similar appearing intracranial cystic lesions. Magn Reson Imaging 19:103–110

Talan-Hranilovic J, Sajko T, Negovetic L, Lupret V, Kalousek M (2002) Cerebral cysticercosis and echinococcosis: a preoperative diagnostic dilemma. Arch Med Res 33:590–594

Torre D, Casari S, Speranza F, et al. (1998) Randomized trial of trimethoprim-sulfamethoxazole versus pyrimethamine-sulfadiazine for therapy of toxoplasmic encephalitis in patients with AIDS. Italian Collaborative Study Group. Antimicrob Agents Chemother 42:1346–1349

Tuzun M, Hekimoglu B (1998) Hydatid disease of the CNS: imaging features. AJR Am J Roentgenol 171:1497–1500

Tuzun M, Altinors N, Arda IS, Hekimoglu B (2002) Cerebral hydatid disease CT and MR findings. Clin Imaging 26:353–357

Vidal JE, Sztajnbok J, Seguro AC (2003) Eosinophilic meningoencephalitis due to Toxocara canis: case report and review of the literature. Am J Trop Med Hyg 69:341–343

Weller PF (1993) Eosinophilic meningitis. Am J Med 95:250–253

White AC Jr (2000) Neurocysticercosis: updates on epidemiology, pathogenesis, diagnosis, and management. Annu Rev Med 51:187–206

White JM, Barker RD, Salisbury JR, et al. (2004) Granulomatous amoebic encephalitis. Lancet 364:220

Wichert-Ana L, Velasco TR, Terra-Bustamante VC, et al. (2004) Surgical treatment for mesial temporal lobe epilepsy in the presence of massive calcified neurocysticercosis. Arch Neurol 61:1117–1119

Wise ME, Sorvillo FJ, Shafir SC, Ash LR, Berlin OG (2005) Severe and fatal central nervous system disease in humans caused by Baylisascaris procyonis, the common roundworm of raccoons: a review of current literature. Microbes Infect 7:317–323

Xinou E, Lefkopoulos A, Gelagoti M, et al. (2003) CT and MR imaging findings in cerebral toxocaral disease. AJNR Am J Neuroradiol 24:714–718

Yoo TW, Mlikotic A, Cornford ME, Beck CK (2004) Concurrent cerebral American trypanosomiasis and toxoplasmosis in a patient with AIDS. Clin Infect Dis 39:e30–e34

Imaging of Parasitic Diseases of the Thorax

3

Santiago Martinez, Carlos S. Restrepo, Jorge A. Carrillo

Contents

3.1 Introduction

A broad spectrum of parasitic infections frequently affects the lungs, mediastinum, and thoracic wall, manifesting with abnormal imaging findings that often make diagnosis challenging. Although most of these infections result in nonspecific abnormalities, familiarity with their imaging features and the diagnostic pathways help the radiologist to formulate an adequate differential diagnosis and to guide diagnosticians in reaching a definitive diagnosis.

3.2 Protozoa

3.2.1 Amebiasis

Entamoeba histolytica is responsible for amebiasis, a parasitosis with a worldwide distribution and an elevated mortality rate, possibly the highest after malaria and schistosomiasis. As much as 1% of the world's population is thought to be infected and up to 100,000 related deaths are reported annually (Mandell et al. 2005; Murray et al. 2005; World Health Organization 1997). The infection is more prevalent among the lower socioeconomic classes in tropical and subtropical climates; other risk factors include immigrants from endemic areas, institutionalized populations (e.g., those with mental retardation), communal living, and promiscuous homosexual males (Ravdin 1988). The most severe cases are often identified among neonates, during pregnancy and postpartum, corticosteroid use, malignancy, and malnutrition (Ravdin 1988).

Cysts remain viable for long periods of time in the environment after being excreted in the feces of human hosts. Humans can become infected by ingestion of these forms that ultimately become trophozoites in the small bowel, constituting the invasive form of the parasite (Barrett-Connor 1982; Botero 2003; Binford and Connor 1976; Hasleton 1996; Travis et al. 2002; Murray et al. 2002; Fishman 1998). The majority of cases develop non-invasive infection in keeping with the natural life cycle of the parasite; in these patients, trophozoites become encysted and excreted again via the feces into the environment (Mandell et al. 2005). While invasive disease may develop by direct invasion of the colonic epithelium, the factor that determines pathogenicity remains unknown (Mandell et al. 2005).

Thoracic disease is the second most common manifestation of extraintestinal amebiasis after liver abscesses (Le Roux 1969; Shamsuzzaman and Hashiguchi 2002). It complicates 7–20% of all cases of hepatic disease and about 2% patients with intestinal disease (Fishman 1998). Thoracic infection may result from several routes: direct extension from a liver abscess to the thorax, which occurs in 6–40% of patients with hepatic compromise; hematogenous spread; and rarely, aspiration (Shamsuzzaman and Hashiguchi 2002). Pericardial compromise is present in less than 2% of all thoracic complications related to amebic hepatic abscesses and is more common in the setting of left hepatic lobe disease. Pain, cardiac tamponade, and sepsis are the most common clinical findings (Le Roux 1969; Ibarra-Perez et al. 1981; Landay et al. 1980).

Thoracic amebiasis is more commonly suspected in patients from endemic areas with a liver abscess. Stool examination is of limited value because cysts or trophozoites are seen in a small proportion of patients with extraintestinal amebiasis (Shamsuzzaman and Hashiguchi 2002), and many pleuropulmonary manifestations may be unrelated to amebiasis, even if parasitic forms are identified in the feces. While "anchovy sauce" content can be obtained from an amebic hepatic abscess or from expectorate from a hepatobronchial fistula, the isolation of parasites in these samples is erratic. Cultures can be obtained only in feces, since the protozoan does not grow in pus. Serologic analysis is helpful for the diagnosis of invasive disease in non-endemic populations (Barrett-Connor 1982; Shamsuzzaman and Hashiguchi 2002).

Pleural effusion is a common finding in thoracic amebiasis. It can be either sterile, as in inflammatory pleural reactions, or a frank empyema if the hepatic abscess happened to rupture into the pleural cavity. Typically, pleuropulmonary findings are preceded by elevation of the right hemidiaphragm (Fig. 3.1). Common parenchymal findings include consolidation (Fig. 3.2) and cavitation (Figs. 3.3, 3.4). When the infection is drained into the airway, a hepatobronchial or bronchobiliary fistula can result. Hematogenous dissemination results in consolidation further away from the diaphragm (Fig. 3.5). Rarely, invasion of the inferior vena cava occurs, eventually resulting in pulmonary thromboembolism. As in pleural disease, pericarditis and pericardial effusion can result from an inflammatory reaction or drainage of a liver abscess into the pericardium or pleura, usually located in the left hepatic lobe (Figs. 3.6, 3.7) (Le Roux 1969; Shamsuzzaman and Hashiguchi 2002; Ibarra-Perez et al. 1981; Landay et al. 1980).

3.2.2 Malaria

The *Anopheles* mosquito is the efficient vector that transmits *Plasmodium* species (*P. falciparum, P. vivax, P. ovale,* and *P. malariae)* to humans, the result being malaria, the most devastating parasitic disease in the world. The 2005 World Malaria Report from the World Health Organiza-

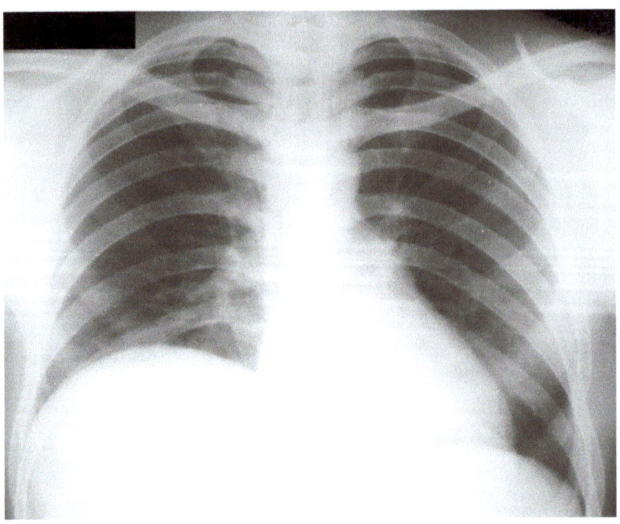

Fig. 3.1 Thoracic amebiasis. Posteroanterior (PA) chest radiograph demonstrates elevation of the right hemidiaphragm, a common finding in the early phase of the thoracic infection

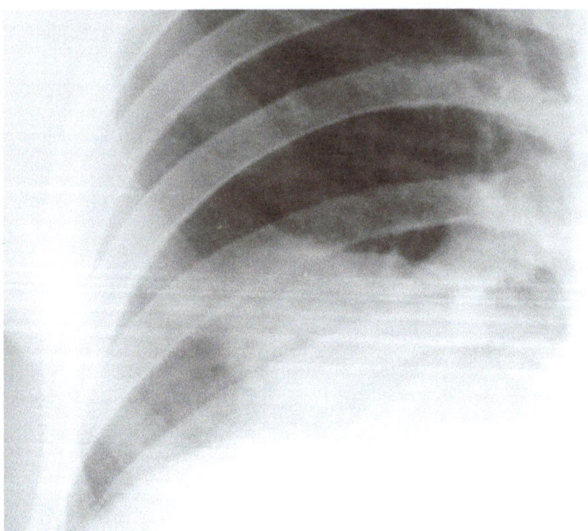

Fig. 3.2 Pulmonary amebiasis. PA chest radiograph, cone view, shows area of consolidation in the right lower lobe

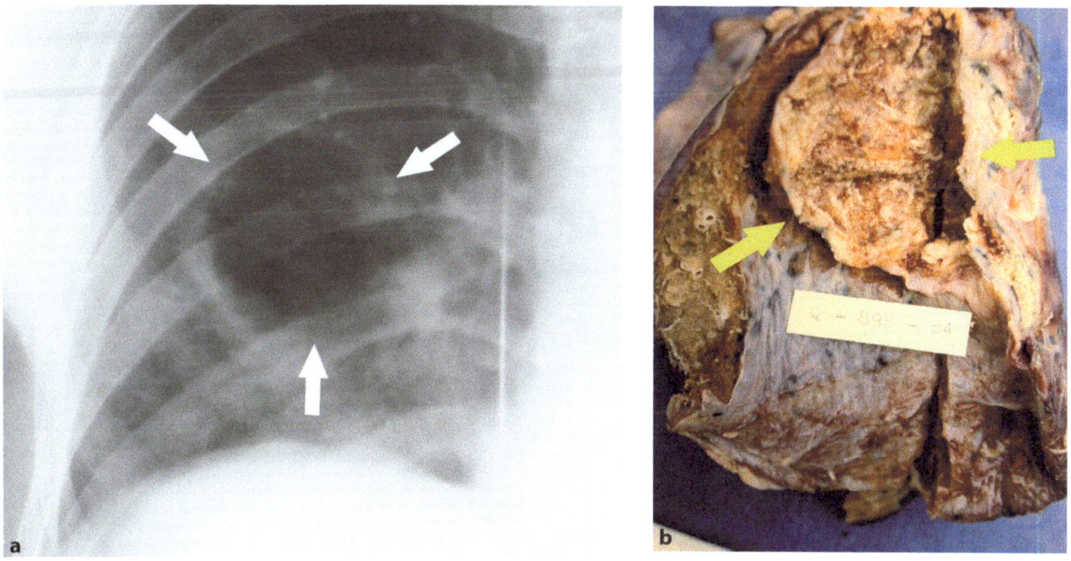

Fig. 3.3 Cavitary pulmonary amebiasis. **a** PA chest radiograph, close-up view, demonstrates cavitation (*arrows*) in the right lower lobe. **b** Macroscopic specimen after autopsy shows an abscess in the right lower lobe (*arrows*) (Reproduced with permission from Radiographics, Martinez et al. 2005)

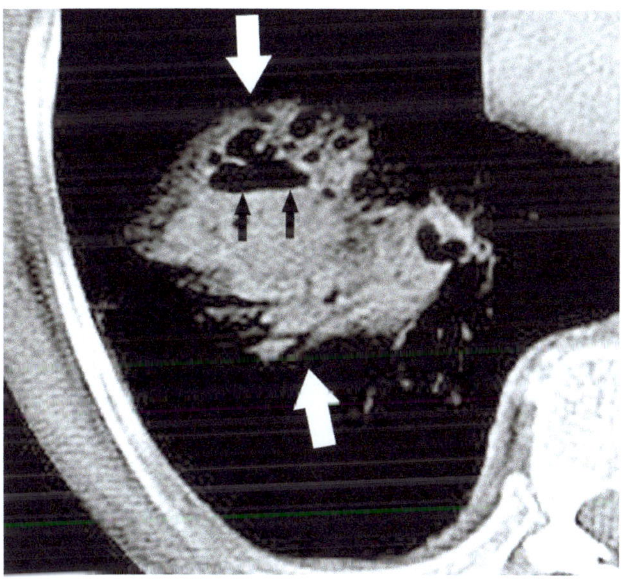

Fig. 3.4 Cavitary pulmonary amebiasis. Close-up view of an axial CT scan of the chest (soft tissue window) shows cavitating consolidation in the right lower lobe (*white arrows*). Note air fluid level (*black arrows*)

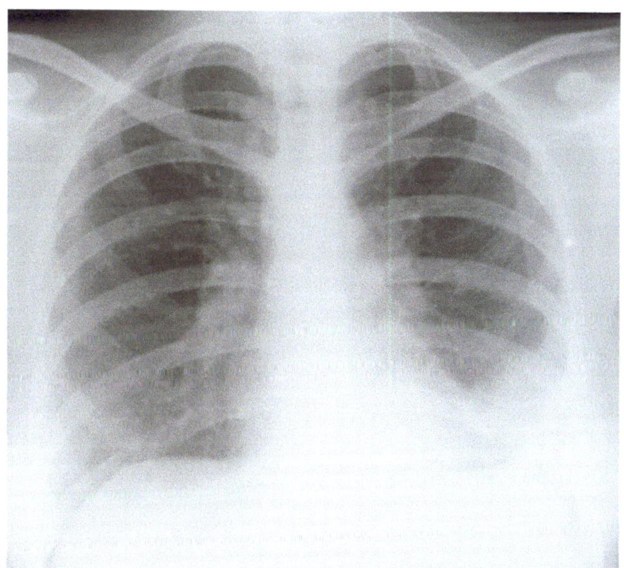

Fig. 3.5 Pulmonary amebiasis. PA chest radiograph demonstrates left lower lobe consolidation and ipsilateral pleural fluid collection. Compromise of areas different from the right lower lobe usually results from hematogenous dissemination

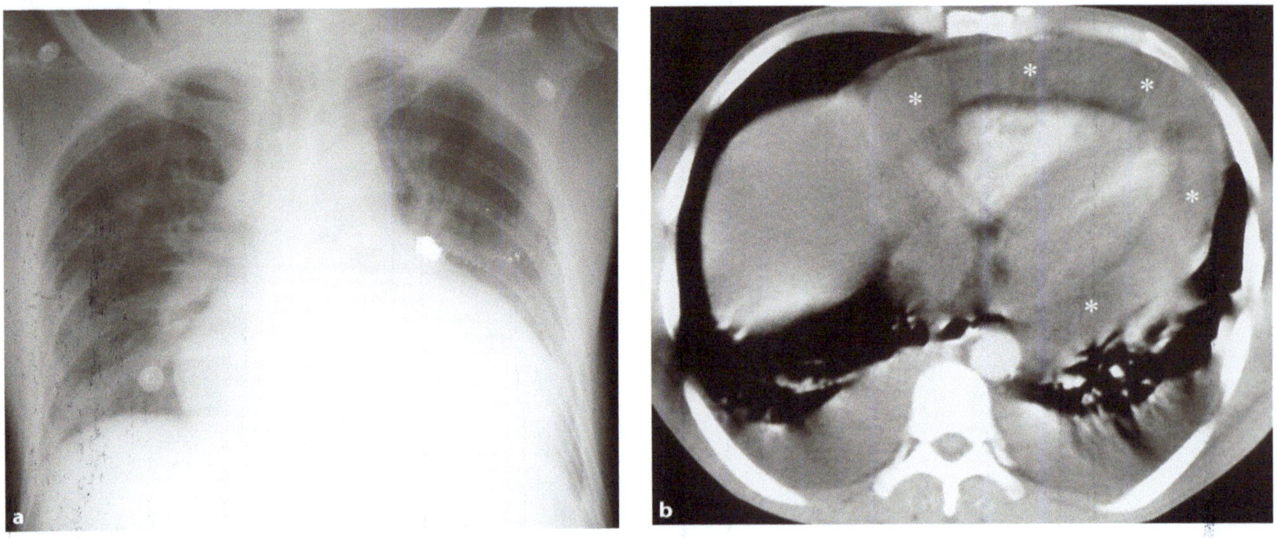

Fig. 3.6 Pericardial amebiasis presenting with cardiac tamponade. **a** PA chest radiograph demonstrates marked enlargement of the cardiomediastinal silhouette. A bullet fragment identified overlying the left cardiac silhouette is located in the paravertebral soft tissues and is unrelated. **b** Axial CT scan of the chest (soft tissue window) shows marked pericardial effusion (*asterisks*). Additionally, there are bilateral pleural effusions. Pericardial fluid resulted from rupture of a left-sided liver lobe abscess (Reproduced with permission from Radiographics, Martinez et al. 2005)

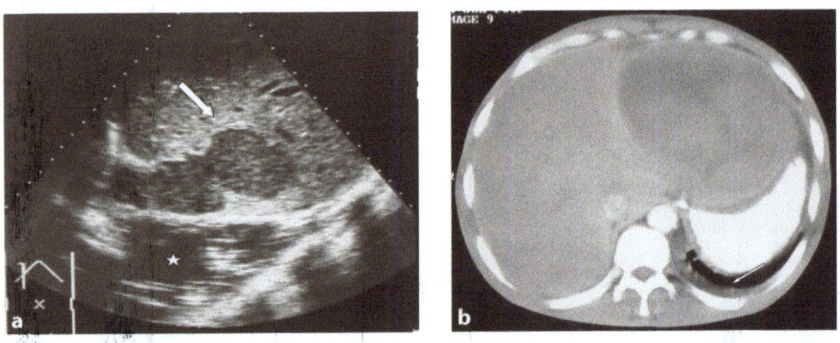

Fig. 3.7 Amebic liver abscess with a pleural reaction. **a** Ultrasound image of the liver showing an amebic liver abscess (*arrow*) and right pleural effusion (*star*). **b** Contrast-enhanced CT scan of the liver demonstrating a left hepatic lobe amebic abscess and left pleural effusion (*arrow*)

tion (WHO) estimated that up to 500 million people had been infected in the previous year (World Health Organization 2005). Consequently, several million deaths in endemic areas such as the tropical areas of South America, Africa, and Southern Asia result every year (Mandell et al. 2005; Murray et al. 2005; Botero 2003). Over 3.2 billion people in 107 countries are at risk of infection (World Health Organization 2005). Children younger than 5 years old, pregnant women and HIV-infected patients are at special risk (Mandell et al. 2005; World Health Organization/Unicef 2005). Of particular concern is *P. falciparum,* which is responsible for the majority of cases of severe malaria, causes more than 1 million deaths each year and exhibits an increasing occurrence of resistance to chloroquine and other antimalarial drugs (World Health Organization 2000a).

Parasites are inoculated into the human blood by the bite of the *Anopheles* mosquito. They mature inside the erythrocytes and are released by hemolysis. The process occurs at certain time intervals that coincide with the periodicity of episodic fever (tertian or quartan) (Murray et al. 2005; World Health Organization 1997; Ravdin 1988; Barrett-Connor 1982; Botero 2003; Murray et al. 2002) and it is specific for each species (Murray et al. 2005; Botero 2003; Binford and Connor 1976; Hasleton 1996; Travis et al. 2002; Fishman et al. 1998; Taylor and White 2002). Thus, malignant tertian fever (*P. falciparum)* manifests with irregular fever spikes, whereas benign tertian fever (*P. vivax, P. ovale*) and quartan fever (*P. malariae*) manifest with fever spikes every 48 and 72 h respectively (Botero 2003).

Clinical findings of malaria include fever with chills, sweating, anemia, leucopenia, and splenomegaly (Murray et al. 2005; Botero 2003; Binford and Connor 1976; Hasleton 1996; Travis et al. 2002; Fishman et al. 1998; Taylor and White 2002). Diagnosis is usually made by identifying trophozoites or other parasitic forms within the erythrocytes in a thin blood smear or parasites in a thick smear. Serologic and nucleic acid amplification tests are also available (Murray et al. 2005; Binford and Connor; Hasleton 1998; Travis et al. 2002; Taylor and White 2002).

The primary thoracic manifestation of malaria is adult respiratory distress syndrome (ARDS). As of 2005, the WHO continued to include ARDS as a criterion for the definition of severe *P. falciparum* malaria (World Health Organization 2000a). In the setting of malaria, ARDS secondary to *P. falciparum* is associated with high mortality of 80% (World Health Organization 2000a). Although the pathophysiologic events related to the development of ARDS remain unclear, available data support the fact that pulmonary edema is rather a high permeability edema secondary to microvascular dysfunction (Cosgriff 1990). Infected erythrocytes sequestrated in the lungs lead to a release of local cytokines that eventually results in pulmonary edema, dyspnea, hypoxic acute lung injury, and ARDS (Mandell et al. 2005; Taylor and White 2002). Although the majority of cases of ARDS are related to the *P. falciparum* infection, association with *P. vivax* and *P. ovale* is also documented in the literature (Lee and Maguire 1999; Munteis et al. 1997; Tanios et al. 2001; Curlin et al. 1999; Carlini et al. 1999). Radiographic and CT findings are consistent with ARDS, i.e., pleural effusions, diffuse interstitial edema, and lobar consolidation (Figs. 3.8, 3.9) (Taylor and White 2002; Cosgriff 1990; Lee and Maguire 1999; Munteis et al. 1997; Tanios et al. 2001; Curlin et al. 1999; Carlini et al. 1981; Cayea et al. 1981; Gachot et al. 1995; Torres et al. 1997). Eosinophilic pneumonia with bilateral heterogeneous opacities has been described in association with the use of the antimalarial drug pyrimethamine (Davidson et al. 1988).

3.2.3 Trypanosomiasis

Trypanosoma cruzi is the etiologic agent of American trypanosomiasis or Chagas' disease. The infection is acquired through the bite of an insect from the *Reduviidae* family (genera *Triatoma, Rhodnius,* and *Panstrongylus*), by the inoculation of trypomastigotes into the human body. The insect usually defecates near to the bite and the inoculation may occur from rubbing the reduviid bug feces over the bite or some other skin defect (Murray et al. 2005). The parasites multiply within the macrophages, which eventually rupture, releasing amastigotes capable of invading diverse organs hematogenously, including the heart and the gastrointestinal tract, but namely the esophagus and colon (Botero 2003; Binford and Connor 1976; Hasleton 1996; Travis et al. 2002; Murray et al. 2002; Fishman et al. 1998).

Chagas' disease is endemic to areas of Central and South America, especially Argentina, Brazil, Bolivia, Chile, Paraguay, and Uruguay. By 2000, the WHO estimated that 16–18 million people were infected in the American countries (World Health Organization 2000b). As many as 45,000 people die yearly due to the disease (Mandell et al. 2005). Starting in 1997 with Uruguay, several countries (i.e., Venezuela, Chile, and Brazil) have reported interruption of vectorial and transfusional transmission of Chagas' disease, with a significant decrease in the incidence of the disease of up to 95% (World Health Organization 1999, 2000b, 2000c). Chagas' disease has also been described in the south-western United States among immigrants from endemic areas (Murray et al. 2002; Hagar and Rahimtoola 1991; Kirchhoff and Neva 1985).

Acute manifestations of trypanosomiasis are rarely clinically detected. Romana's sign is a classic manifestation that includes fever and facial or unilateral

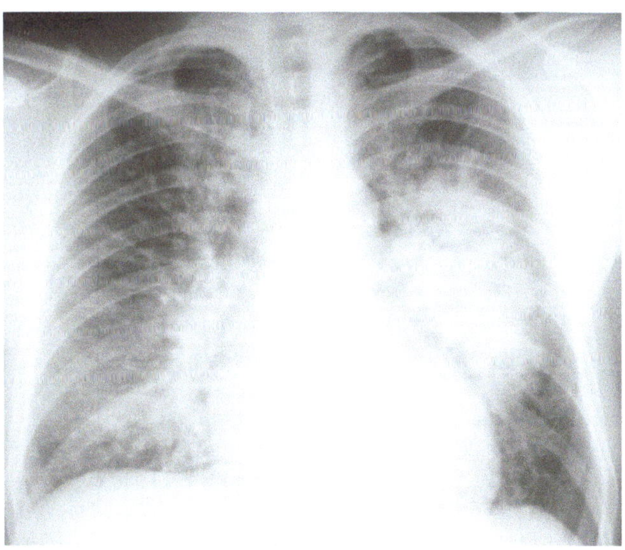

Fig. 3.8 Acute respiratory distress syndrome (ARDS) in a young patient with *P. falciparum* malaria. PA chest radiograph demonstrates bilateral and diffuse heterogeneous opacities in all four quadrants of the lungs. Further clinical criteria for ARDS were positive. Parasitic forms of *P. falciparum* were identified in the thin peripheral blood smear

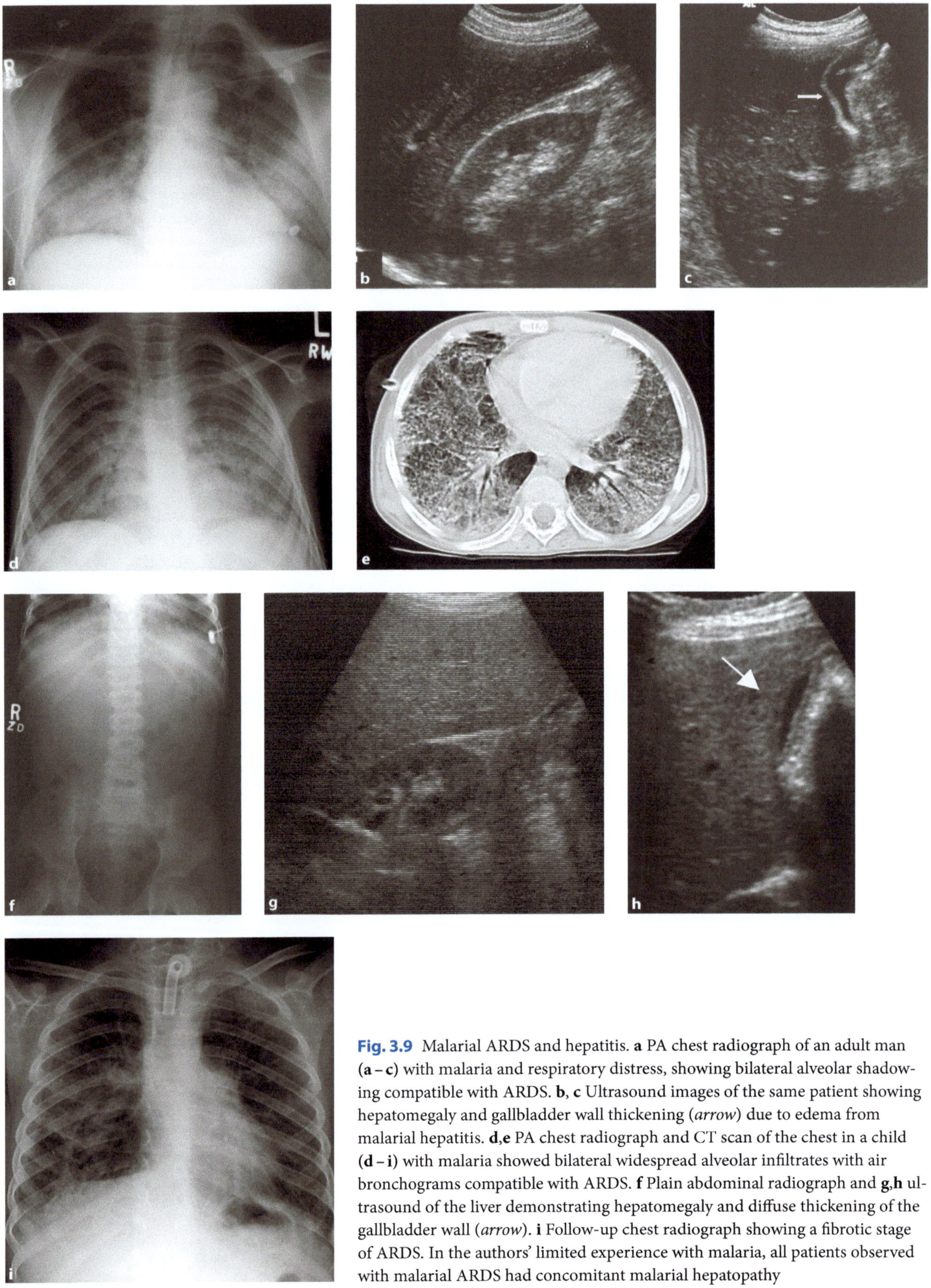

Fig. 3.9 Malarial ARDS and hepatitis. **a** PA chest radiograph of an adult man (**a – c**) with malaria and respiratory distress, showing bilateral alveolar shadowing compatible with ARDS. **b, c** Ultrasound images of the same patient showing hepatomegaly and gallbladder wall thickening (*arrow*) due to edema from malarial hepatitis. **d,e** PA chest radiograph and CT scan of the chest in a child (**d – i**) with malaria showed bilateral widespread alveolar infiltrates with air bronchograms compatible with ARDS. **f** Plain abdominal radiograph and **g,h** ultrasound of the liver demonstrating hepatomegaly and diffuse thickening of the gallbladder wall (*arrow*). **i** Follow-up chest radiograph showing a fibrotic stage of ARDS. In the authors' limited experience with malaria, all patients observed with malarial ARDS had concomitant malarial hepatopathy

palpebral edema. Signs and symptoms of acute myocarditis and meningoencephalitis have sometimes been described (Mandell et al. 2005). Although detection of trypomastigotes in the blood smear, culture, and xenodiagnosis are the most common methods used to establish the diagnosis, their sensitivity is not greater than 50% (Mandell et al. 2005). Polymerase chain reaction (PCR) techniques appear to be promising, especially in persons with borderline serology, infected patients who have received specific treatment, and acute or congenital disease not detected in the blood smear (Mandell et al. 2005). Radiographically, acute myocarditis can present with acute heart failure (Fig. 3.10).

Patients are more commonly diagnosed in the chronic phase. Late cardiac manifestations include chronic myocarditis with focal and diffuse loss of myocytes, fibrosis, and focal atrophy, as well as involvement of the conduction system with a bundle branch block, which can progress to a complete atrioventricular block. Late gastrointestinal compromise is related to neuronal damage of the myenteric plexus, with development of achalasia and megacolon (Botero 2003; Hagar and Rahimtoola 1991; Kirchhoff and Neva 1985; Camara et al. 1993; Prata 1994; Umezawa et al. 2001). Although bronchopathy has rarely been described due to denervation of the bronchial walls, it appears not to have significant clinical impact (Lemle 1999). Serologic tests are preferred for the diagnosis of chronic forms.

Radiologic findings reflect the aforementioned clinical features. Severe cardiomegaly, usually with evidence of venous hypertension (e.g., septal lines, pulmonary edema, pleural effusion), is often seen in chronic dilated cardiomyopathy (Fig. 3.11) (Hagar and Rahimtoola 1991; Kirchhoff and Neva 1985; Camara et al. 1993; Prata 1994; Umezawa et al. 2001). Achalasia (Fig. 3.12) and megacolon are usually confirmed with barium studies (Botero 2003; Camara et al. 1993).

The role of MR in cardiac Chagas' disease has recently been described. Areas of myocardial fibrosis are identified as myocardial delayed enhancement in inversion recovery gradient-echo sequences 10–20 min after the intravenous injection of gadolinium-based contrast (Fig. 3.13). These hyperintense areas, which can be transmural, subendocardial, along the midwall, and subepicardial, are more prone to being identified toward the apex, inferior, and inferolateral walls. Although often indistinguishable from myocardial fibrosis due to coronary artery disease, the finding could be a helpful marker of disease severity among seropositive patients, especially those who are asymptomatic (Society for Cardiovascular Magnetic Resonance 2003; Mahrholdt et al. 2005; Rochitte et al. 2005).

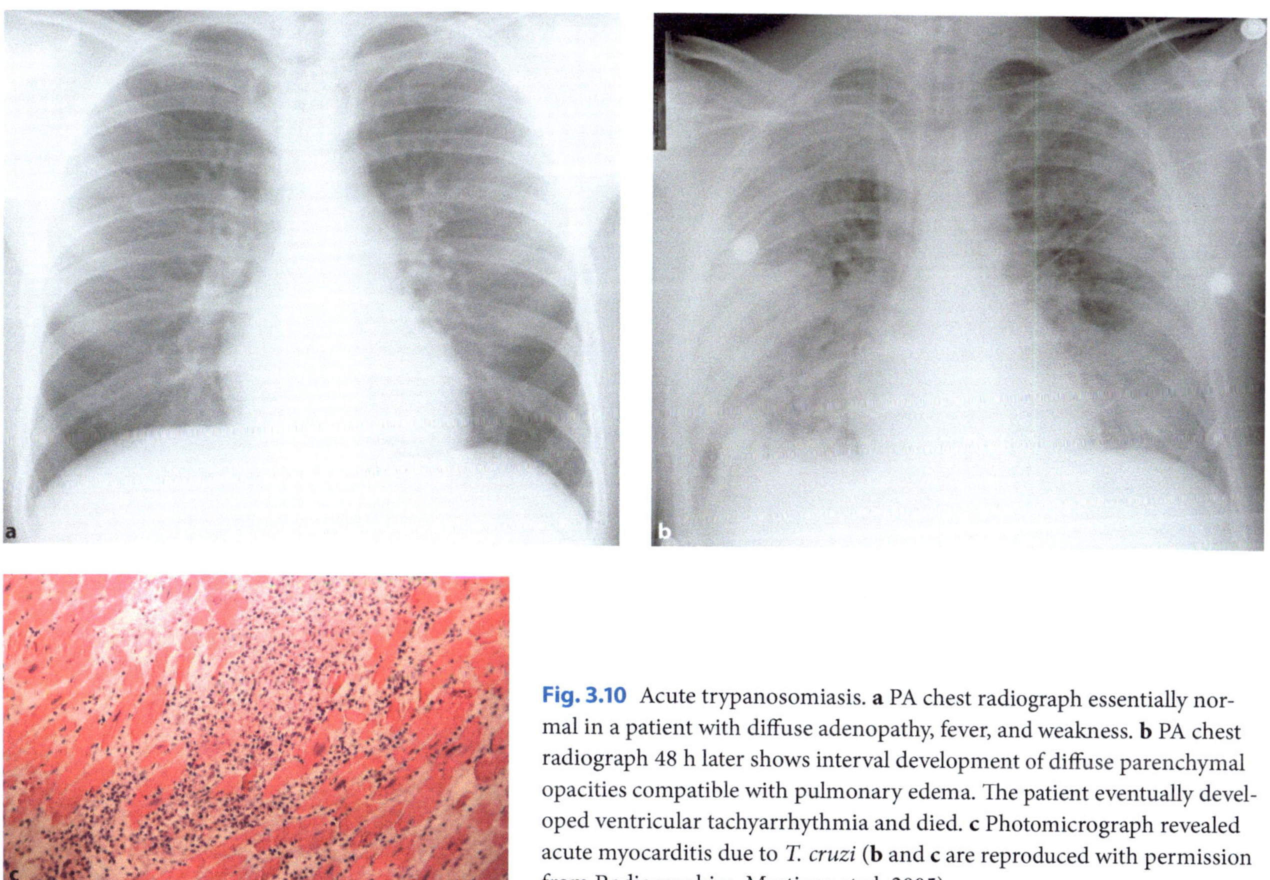

Fig. 3.10 Acute trypanosomiasis. **a** PA chest radiograph essentially normal in a patient with diffuse adenopathy, fever, and weakness. **b** PA chest radiograph 48 h later shows interval development of diffuse parenchymal opacities compatible with pulmonary edema. The patient eventually developed ventricular tachyarrhythmia and died. **c** Photomicrograph revealed acute myocarditis due to *T. cruzi* (**b** and **c** are reproduced with permission from Radiographics, Martinez et al. 2005)

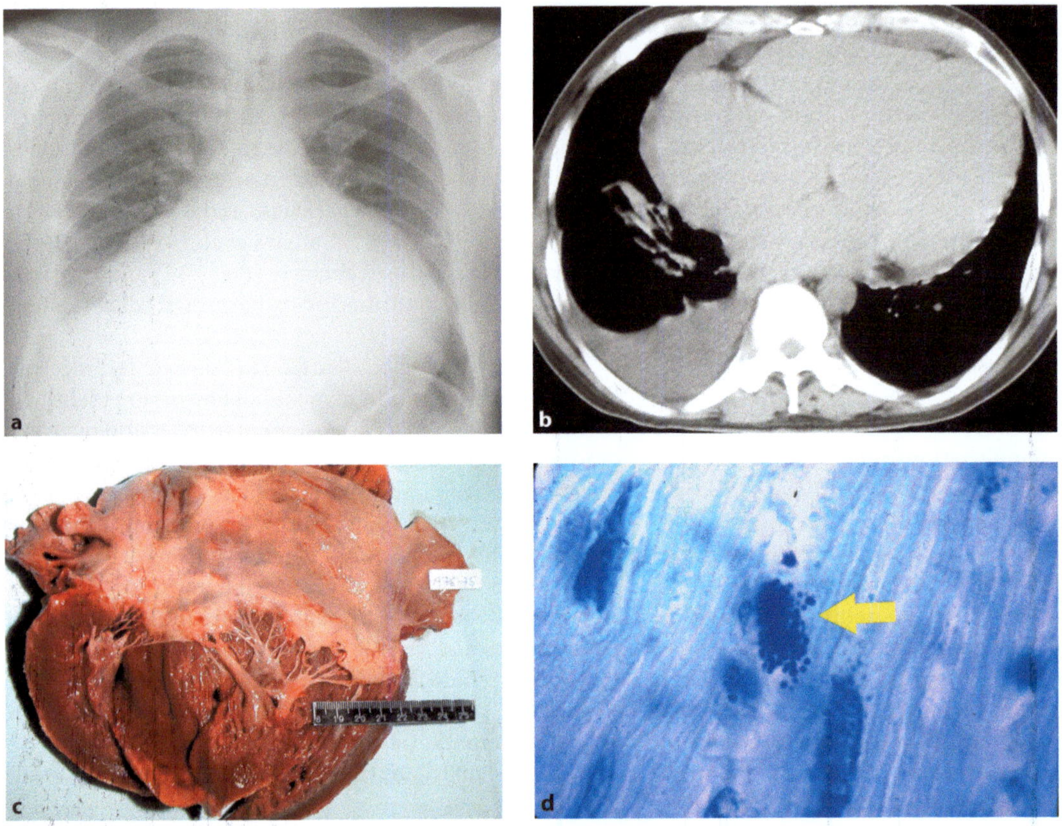

Fig. 3.11 Chronic myocarditis due to Chagas' disease. **a** PA chest radiograph shows severe and diffuse enlargement of the cardiac silhouette, vascular redistribution in the upper lobes, and right-sided pleural effusion. **b** Axial CT of the chest (mediastinal window) demonstrates marked dilatation of all cardiac chambers and right-sided pleural effusion. **c** Macroscopic specimen exhibits marked cardiomegaly and thickening of the ventricular wall. **d** Photomicrograph (Giemsa stain, ×10) shows *T. cruzi* amastigotes within a myocardial fiber (*arrow*) (**a**,**c**, and **d** are reproduced with permission from Radiographics, Martinez et al. 2005)

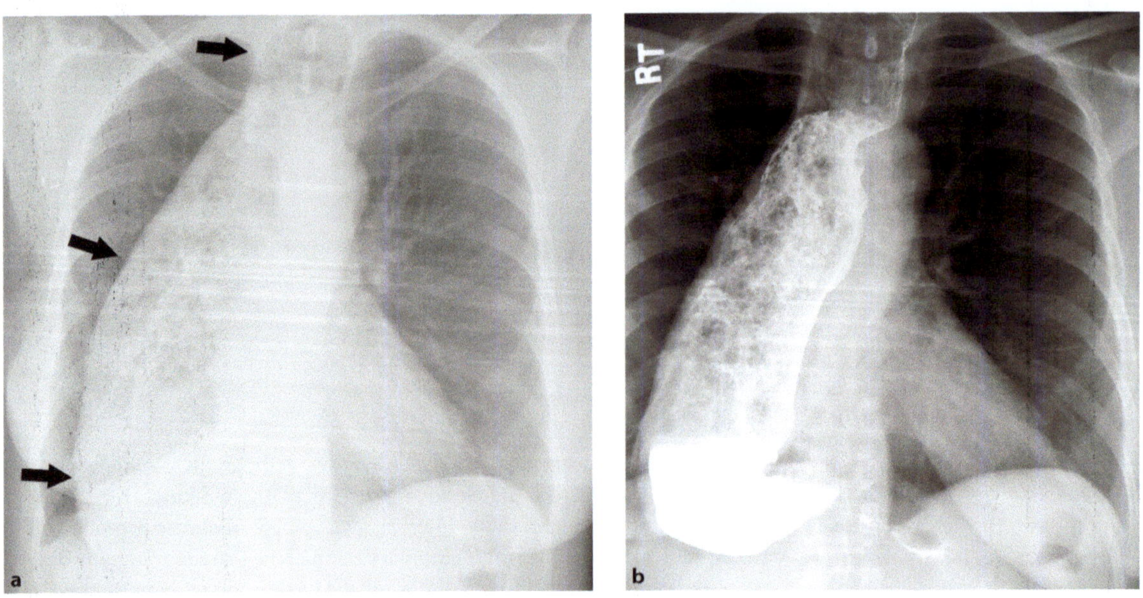

Fig. 3.12 Achalasia secondary to Chagas' disease. **a** PA chest radiograph demonstrates a right-sided tubular paramediastinal soft tissue mass (*arrows*). **b** Barium swallow shows massive dilatation of the esophagus compatible with a Chagasic megaesophagus

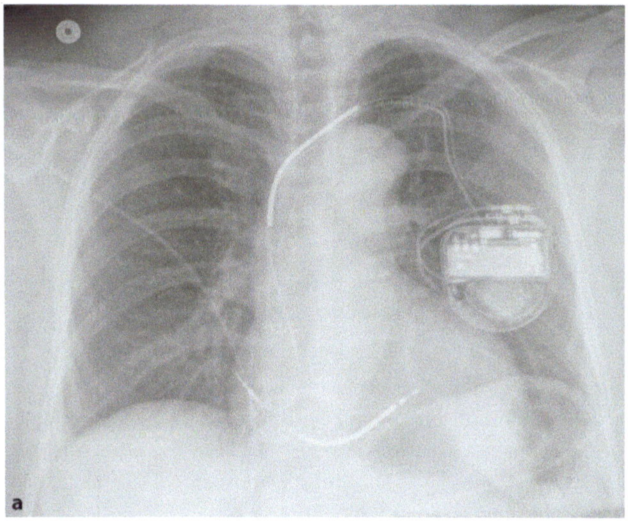

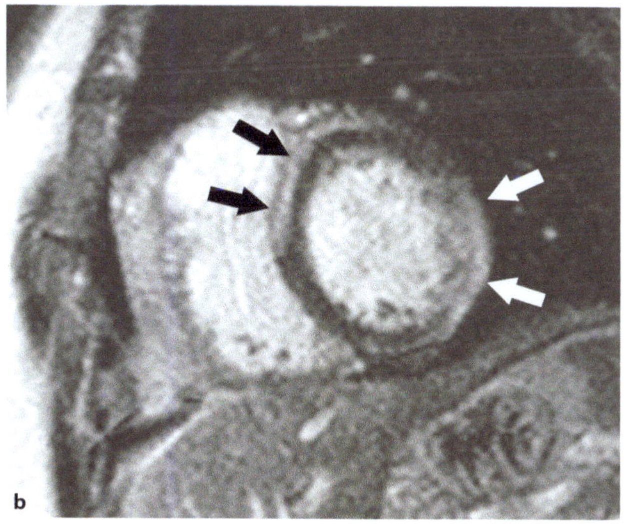

Fig. 3.13 Cardiac Chagas' disease. **a** PA chest radiograph demonstrates mild enlargement of the cardiac silhouette. There is a dual-lead automatic implantable cardioverter defibrillator in the correct position. **b** Double inversion recovery MR image obtained 10 min after intravenous injection of gadolinium. In the anterior and anteroseptal wall, there is epicardial enhancement with sparing of the endocardium and myocardium (*black arrows*) An additional focus of transmural enhancement is present in the lateral wall (*white arrows*)

3.2.4 Toxoplasmosis

Human toxoplasmosis results from infection with *Toxoplasma gondii,* an intracellular protozoan found in a variety of animals such as birds and humans, whose ultimate reservoir is felines (Mariuz et al. 1997; Wallace 1973). The infection has worldwide distribution and although it may infect inmmunocompetent patients, most affected individuals have a cell-mediated immunodeficiency such as AIDS (Mariuz et al. 1997), usually with a CD4 count below 200/mm^3 (Crowe et al. 1991). Infection is acquired through the ingestion of either contaminated food/beverages or meat with tissular forms from intermediate hosts. Transplacental infection is also a well-known route resulting in congenital toxoplasmosis (Mariuz et al. 1997).

The lungs and heart are the most frequently affected organ after the central nervous system (Hofman et al. 1993a; Roldan et al. 1987; Hofman et al. 1993b; Hollman 1988). The lung can be affected either primarily or as the result of dissemination from a CNS infection. Clinical manifestations of *Toxoplasma* pneumonia include fever, coughing, and dyspnea (Rabaud et al. 1996); however, it can be asymptomatic or minimally symptomatic. Myocardial involvement includes arrhythmias (atrial and ventricular), sudden death, AV block, pericarditis, and heart failure (Hofman et al. 1993b; Mariani et al. 2006; Duffield et al. 1996; Sahasrabudhe et al. 2003). Diagnosis is usually made by identifying parasites in the bronchoalveolar lavage and lung biopsy (Bonilla and Rosa 1994; Oksenhendler et al. 1990), or in cardiac tissues of patients with acute myocarditis (Hofman et al. 1993b). Serologic and PCR techniques are also available (Mariuz et al. 1997; Lavrard et al. 1995). Despite appropriate treatment, relapse and mortality remain high among HIV patients (Rabaud et al. 1996; Pomeroy and Filice 1992).

Radiographic manifestations are nonspecific and rather similar to other opportunistic diseases in the HIV patient (Schnapp et al. 1992). The most common radiological manifestations include diffuse and bilateral reticulonodular or nodular opacities (Fig. 3.14) (Goodman and Schnapp 1992). Other less common findings include consolidation with or without air bronchogram formation (Figs. 3.15, 3.16), micronodules, cavitations (Fig. 3.17), pleural effusion, and pneumothorax (Rabaud et al. 1996; Pomeroy and Filice 1992; Mendelson et al. 1987; Tawney et al. 1986; Libanore et al. 1991). Radiographic signs of pulmonary edema can be seen in the setting of acute myocarditis (Fig. 3.18).

3.3 Nematodes (Roundworms)

3.3.1 Ascariasis

Infection with *Ascaris lumbricoides* (Fig. 3.19) is among the most common worldwide parasitic infections. Human infection is thought to be present in one-fourth of the world's population (World Health Organization 2002) with an estimated mortality between 20,000 and 60,000 per year (Mandell et al. 2005; Sarinas and Chitkara 1997), primarily as a consequence of intestinal obstruction (Sarinas and Chitkara 1997). The parasite has worldwide distribution; however, tropical and subtropical climates in Southeast Asia, Africa, and Central/South America

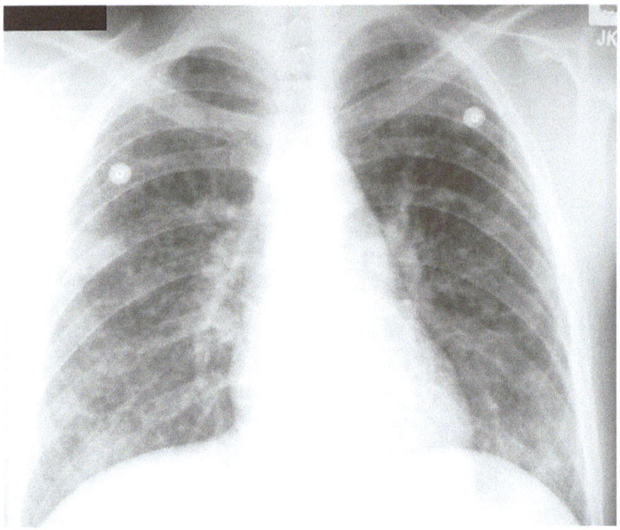

Fig. 3.14 Pulmonary toxoplasmosis in a patient with AIDS. PA chest radiograph demonstrates diffuse and bilateral reticulonodular opacities. Parasites were isolated in the bronchoalveolar lavage (Courtesy of Dr. Philip Goodman – Duke University Medical Center, Durham, NC, USA)

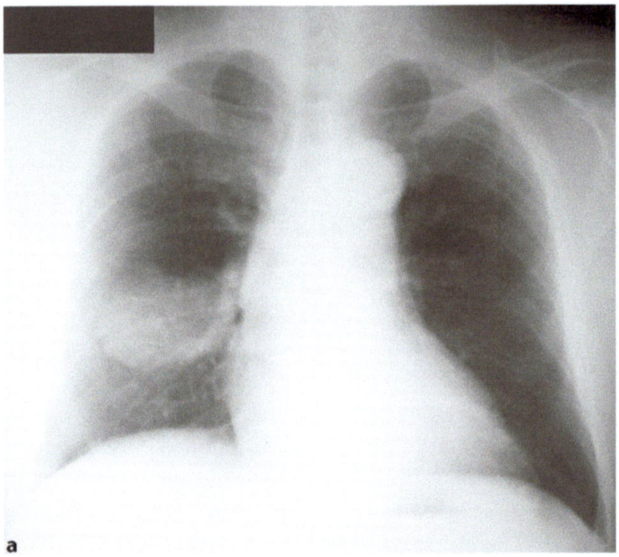

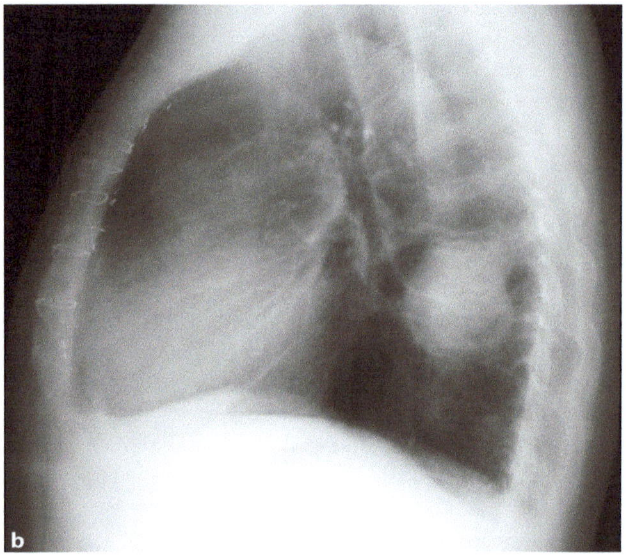

Fig. 3.15 Pulmonary toxoplasmosis in a patient with AIDS. **a** PA chest radiograph shows a round homogenous consolidation in the right lower lung. **b** Lateral chest radiograph helps further localization of the infection in the right lower lobe. Diagnosis was proven pathologically (Courtesy of Dr. Philip Goodman – Duke University Medical Center, Durham, NC, USA)

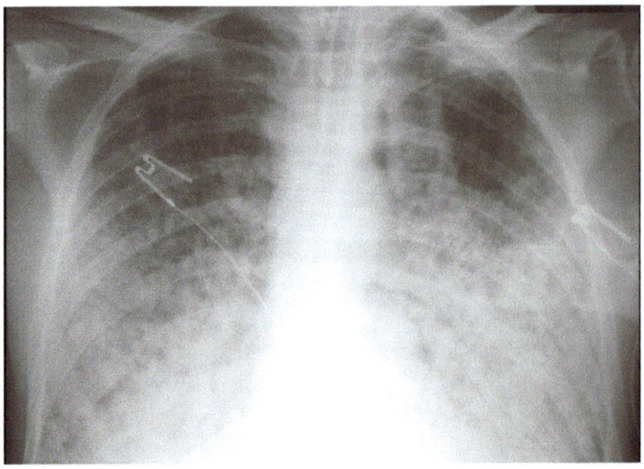

Fig. 3.16 Pulmonary toxoplasmosis in a patient with AIDS. PA chest radiograph demonstrates extensive consolidation and nodular opacities throughout the lungs. Diagnosis was proven pathologically. (Courtesy of Dr. Philip Goodman – Duke University Medical Center, Durham, NC, USA)

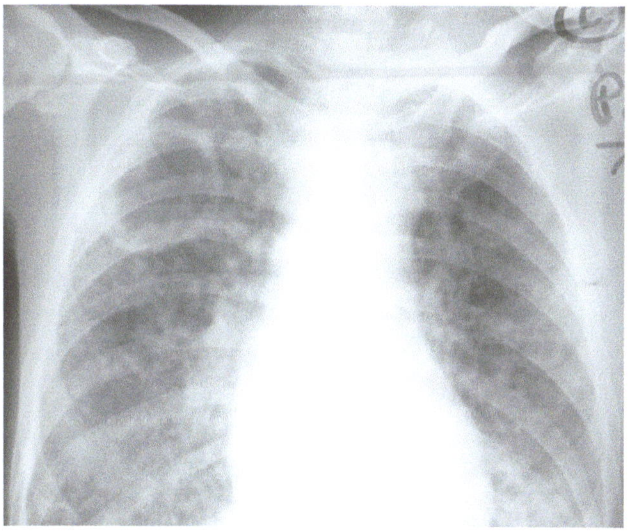

Fig. 3.17 Cavitary pulmonary toxoplasmosis in a patient with AIDS. PA chest radiograph demonstrates bilateral diffuse nodular opacities. In addition, there is a cavitary lesion in the right upper lobe. Diagnosis after resection demonstrated the presence of *T. gondii* as the causative agent (Courtesy of Dr. Philip Goodman – Duke University Medical Center, Durham, NC, USA)

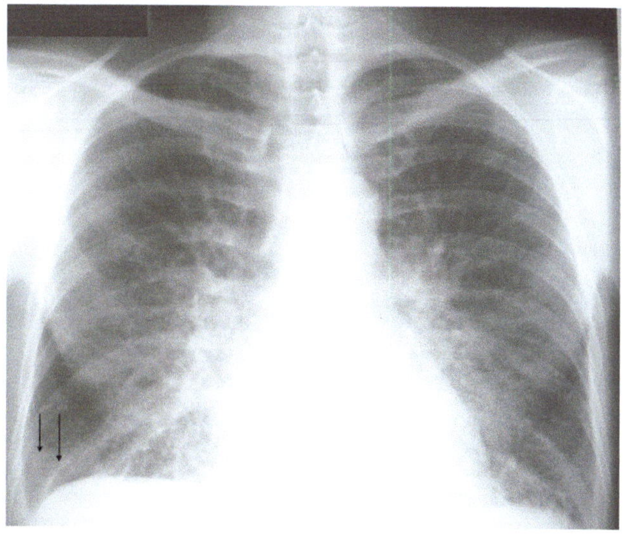

Fig. 3.18 Pulmonary edema in the setting of acute myocarditis due to *T. gondii*. PA chest radiograph showing a normal heart size, bilateral and symmetrical perihilar shadowing with basal septal B lines of Kerley (*arrows*), and bilateral small pleural effusions consistent with cardiogenic edema (Courtesy of Dr. Philip Goodman – Duke University Medical Center, Durham, NC, USA)

account for the majority of people infected (Sarinas and Chitkara 1997). Under certain unusual circumstances, *Ascaris suum*, a large roundworm endemic to pigs, can infect humans (see visceral larva migrans) (Maruyama et al. 1996; Sakakibara et al. 2002).

The parasite is acquired by ingestion of embryonated eggs, usually present in contaminated foods or fluids (Fishman 1998). For completing their natural cycle, parasitic larvae migrate from the small intestine to the pulmonary arterial circulation 4 days after the ingestion of the eggs (Mandell et al. 2005). After 6–10 days of growing, larvae break into the alveoli and eventually are ingested; once in the intestine and after 2 months, mature worms produce eggs that are excreted in human feces, completing the cycle. Larvae in the lungs produce an inflammatory reaction with destruction of capillaries and alveolar walls, subsequent edema, hemorrhage, and epithelial cell desquamation, causing chemotaxis of neutrophils and eosinophils (Botero 2003; Binford and Connor 1976; Hasleton 1996; Travis et al. 2002; Murray et al. 2002; Fishman et al. 1998).

Although ascariasis is usually asymptomatic, up to 15% of infected patients may experience clinical symptoms (Mandell et al. 2005). Lung disease is usually asymptomatic, but as many as 20% of patients (Spillmann 1975) will present with fever, coughing, expectoration, and peripheral blood eosinophilia (Mandell et al. 2005; Sarinas and Chitkara 1997), sometimes recognized as Loeffler's-like syndrome (Fishman 1998). Asthma has also been described in the setting of ascariasis (Crompton 2001). Eosinophils and Charcot-Leyden crystals are often identified in the sputum (Sarinas and Chitkara 1997). Confirmation requires identification of larvae in the sputum or gastric aspirates (Murray et al. 2005; Fishman 1998; Proffitt and Walton 1962). In patients from non-endemic areas who present with pulmonary symptoms, the diagnosis is suggested when eggs are present in the stool (Botero 2003; Zumba and James 2002).

Chest radiography and CT may demonstrate migratory, ground-glass, and alveolar opacities that characteristically clear within days to weeks (Figs. 3.20, 3.21). Lobar consolidation and alveolar hemorrhage have also been described (Barrett-Connor 1982; Botero 2003; Proffitt and Walton 1962; Zumla and James 2002).

3.3.2 Strongyloidiasis

Humans are the primary host of the microscopic nematode *Strongyloides stercoralis* (Barrett-Connor 1982; Botero 2003; Binford and Connor 1976; Hasleton 1996; Travis et al. 2002; Murray et al. 2002; Fishman et al. 1998). Although reports on the global prevalence of the disease are highly dissimilar (ranging from 1 to 100 million people worldwide), it appears clear that strongyloidiasis is not as frequent as infection with other nematodes (e.g., *Ascaris lumbricoides* or *Trichuris trichiura)* (Mandell et al. 2005; Murray et al. 2002). The parasite is found in all tropical and subtropical regions (Mandell et al. 2005; Murray et al. 2002).

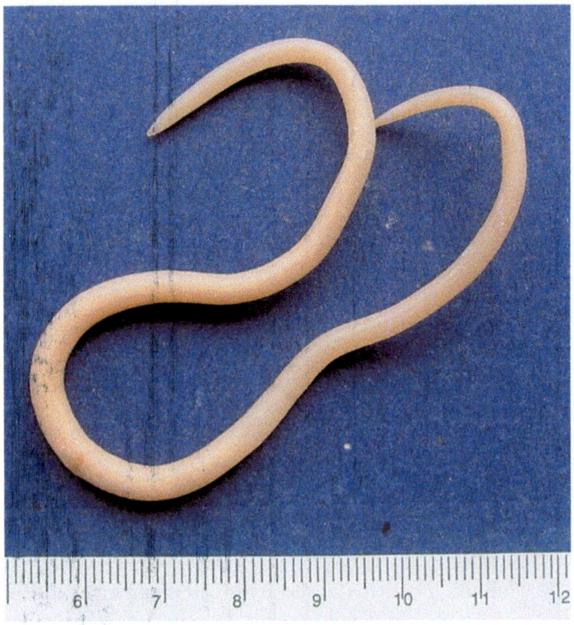

Fig. 3.19 Photograph of an *Ascaris lumbricoides* worm

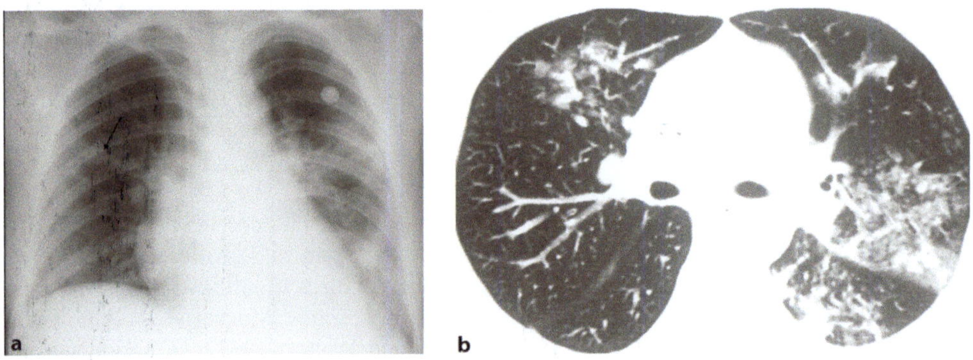

Fig. 3.20 Pulmonary ascariasis. **a** PA chest radiograph demonstrates heterogeneous opacities in the left lung and to a lesser extent in the right lung (*arrow*). **b** Axial chest CT (lung window) shows ill-defined areas of ground-glass opacity and consolidation in both lungs

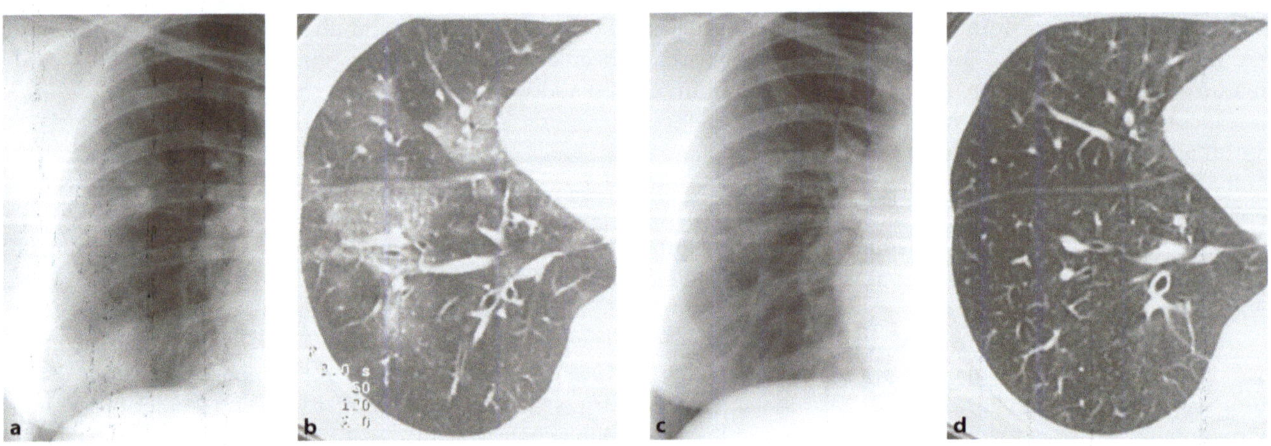

Fig. 3.21 Pulmonary ascariasis. **a** PA chest radiograph shows subtle opacities in the right mid and lower zones. **b** A close-up view of an axial CT scan of the chest (lung window) demonstrates ground-glass opacities in the right middle and lower lobes. **c,d** Follow-up examinations demonstrating complete resolution of the abnormalities after a period of 2 weeks (**a** and **b** are reproduced with permission from Radiographics, Martinez et al. 2005)

Infective filariform larvae are capable of invading the skin from the contaminated soil (Murray et al. 2005). Larvae migrate hematogenously to the lungs where they mature and are eventually coughed up and swallowed. In the small intestine adults produce eggs, which generate rhabditiform larvae that can be either excreted into the environment in human feces, completing the cycle, or become filariform larvae (Murray et al. 2005; Barrett-Connor 1982; Botero 2003; Binford and Connor 1976; Travis et al. 2002; Murray et al. 2002; Fishman 1998) capable of autoinfection to perpetuate the cycle. This chronic pathway of continuous autoinfection can lead to a massive and life-threatening parasitic infestation (the so-called hyperinfection syndrome), especially in AIDS patients and in patients who are receiving glucocorticoid therapy (Chu et al. 1990). Hyperinfection syndrome is associated with a mortality rate close to 100% without treatment and perhaps higher than 25% when treated (Mandell et al. 2005).

Diagnosis can be suggested clinically in patients from – or those who have traveled to – endemic areas, who present with peripheral blood eosinophilia, pulmonary symptoms, and abdominal pain/diarrhea. On the other hand, hyperinfection syndrome usually presents with systemic inflammatory response syndrome in the setting of an immunocompromised patient. Eosinophilia is often absent. Definitive diagnosis is made by identifying larvae in the sputum, bronchoalveolar lavage or lung biopsy (Mandell et al. 2005; Barrett-Connor 1982; Botero 2003; Binford and Connor 1976; Chu et al.1990).

Radiologic findings include ill-defined and migratory opacities that typically resolve in 1–2 weeks. Hyperinfection syndrome can manifest with extensive consolidation, which can be infectious, hemorrhagic (Fig. 3.22), due to noncardiogenic edema, or a mixture (Woodring et al. 1994). A miliary pattern and reticular opacities can be better depicted on the CT scan (Fig. 3.23) (Woodring et al. 1994; Krysl et al. 1991; Reeder and Palmer 1980).

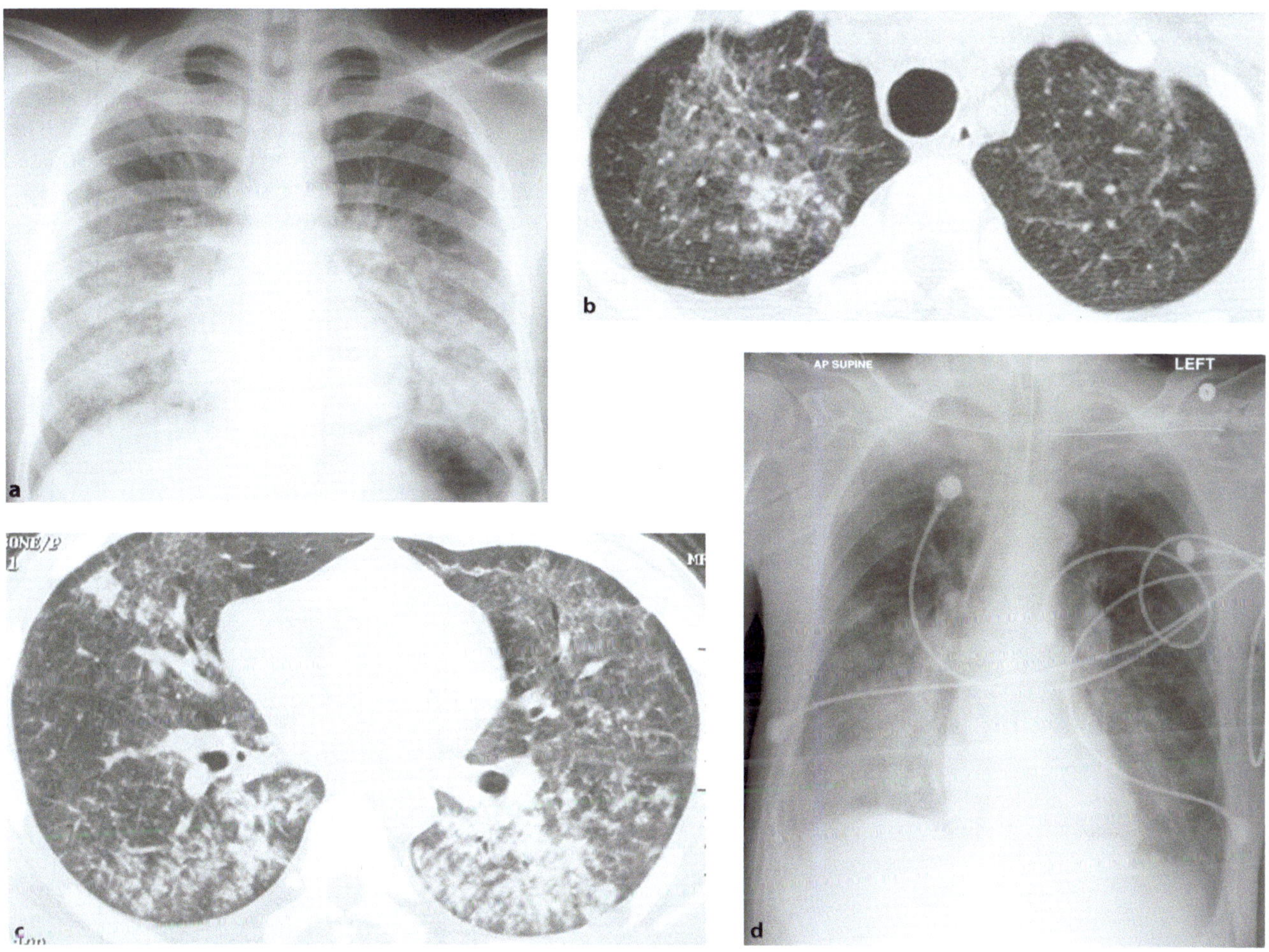

Fig. 3.22 Pulmonary strongyloidiasis. **a** PA chest radiograph demonstrates bilateral widespread opacities throughout the lungs with perihilar and basilar predominance. **b** Axial CT scan of the chest (lung windows) shows bilateral apical ground-glass opacities. **c** Axial CT scan of the chest (lung windows) section at the level of the lung bases showing more coalescent opacities. **d** Plain radiograph of the chest of another patient with pulmonary strongyloidiasis, showing bilateral perihilar and basal confluent infiltrates. (**a** and **c** are reproduced with permission from Radiographics, Martinez et al. 2005)

Superimposed bacterial infection with cavitation and abscess formation is not an uncommon finding (Chu et al. 1990; Woodring et al. 1994; Berk et al. 1987; Cook et al. 1987; Davidson 1992; Makris et al. 1993; Simpson et al. 1993; Ford et al. 1981; Ali-Munive et al. 2002). Rarely, larvae can migrate to the pleura and pericardium causing pleural and pericardial effusion (Barrett-Connor 1982; Woodring et al. 1994; Reeder and Palmer 1980; Davidson 1992; Bruno et al. 1982; Froes 1930).

3.3.3 Hookworms

Hookworm infection is caused by *Ancylostoma duodenale* and *Necator Americanus.* Hookworms share several characteristics with *A. lumbricoides* including worldwide distribution, especially in the tropical and subtropical regions, and the necessity of a maturation phase in the lungs. The infection is thought to occur in about 25% of the world's population (Murray et al. 2005; Sarinas and Chitkara 1997; Hotez and Pritchard 1995). As opposed to ascariasis, hookworm infection is acquired by the percutaneous penetration of larvae from the soil. Parasites migrate to the lungs where they ultimately penetrate the alveolar walls, ascend through the trachea and eventually are swallowed up into the small intestine (Mandell et al. 2005).

Pulmonary disease is related to the migration of parasites to the lungs, which causes eosinophilic pleural effusion (Yassin et al. 2007) or transient pneumonitis (Loeffler's-like syndrome), pathophysiologically and clinically similar to ascariasis (Sarinas and Chitkara 1997), though less frequent and severe (Mandell et al. 2005). Peripheral blood eosinophilia is common (Sarinas and Chitkara 1997). Radiographic manifestations are thought to be similar to those of ascariasis (Sarinas and Chitkara 1997); however, there are not enough data available in the radiologic literature. Diagnosis is confirmed by demonstrating the parasite in respiratory, gastric or duodenal secretions (Sarinas and Chitkara 1997). The presence of eggs is not helpful during pulmonary disease, since this event is expected to occur 2 months after the dermal penetration (Sarinas and Chitkara 1997), i.e., after the parasite's pulmonary phase (Mandell et al. 2005).

3.3.4 Visceral Larva Migrans/Loeffler's Syndrome

Visceral larva migrans (VLM), or Loeffler's syndrome, is an infection classically caused by *Toxocara canis* and *Toxocara catis* (Beaver et al. 1952; Dent et al. 1956); however, association with *Ascaris suum* has also been described (Maruyama et al. 1996; Sakakibara et al. 2002; Sakai et al. 2006; Van Knapen et al. 1992). In all three species, the infection is usually acquired by ingestion of contaminated products (Mandell et al. 2005; Chitkara and Sarinas 1997; Phills et al. 1972). Once in the intestinal mucosa, larvae

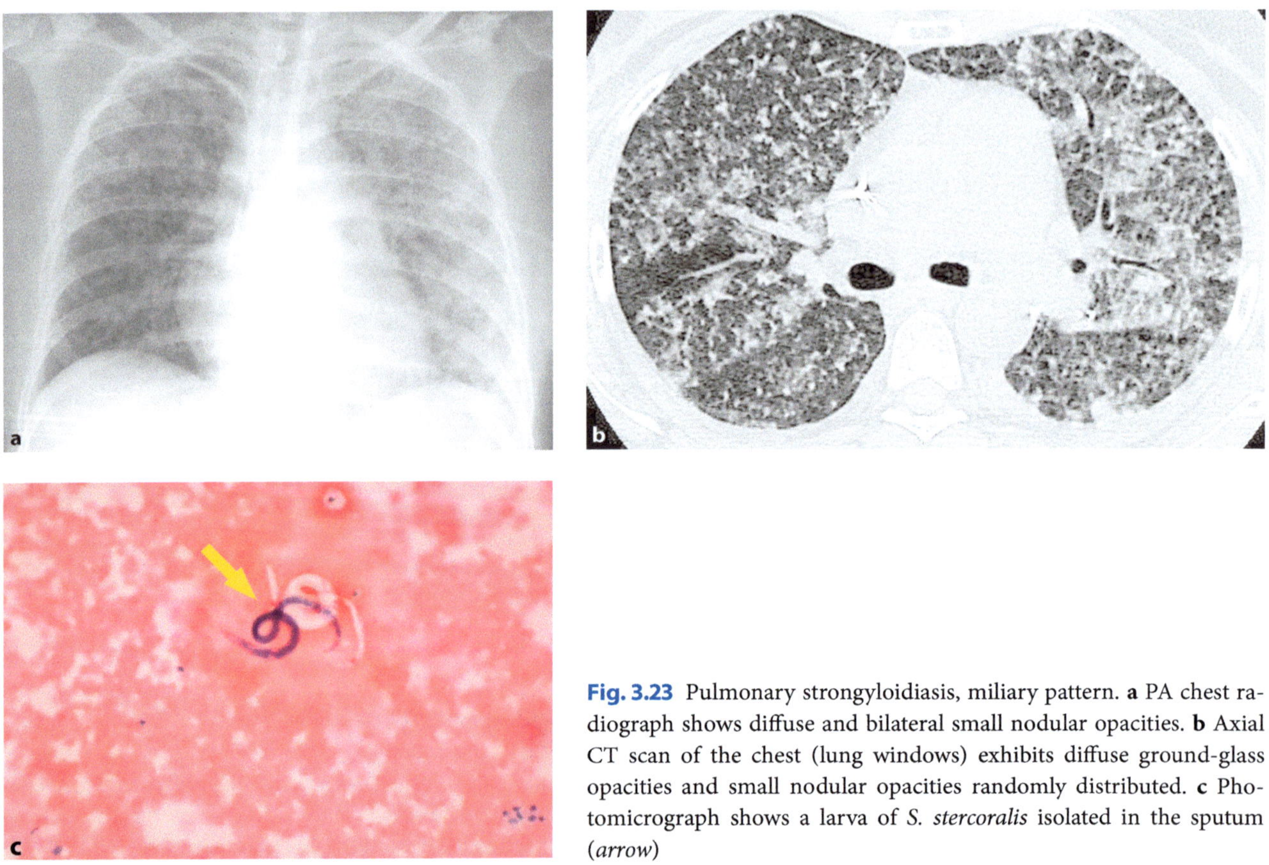

Fig. 3.23 Pulmonary strongyloidiasis, miliary pattern. **a** PA chest radiograph shows diffuse and bilateral small nodular opacities. **b** Axial CT scan of the chest (lung windows) exhibits diffuse ground-glass opacities and small nodular opacities randomly distributed. **c** Photomicrograph shows a larva of *S. stercoralis* isolated in the sputum (*arrow*)

can migrate to a variety of organs including lymphatics, liver, lungs, and less frequently the heart, central nervous system, eye, and other organs (Chitkara and Sarinas 1997). *T. canis* and *T. catis* have worldwide distribution wherever dogs and cats, respectively, are present (Murray et al. 2005). Children are at higher risk due to pica, proximity with pets, and outdoor play (Chitkara and Sarinas 1997). Infection with *A. suum* was reproduced experimentally in humans in the 1970s (Phills et al. 1972); however, outbreaks have been described in Japan since then (Maruyama et al. 1996; Sakakibara et al. 2002; Sakai et al. 2006).

Larvae of these species are unable to grow into mature adults in humans and thus eggs or worms are not detected in feces (Sakai et al. 2006). VLM due to *T. canis* and *T. catis* can cause pulmonary disease in 25–85%. Clinical manifestations include mild forms with coughing and wheezing, severe bronchiolitis, asthma, and acute/chronic eosinophilic pneumonia with respiratory failure (Chitkara and Sarinas 1997; Bartelink et al. 1993; Inoue et al. 2002), usually with associated peripheral blood eosinophilia (Fishman 1998; Chitkara and Sarinas 1997). The pulmonary migration of *A. suum* triggers an inflammatory reaction similar to that elicited by *A. lumbricoides* (Phills et al. 1972). Clinical forms of infection with *A. suum* are similar to other presentations of VLM (Sakai et al. 2006; Phills et al. 1972). Diagnosis of VLM is achieved by the detection of antibodies by enzyme-linked immunosorbent assay (ELISA) (Sakai et al. 2006; Chitkara and Sarinas 1997). Larvae of *A. suum* can be isolated in respiratory secretions and gastric aspirates during the pulmonary phase (Phills et al. 1972).

Scant information regarding radiologic manifestations of VLM due to *T. canis* and *T. catis* is available in the literature. Among children, abnormal chest radiograph is identified in approximately 40% of cases, most commonly perihilar reticular opacities (Snyder 1961); some data support that abnormalities can resolve within days (Beshear and Hendley 1973). Isolated case reports have shown other characteristics like mediastinal and retroperitoneal adenopathy evident on the CT scan (Wolach et al. 1995). In adults, radiographic manifestations include scattered bilateral reticular or heterogeneous opacities that can be migratory (Chitkara and Sarinas 1997; Bartelink et al. 1993) and less commonly, nodules and segmental consolidations that can resolve within days (Chitkara and Sarinas 1997; Inoue et al. 2002; Feldman and Parker 1992; Sane and Barber 1997). Bacterial superimposed infection has been documented in immunosuppressed patients (Kremery et al. 1992). Limited information is available regarding CT findings (Fig. 3.24). Isolated case reports in adults demonstrated peripheral alveolar and ground-glass opacities (Inoue et al. 2002) and small ill-defined ground-glass and solid nodules (Sane and Barber 1997; Roig et al. 1992). Radiologic characteristics of infection due to *A. suum* appear to be similar to other forms of VLM, including bilateral reticulonodular opacities on chest radiographs and bilateral nodules with halo or ill-defined ground-glass opacities on CT scans, which may be associated with multiple low attenuation lesions in the liver (Maruyama et al. 1996; Sakakibara et al. 2002; Sakai et al. 2006).

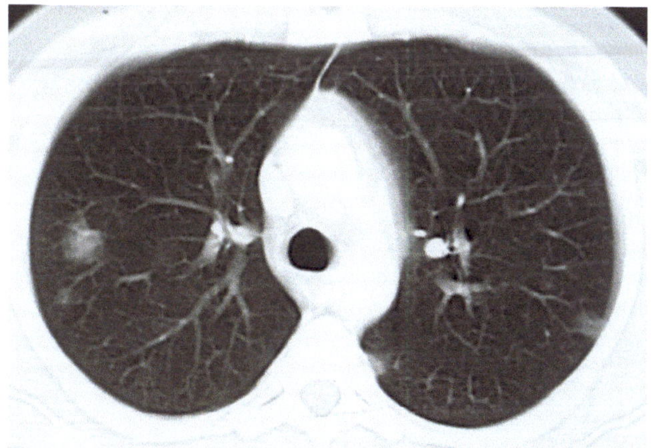

Fig. 3.24 Computed tomography scan of the chest showing bilateral patches of peripheral pulmonary infiltrates in a patient with eosinophilia and proven toxocariasis by positive blood serology test. The pulmonary changes healed completely following antiparasitic drug treatment

3.3.5 Dirofilariasis

As the prevalence of the dog heartworm among canines appears to be rising, human dirofilariasis is increasingly being reported (Chitkara and Sarinas 1997; Asimacopoulos et al. 1992; Richert and Krakaur 1959; Roy et al. 1993). The disease has been sporadically reported worldwide, with many cases emanating from the East Coast and South of the United States (Mandell et al. 2005; Asimacopoulos et al. 1992). It is caused by *Dirofilaria immitis*, a filarial nematode that is transmitted from dogs to humans by mosquitoes. An immature adult worm, unable to mature in the accidental human host, can reach a peripheral vein and travel in the bloodstream until it lodges in the arterial pulmonary circulation where it dies, causing local vasculitis and eventually an infarct (Mandell et al. 2005; Botero 2003; Murray et al. 2002).

The infection is frequently asymptomatic and becomes evident due to the incidental detection of a solitary pulmonary nodule (Mandell et al. 2005; Murray et al. 2005; Fishman 1998). Patients can sometimes present with coughing, pain, and hemoptysis, most likely due to pulmonary infarct (Mandell et al. 2005; Fishman 1998). Eosinophilia is present in less than 15% of cases (Mandell et al. 2005).

Although a solitary pulmonary nodule, 3 cm or less in diameter (the so-called coin-shaped lesion), represents the classic radiologic presentation of the infection (Figs. 3.25, 3.26) (Asimacopoulos et al. 1992; Levinson et al. 1979; Shah 1999), other findings such as multifocal heterogeneous opacities that resolve after several weeks and evolve into multiple nodules have also been described (Mandell et al. 2005; Kochar 1985). Despite serologic tests being available, they are not considered to be helpful because these lesions are worrisome for malignancy and thus usually excised (Mandell et al. 2005). Like other infectious nodules, pulmonary nodules in dirofilariasis can show increased uptake on PET scan (Moore and Franceschi 2005), so they cannot be differentiated from malignant pulmonary nodules. Definitive diagnosis is usually made based on the histopathology of the excised nodule and, sporadically, with needle aspiration biopsy of the nodule and demonstration of fragments of the parasite (Fishman et al. 1998; Asimacopoulos et al. 1992).

3.3.6 Microfilariae (Tropical Pulmonary Eosinophilia)

Tropical pulmonary eosinophilia (TPE) is a rare parasitic infection caused by microfilariae of the lymphatic-dwelling organisms *Wuchereria bancrofti* and *Brugia malayi*, affecting people living in India and Southeast Asia. Humans contract the disease when they are bitten by mosquitoes that carry infective larvae.

Clinically, patients present with an asthma-like syndrome. Peripheral blood eosinophilia and elevated serum IgE levels are present. Radiographically, reticulonodular infiltrates or a miliary pattern are seen on chest radiographs. The differential diagnosis includes sarcoidosis, miliary tuberculosis, and bronchial asthma. A dilated

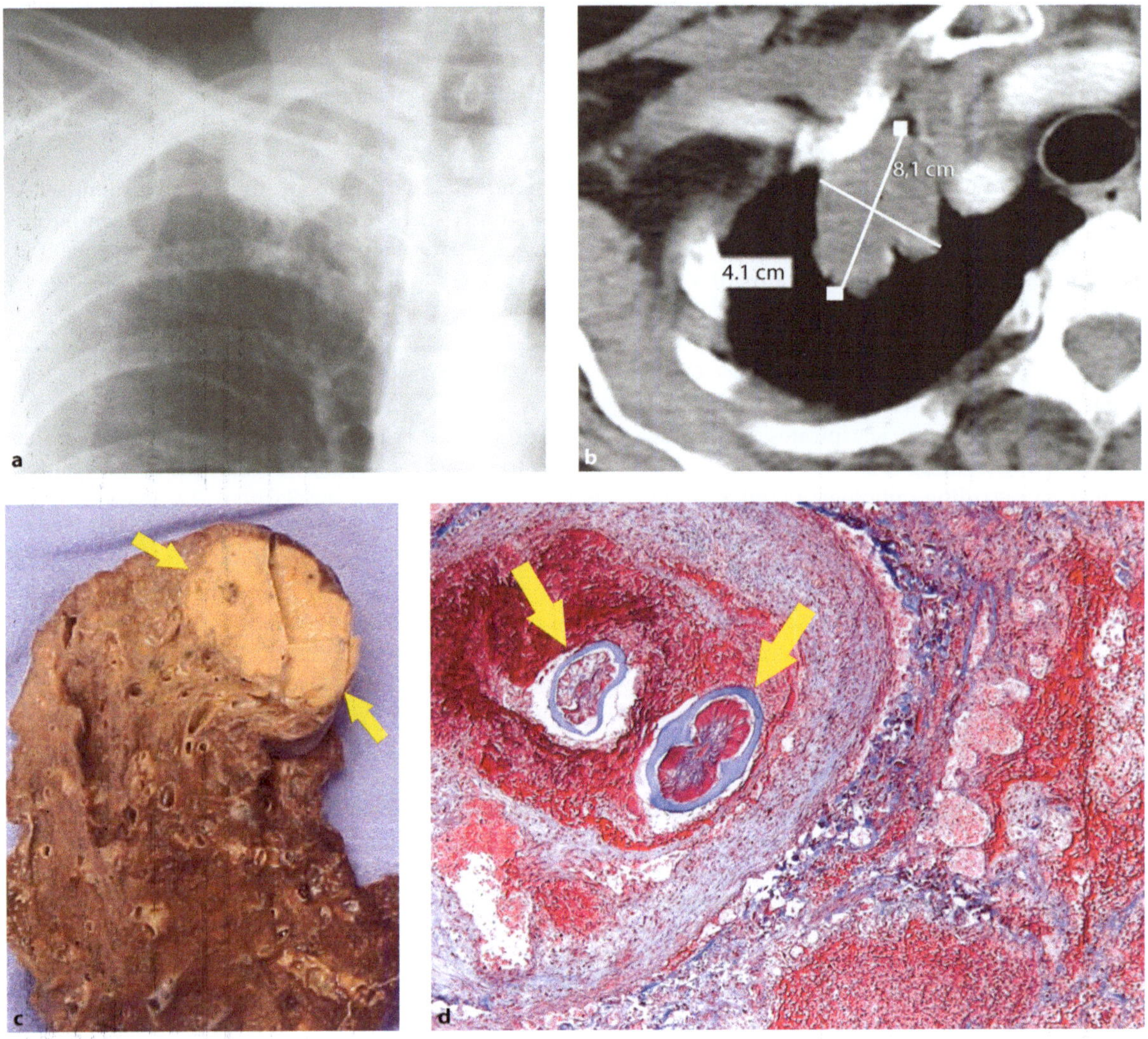

Fig. 3.25 Pulmonary dirofilariasis presenting as a lung mass. **a** Close-up PA chest radiograph demonstrates a round mass in the right apical area, the so-called coin-shaped lesion. **b** Axial CT of the chest (soft tissue window) further characterizes the mass, showing well-defined borders. The patient underwent lobectomy. **c** Macroscopic specimen demonstrates a round mass in the right upper lobe (*arrows*). **d** Photomicrograph shows arterial thrombosis with parasitic fragments inside the pulmonary artery (*arrows*) as well as intense inflammatory reaction. (Courtesy of Dr. Fortunato Juarez, INER, Mexico DF, Mexico)

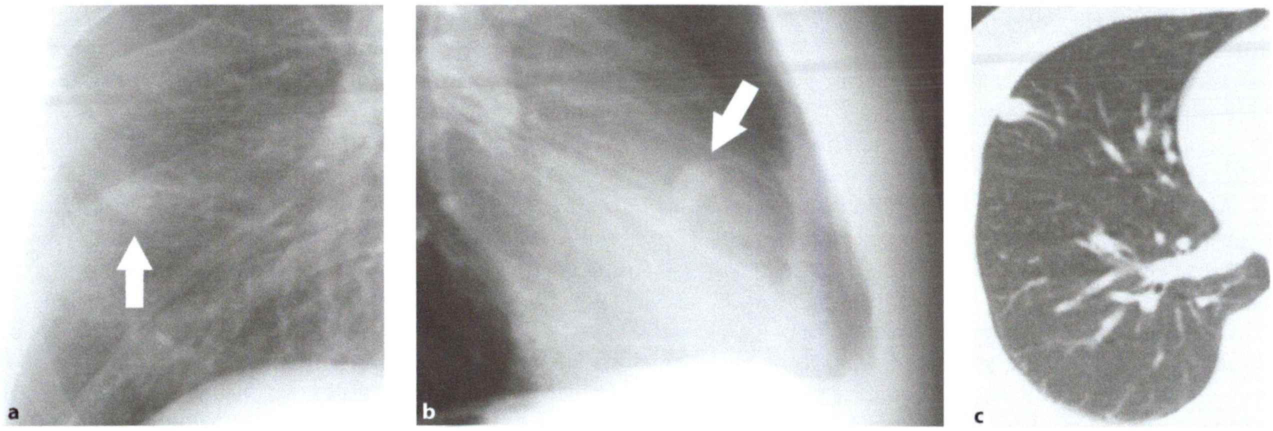

Fig. 3.26 Dirofilariasis presenting as a solitary pulmonary nodule. **a,b** PA and lateral chest radiographs, cone views, demonstrate a small soft tissue nodule in the right middle lobe (*arrows*). **c** Axial CT scan of the chest (lung window) shows a small nodule in the periphery of the right middle lobe (Courtesy of Dr. Edward Patz – Duke University Medical Center, Durham, NC, USA)

thoracic duct in the chest and diffuse lymphangiectasia in the abdomen and pelvis were reported by Ahn et al. (2005) on a CT scan of the body; this finding gives a clue to the diagnosis of filariasis. Diagnosis is confirmed by identification of microfilaria in lymph nodes or pulmonary nodules, and by specific serology tests. However, often microfilariae cannot be identified on microscopic examination; then a favorable response to treatment with diethylcarbamazine is diagnostic (Kuznen 2006; Lahiri 1993).

3.3.7 Gnathostomiasis

Gnathostomiasis, caused by *Gnathostoma spinigerum*, is a food-borne parasitic zoonosis caused by ingestion of the uncooked or undercooked flesh of freshwater fishes, with predominantly cutaneous manifestations. Although four distinct species of the genus *Gnathostoma* were identified as the causative agents for human gnathostomiasis, human infections with *G. doloresi* have been found in Japan, concentrated in the Miyazaki Prefecture. Lung involvement is very rare, and few case reports have been reported in the medical literature (Charoensatanakul 1997; Prijyanonda et al. 1955).

3.4 Cestodes (Tapeworms)

At least four species of *Echinococcus* can infect humans: *E. granulosus*, *E. multilocularis*, *E. vogeli* and *E. oligarthrus*. Infection is acquired by ingesting food/beverages contaminated with eggs. Larvae penetrate the bowel wall and migrate primarily to the liver. *E. granulosus*, the most common *Echinococcus* to cause disease, is seen the Mediterranean region, Eastern Europe, Africa, South America, the Middle East, Australia, and New Zealand (Murray et al. 2005; Botero 2003; Binford and Connor 1976; Hasleton 1996; Travis et al. 2002; Fishman et al. 1998). *E. multilocularis* has a holo-arctic distribution (Alaska, Canada, the entire tundra region) and in some regions of Asia (Russia, China, Japan) and northern Europe (central and eastern France, Switzerland, Austria, Germany) (Gottstein and Reichen 2002). *E. vogeli* and *E. oligarthrus* are endemic in the tropical regions of South America (Botero 2003; D'Alessandro 1997; Rodrigues-Silva et al. 2002). An estimated 65 million people in endemic areas are infected (Murray et al. 2005).

3.4.1 Unilocular Cystic Echinococcosis

Unilocular cystic echinococcosis is caused by *E. granulosus*. Overall, the liver is the most commonly affected organ; however, thoracic disease is a very common presentation among adults (Beggs 1985; Bonakdarpour 1967; Polat et al. 2003) and perhaps the most common among children (Slim et al. 1971; Bloomfield 1980). Diverse organs in the chest can be affected by the disease either by growing cysts from the liver that traverse the diaphragm or by hematogenous spread (Gottstein and Reichen 2002). Although the lungs are affected in most cases of thoracic hydatid disease, other thoracic organs can be affected (pleural fissures, parietal pleura, chest wall, mediastinum, diaphragm and heart) (Kilic et al. 2006; Oguzkaya et al. 1997; Qian 1988).

Pulmonary hydatid disease can remain asymptomatic for long periods of time (months to years) or manifest with diverse symptoms including coughing, hemoptysis, bilioptysis, pneumothorax, pleuritis, lung abscess, parasitic pulmonary embolism, anaphylaxis secondary to cyst rupture, or cyst superinfection (Gottstein and Reichen

2002; Polat et al. 2003). Pathologically, cysts consist of three layers:

1. The pericyst, composed of fibroblasts, giant cells, and eosinophils, which form a rigid layer
2. An acellular, middle laminated membrane with nutrient functions
3. A thin, translucent inner germinal layer, containing various scolices and generating daughter cysts (Pedrosa et al. 2000)

Eosinophilia is present in less than 15% of cases and generally occurs in the setting of leakage of antigenic material, i.e., cyst rupture. Although a variety of serologic studies are available, high false-negative and false-positive results have been described (Morar and Feldman 2003). Indirect hemagglutination and ELISA tests in association with abdominal ultrasonography can be used as screening tests in high-risk populations (Gottstein and Reichen 2002; Shambesh et al. 1999; MacPherson et al. 1987). Definitive diagnosis relies on the histopathology (Gottstein and Reichen 2002).

Radiographic and CT findings demonstrate cystic lesions, which can be solitary (60% of cases) or multiple (Fig. 3.27), unilateral or bilateral (20–50%). Lesions are predominantly identified in the lower lobes (60%) and can exhibit diameters between 1 and 20 cm. The coexistence of liver and lung disease is present in only 6% of patients (Polat et al. 2003). Uncomplicated cysts, the most common presentation (Saksouk et al. 1986), may be seen as round or oval masses that have well-defined borders (Fig. 3.28), do not enhance after contrast material injection, whilst the pericyst enhances if infected, and have a hypoattenuating content relative to the capsule. On MRI, the cyst content appears characteristically hypointense on T1- and hyperintense on T2-weighted images with a well-defined wall that is isointense and hypointense respectively (Von Sinner et al. 1990, 1991). The development of daughter cysts inside the mother cyst is an early sign of degeneration. On MRI the contents of the mother cyst tend to be more intense with hypointense, viable daughter cysts on T1- and both the mother and the daughter cysts are isointense on T2-weighted images (Von Sinner et al. 1990, 1991). The "meniscus sign" or "crescent sign," which is characterized by the presence of air between the pericyst and the laminated membrane, appears as growth continues and the cysts erode adjacent bronchioles (Figs. 3.29, 3.30). It is considered to be a sign of impending rupture. Cystic rupture may result in different radiologic signs. The "double arch," "cumbo sign," or "onion peel sign," defined as the presence of the meniscus sign and an air–fluid level within the endocyst. The "water lily sign" represents an endocyst floating in a partially fluid-filled cyst (Fig. 3.31), whereas an endocyst floating in a cyst with no fluid is recognized as the "mass within the cavity" appearance (Beggs 1985; Bonakdarpour 1967; Polat et al. 2003; Pedrosa et al. 2000; Balikian and Mudarris 1974). Rupture can be associated with consolidation adjacent to the cyst (Saksouk et al. 1986). Atypical manifestations of cysts are less frequent, but have certainly been described (Koul et al. 2000). Radiographic and CT findings in transdiaphragmatic dissemination (Fig. 3.32) include pleural effusion, hemidiaphragm elevation, pulmonary consolidation, laminar basal atelectasis, pleural cysts, hydropneumothorax, bronchobiliary fistula and empyema (Balikian and Mudarris 1974; Koul et al. 2000; Bhatia 1997; Gouliamos et al. 1991; Ramos

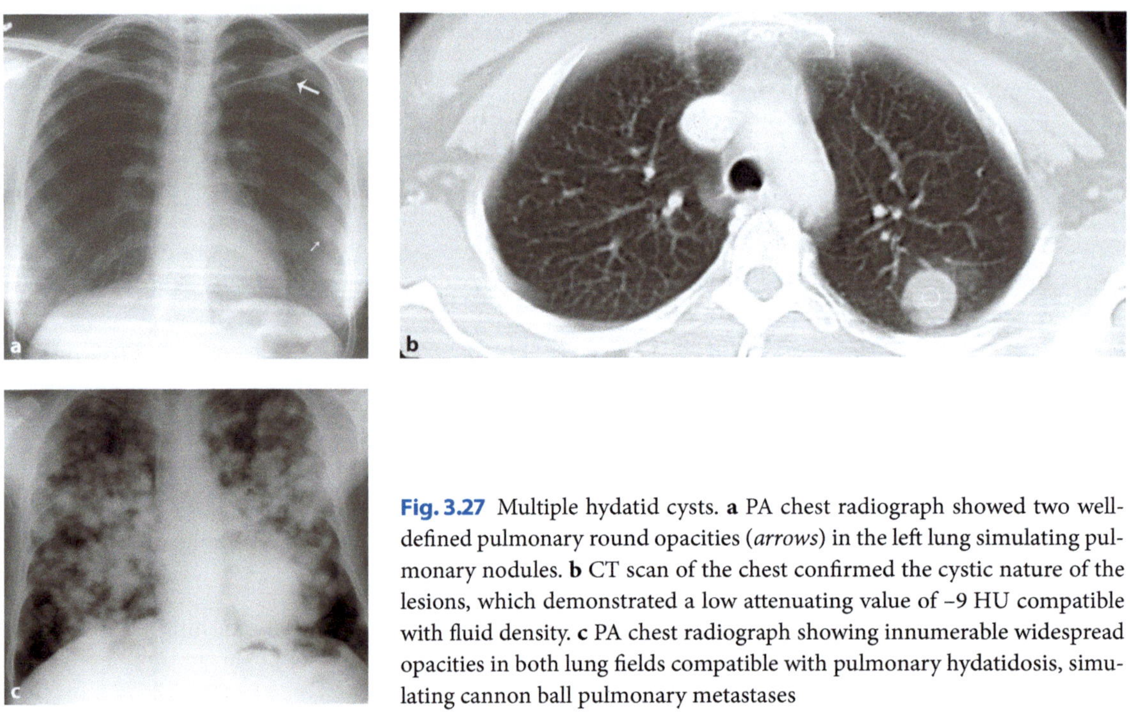

Fig. 3.27 Multiple hydatid cysts. **a** PA chest radiograph showed two well-defined pulmonary round opacities (*arrows*) in the left lung simulating pulmonary nodules. **b** CT scan of the chest confirmed the cystic nature of the lesions, which demonstrated a low attenuating value of –9 HU compatible with fluid density. **c** PA chest radiograph showing innumerable widespread opacities in both lung fields compatible with pulmonary hydatidosis, simulating cannon ball pulmonary metastases

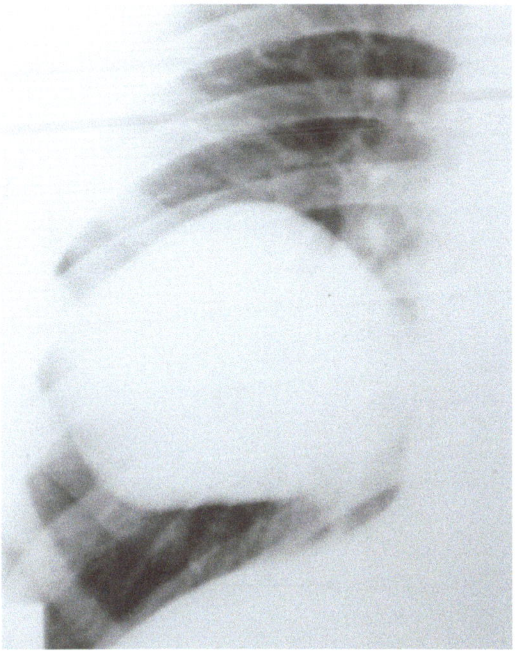

Fig. 3.28 Hydatid disease (*E. granulosus*). PA chest radiograph, close-up view, shows a large cyst in the right lower lung. (Reproduced with permission from Radiographics, Martinez et al. 2005)

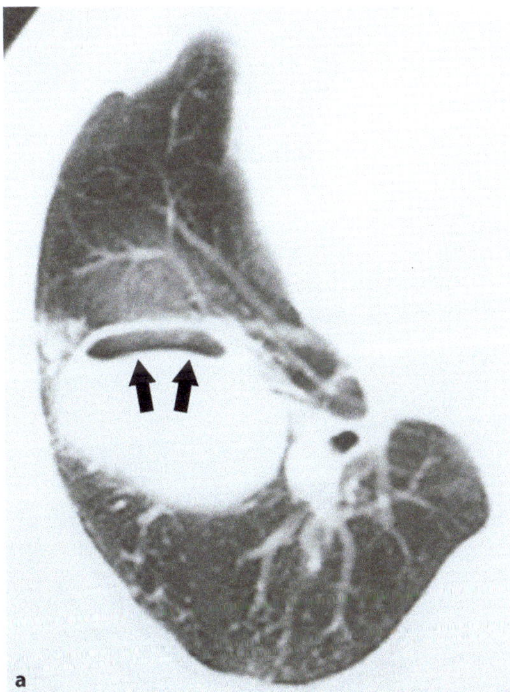

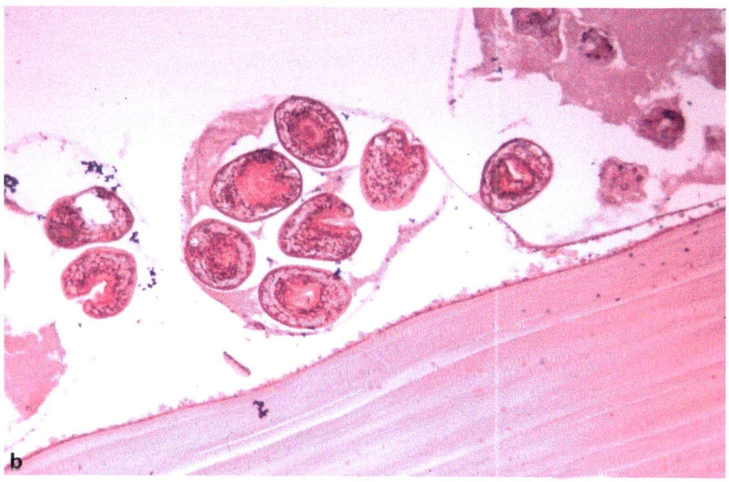

Fig. 3.29 Pulmonary hydatid disease (*E. granulosus*). **a** Axial CT scan of the chest (lung window) shows a hypoattenuating crescent sign, the so called meniscus sign (*arrows*). **b** Photomicrograph (HE, ×40) obtained after surgical resection demonstrates the inner germinal layer, to which several daughter protoscolices of *E. granulosus* are attached (Reproduced with permission from Radiographics, Martinez et al. 2005)

et al. 1975; Von Sinner 1990a; Kurkcuoglu et al. 2002a; Kabiri et al. 2001; Sahin et al. 2006; Nadir et al. 2005). Pulmonary cysts do not or very rarely calcify (Bonakdarpour 1967; Polat et al. 2003). Similar radiologic findings have been reported in other intrathoracic extrapulmonary cysts, e.g., mediastinum, pericardium, hila, chest wall (Nadir et al. 2005; Cantoni et al. 1993; Dahniya et al. 2001; Marcos et al. 1969; Ozdemir et al. 1994; Tuzun and Hekimoglu 2001), cardiovascular system (Fig. 3.33) (Cantoni et al. 1993; Miralles et al. 1994; Malouf et al. 1985; Tercan et al. 2005; Odev et al. 2002; Franquet et al. 1999). In contrast to pulmonary hydatid cysts, mediastinal hydatid cysts do calcify at the periphery, i.e., they show pericystic calcifications (Fig. 3.33) (Zidi et al. 2006). In some patients with cardiac hydatid disease, cyst rupture may occur, leading to hydatid embolism to the pulmonary arteries (Fig. 3.34), or to the brain, causing a stroke.

In patients with peripheral intrapulmonary solitary or multiple coin lesions adjacent to the pleura and chest

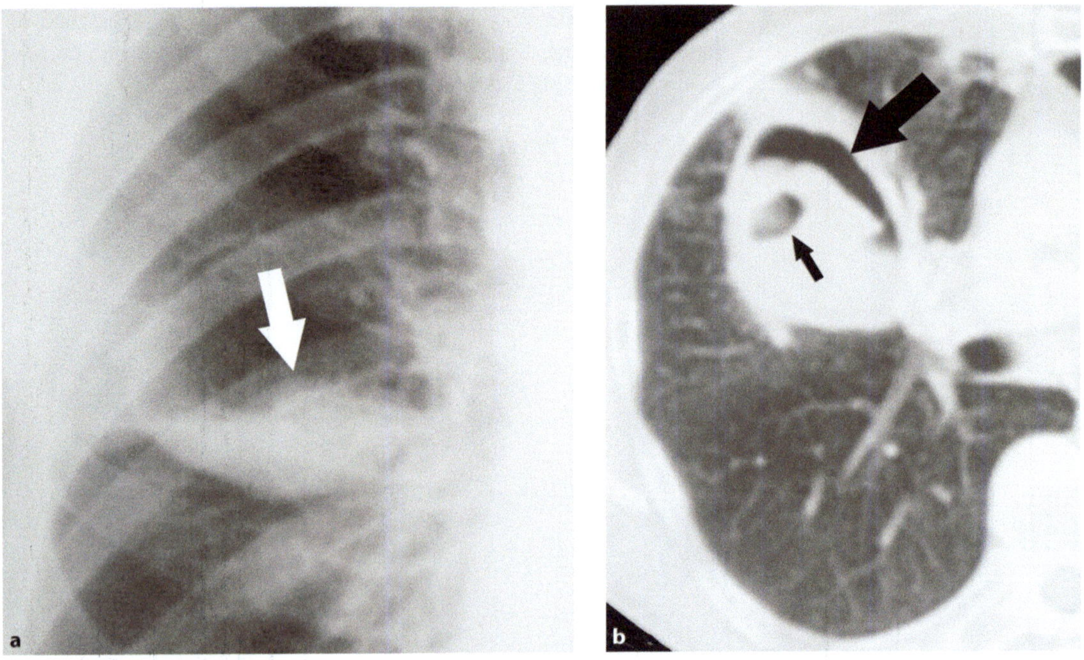

Fig. 3.30 Pulmonary hydatid disease (*E. granulosus*). **a** PA chest radiograph, cone view, shows cavitation with dependent floating soft tissue (*arrow*). **b** Axial CT scan of the chest (lung window) better characterizes the findings. There is air surrounding the pericyst (*thick arrow*) and inside the endocyst (*thin arrow*)

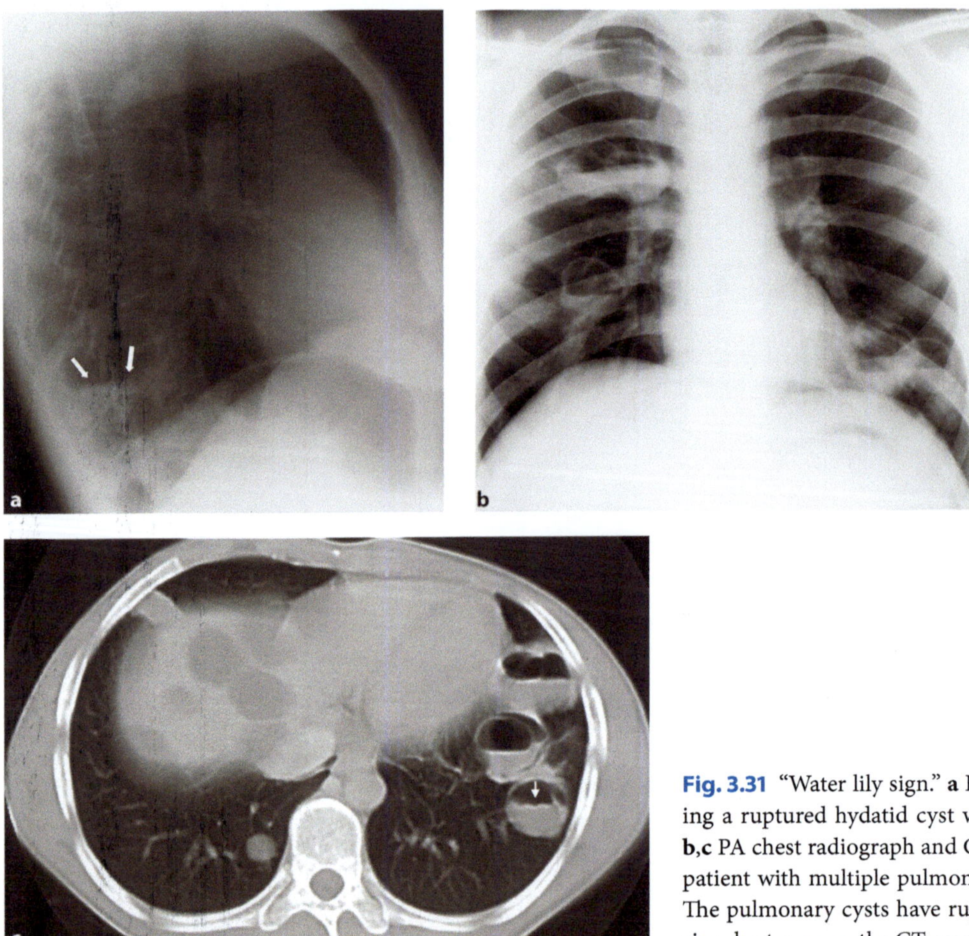

Fig. 3.31 "Water lily sign." **a** Lateral chest radiograph showing a ruptured hydatid cyst with a water lily sign (*arrows*). **b,c** PA chest radiograph and CT scan of the chest of another patient with multiple pulmonary and hepatic hydatid cysts. The pulmonary cysts have ruptured and exhibit a water lily sign, best seen on the CT scan (*arrow*)

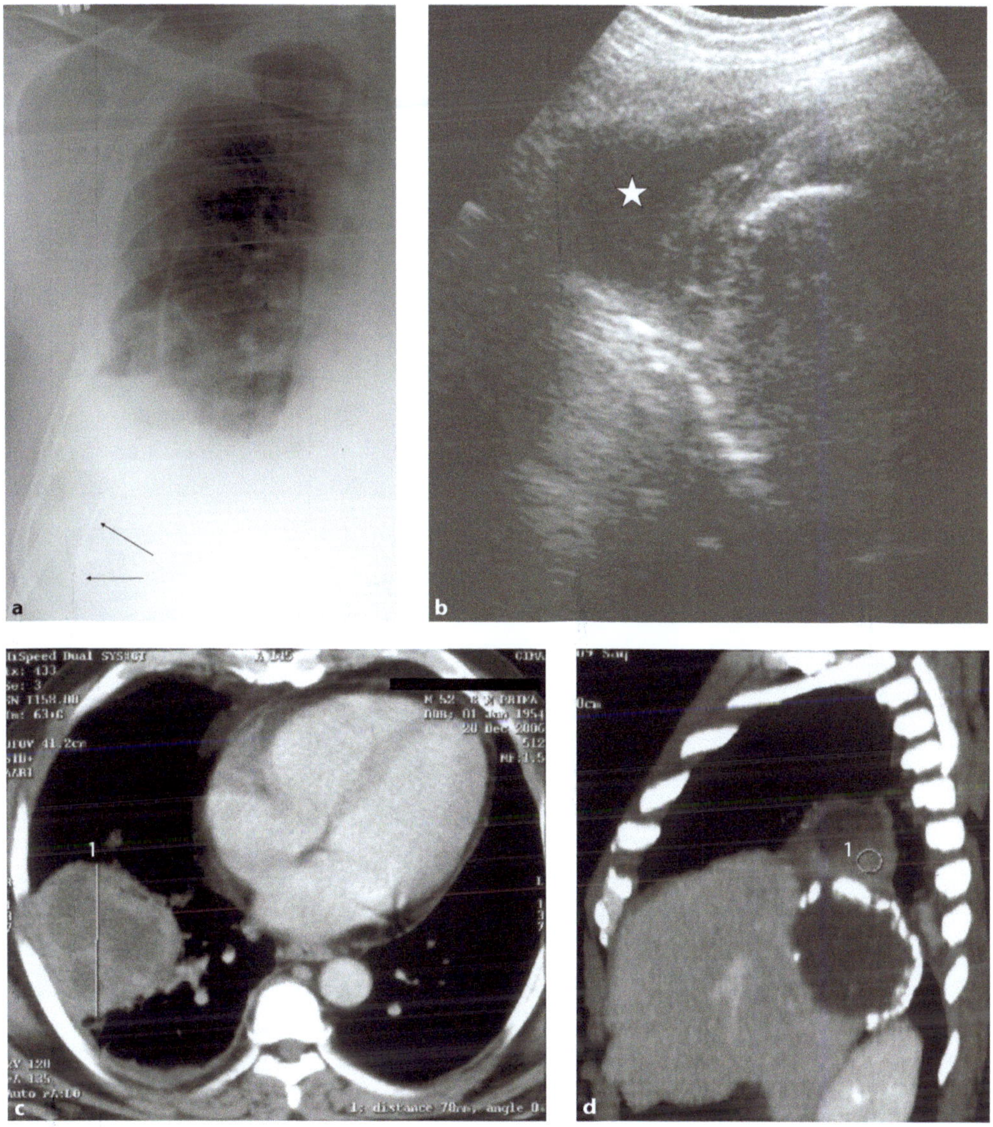

Fig. 3.32 Transdiaphragmatic dissemination of a hepatic hydatid cyst. **a** PA chest radiograph, cone view, showing right lower lobe consolidation and egg-shell calcification in the liver (*arrows*). **b–d** Ultrasound and CT images confirming the presence of a hepatic hydatid cyst that has ruptured through the diaphragm into the right pleural cavity (*star*) (Courtesy of Dr. Nadim Kanj, Department of Internal Medicine, American University of Beirut Medical Center, Beirut, Lebanon)

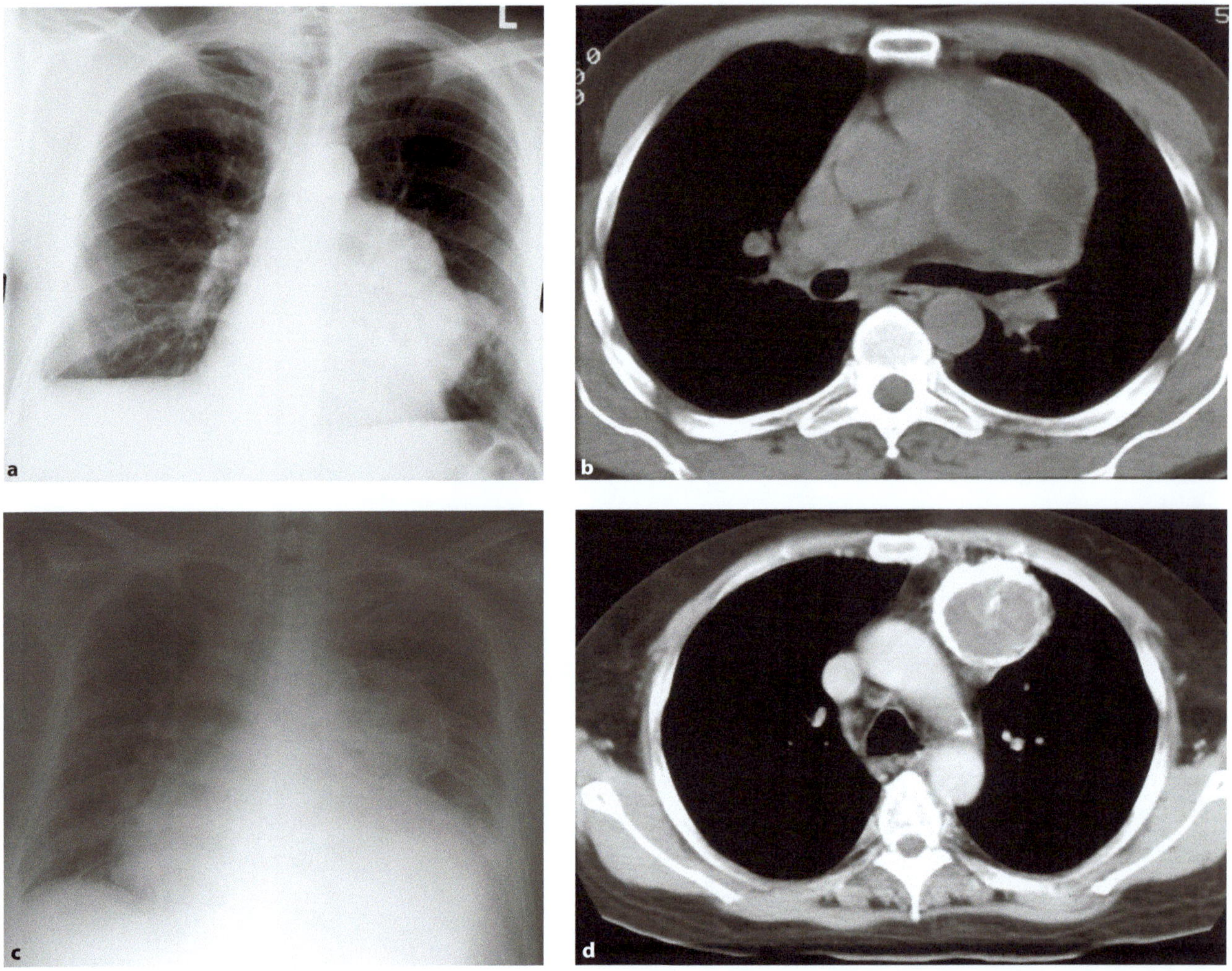

Fig. 3.33 Pericardial and mediastinal hydatid cysts. **a** PA chest radiograph showing a left paracardiac lobulated mass. **b** Non-enhanced CT scan of the chest showed a pericardial hydatid cyst containing daughter cysts. **c,d** Portable chest radiograph and CT scan of the chest demonstrate a calcified inactive hydatid cyst in the anterior mediastinum

wall, ultrasound is helpful in demonstrating the cystic nature of the lesion (Fig. 3.35), thus suspecting hydatid disease. MRI and CT have been used to evaluate response to medical treatment (i.e., albendazole and praziquantel, etc.) in hepatic disease (Von Sinner et al. 1991; Von Sinner 1990b). The use of medical treatment in thoracic disease is controversial; however, it has been attempted with variable success [i.e., a cure rate of up to 30% (Fig. 3.36), persistence of disease in about 50%, and recurrence in up to 20% of all cases] in advanced disease, inoperable cases or patients who do not accept surgical treatment. Improvement is identified as disappearance or decrease in size of cysts as well as a decrease in surrounding inflammatory changes (Morar and Feldman 2003; Kurkcuoglu et al. 2002b; Morris et al. 1985; Horton 1989; Teggi et al. 1993; Kuzucu et al. 2004).

3.4.2 Alveolar Echinococcosis

This parasitosis of unknown incidence, caused by *E. multilocularis,* is less frequent than *E. granulosus* (Morar and Feldman 2003), but more aggressive. It is prevalent in Central Europe, Russia, western China, northern Japan, North America, particularly Alaska and Canada, and North Africa (Morar and Feldman 2003). Intermediate hosts include foxes and small rodents. Definitive hosts are dogs and cats. Humans become infected by accidentally ingesting the eggs of the tapeworm, excreted by the final hosts or during normal feeding by a variety of rodents and small lagomorphs (Vuitton et al. 2003). The infection behaves like a malignant liver tumor, invading and metastasizing to the brain, lungs and other organs (Mandell et al. 2005; Morar and Feldman 2003). If left

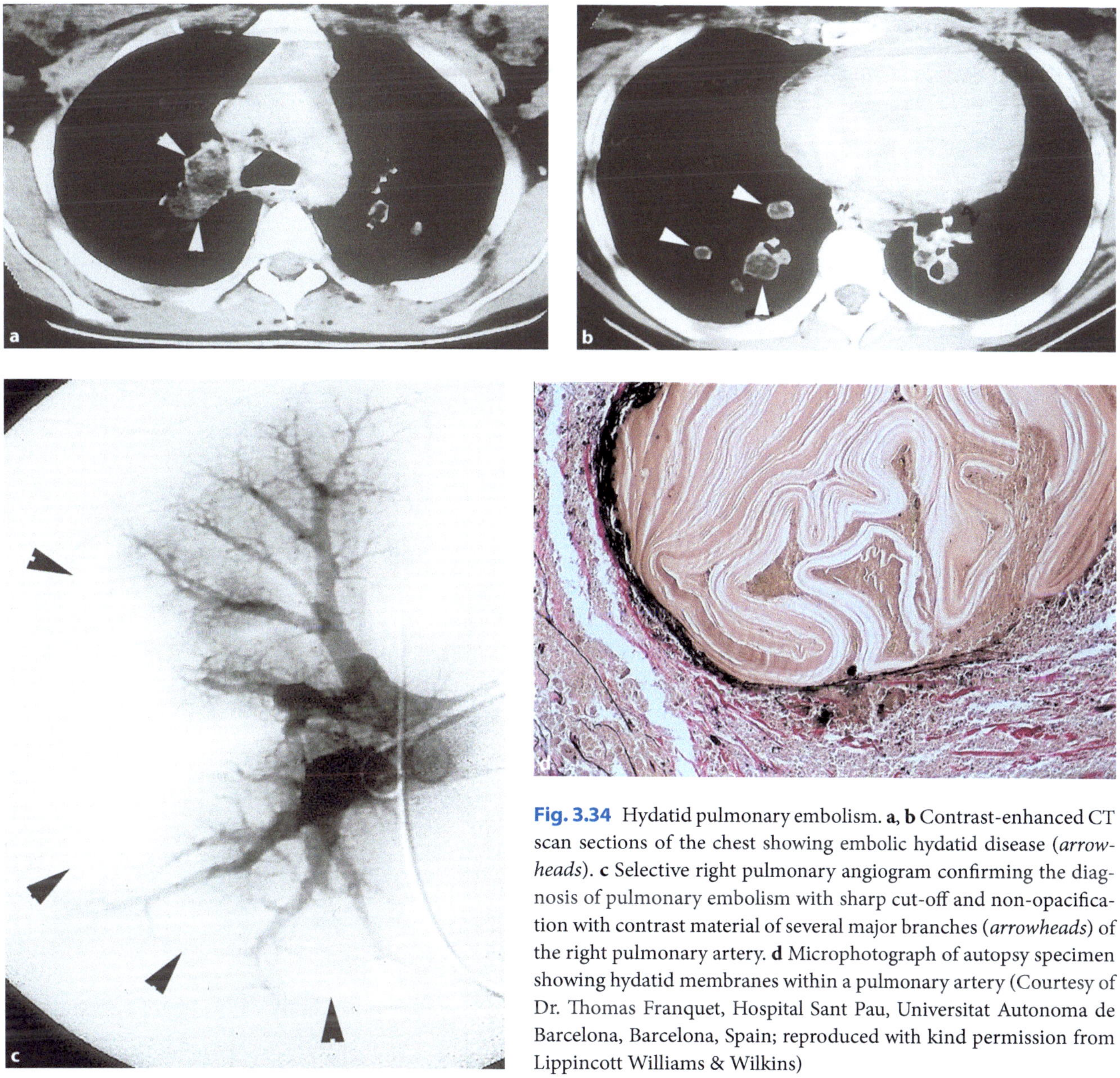

Fig. 3.34 Hydatid pulmonary embolism. **a, b** Contrast-enhanced CT scan sections of the chest showing embolic hydatid disease (*arrowheads*). **c** Selective right pulmonary angiogram confirming the diagnosis of pulmonary embolism with sharp cut-off and non-opacification with contrast material of several major branches (*arrowheads*) of the right pulmonary artery. **d** Microphotograph of autopsy specimen showing hydatid membranes within a pulmonary artery (Courtesy of Dr. Thomas Franquet, Hospital Sant Pau, Universitat Autonoma de Barcelona, Barcelona, Spain; reproduced with kind permission from Lippincott Williams & Wilkins)

untreated, virtually 100% of patients will ultimately die within 15 years (Morar and Feldman 2003; Wilson et al. 1995; Ammann and Eckert 1996).

Clinical manifestations include fatigue, weight loss, coughing, and hemoptysis. According to the European Echinococcosis Registry, thoracic compromise, very often associated with liver disease, occurs by direct extension to the diaphragm, lungs, and pleura (12% of all cases) or metastatic spread to the lungs (~6% of all cases) (Ammann and Eckert 1996; Akinoglu et al. 1991; Kern et al. 2003). Metastasis to the right atrium (Etievent et al. 1986) and thoracic spine have also been described (Reuter et al. 2000). Definitive diagnosis can be achieved by immunohistochemical and histological analysis. Serologic tests, also available, are important in the early detection of asymptomatic cases (Gottstein and Reichen 2002).

Metastases to the lungs appear as multiple, peripherally located, small, ill-defined, irregular lesions, less than 3 cm in diameter, which may or may not exhibit stippled or peripheral calcifications (Tuzan and Hekimoglu 2001; Jiang 2002; Treugut et al. 1980; Reittner et al. 1996). Variable changes in the right lung base occur when a liver mass invades the diaphragm and extends into the chest, including pleural effusion, empyema, and right lower lobe parenchymal nodules or masses due to cysts (Treugut et

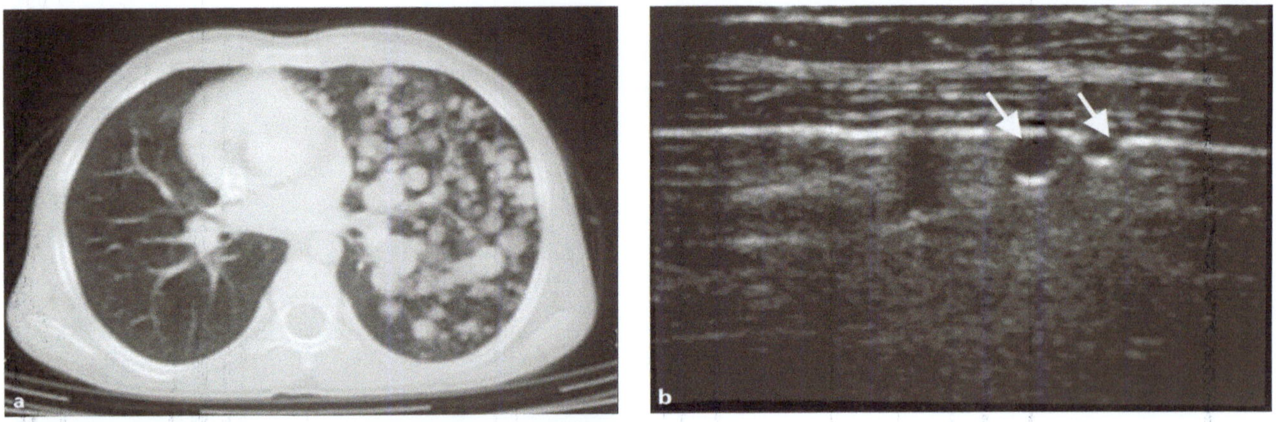

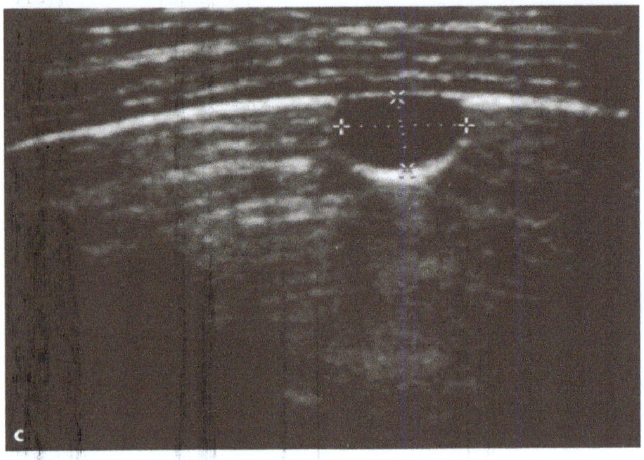

Fig. 3.35 Usefulness of ultrasound. **a** CT scan of the chest in a 10-year-old boy with multiple round opacities involving the left lung. The right lung is clear. **b,c** Ultrasound of the chest demonstrated the cystic nature of these lesions (*arrows*) (Courtesy of Dr. Nadim Kanj, Department of Internal Medicine, American University of Beirut Medical Center, Beirut, Lebanon)

al. 1980). Bronchobiliary fistula is a complication of direct extension. It can be suspected on CT examination by the coexistence of a liver mass extending through the diaphragm with clustered calcifications and air, and associated continuity with air bronchograms in the right lower lobe. The fistulous tracts can be identified on MR cholangiographic sequences. The diagnosis can be confirmed by demonstrating passage of the radiotracer or contrast material to the tracheobronchial tree on a Tc-HIDA hepatobiliary scintigraphy scan or endoscopic retrograde cholangiography respectively (Senturk et al. 1998).

Response to medical treatment with benzimidazoles, particularly in liver disease, has been demonstrated by imaging techniques (e.g., conventional radiographs, ultrasound, and CT scanning) in animal models (Taylor et al. 1989) and humans (Senturk et al. 1998; Wilson et al. 1992; Reuter et al. 2000; Ammann et al. 1994).

3.4.3 Polycystic Echinococcosis

Echinococcus vogeli causes polycystic echinococcosis, a relatively recently described echinococcosis endemic in the tropical areas of Central and South America. Humans become infected after a complex cycle by ingestion of fluid/food contaminated with parasite eggs shed in bush dogs' feces. Polycystic echinococcosis shares several similarities with alveolar echinococcosis:

1. The liver is the target organ and thus the most commonly affected
2. It can affect the thoracic organs either by direct extension or hematogenous spread (metastasis) (D'Alessandro 1997; Martinez et al. 2005)

By the late 1990s, at least 86 cases had been recognized in the literature (D'Alessandro 1997), and today around 200 cases have been identified, but are thought to be only the tip of the iceberg (Dr. A. D'Alessandro, personal communication).

In hematogenous spread, solitary or multiple soft tissue nodules, rarely calcified, can be identified on the chest radiograph (Fig. 3.37). Mediastinal cysts, which can calcify, can manifest as mediastinal widening, and are better evaluated by CT scanning. Direct extension from liver disease usually demonstrates pleural effusion, pleural cysts, and right lower lobe parenchymal cysts. Con-

Fig. 3.36 Successful medical treatment of a small pulmonary hydatid cyst. **a** Initial PA chest radiograph, cone view, at presentation showing a round lesion in the left mid lung field. **b** CT scan of the chest showed a small crescent of air within the lesion compatible with a hydatid cyst. **c** Follow-up chest radiograph, cone view, obtained after medical therapy, showed a larger crescent of air compatible with degeneration of the cyst. **d** Further follow-up chest radiograph, cone view, obtained after a 2-year interval showed complete healing with a residual linear scar at the site of the cyst

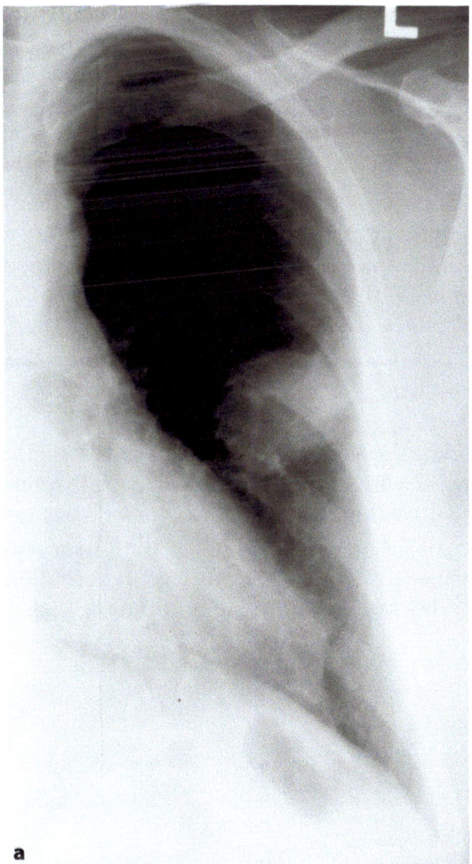

a

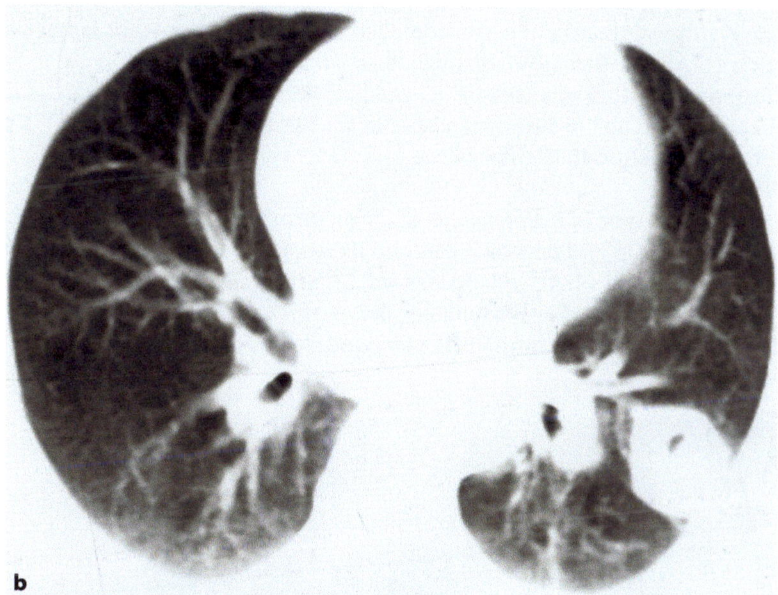

b

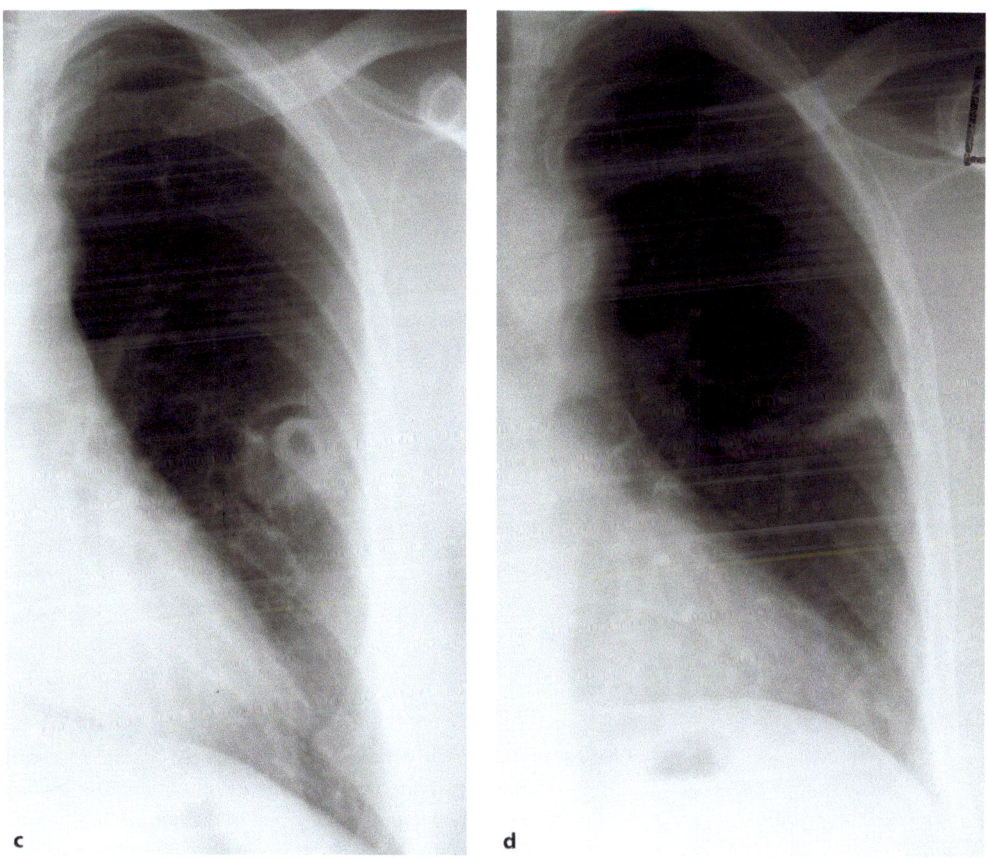

c d

solidation surrounding parenchymal cysts is sometimes identified (Fig. 3.38). Infection of the thoracic wall demonstrates cystic expansion of the ribs and surrounding soft tissues (Fig. 3.39) (D'Alessandro 1997; Rodrigues-Silva et al. 2002; Martinez et al. 2005; Meneghelli et al. 1992a, 1986; D'Alessandro et al. 1979).

Awareness of this particular type of echinococcosis is important in endemic regions, since it shows an effective response to albendazole and, in contrast to hydatid disease, surgical treatment is considered as a second line option (D'Alessandro 1997; Meneghelli et al. 1986, 1992b). Response of thoracic disease to medical treatment has been verified by CT scanning, either as the disappearance of or a reduction in the size of the cysts (Meneghelli et al. 1992b).

A fourth type of *Echinococcus* (*E. oligarthrus*) has been isolated in wild and domestic cats and its larvae are found in agouties and other rodents. The distribution is similar to that of *E. vogeli*. Fortunately, only a few cases have been documented in humans (D'Alessandro 1997; Basset et al. 1998; D'Alessandro et al. 1995; Lopera et al. 1989; Salinas-Lopez et al. 1996).

3.4.4 Sparganosis

Spirometra species occasionally induce eosinophilic pleuritis, or eosinophilic pulmonary granuloma simulating a malignant pulmonary nodule, in a few patients identified in Japan (Ishi et al. 2001; Iwatani et al. 2006).

3.4.5 Cysticercosis

The central nervous system and muscles are the major site of involvement with cysticercosis; a case of disseminated cysticercosis with pulmonary involvement was reported from Brazil (Mamere et al. 2004). Pulmonary and chest wall musculature nodular lesions were detected on imaging by CT and MRI in the brain and thorax. Calci-

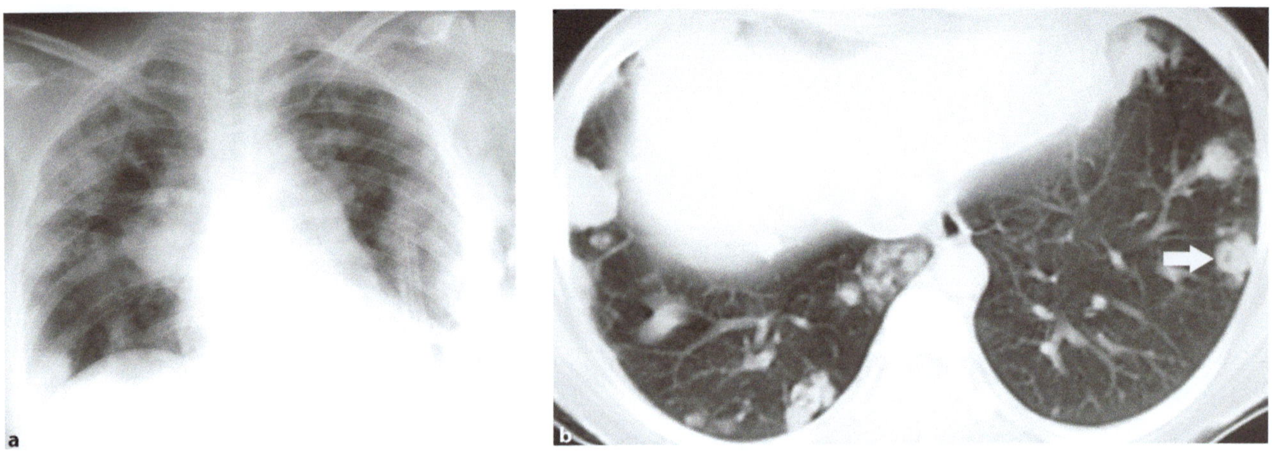

Fig. 3.37 Polycystic echinococcosis *(E. vogeli)*. **a** PA chest radiograph shows multiple bilateral soft tissue pulmonary nodules. **b** Axial CT scan of the chest (lung window) depicts multiple pulmonary nodules. A cavitated nodule in the left lower lobe (*arrow*) reveals the cystic nature of nodules. *E. vogeli* was proven to be the causative agent

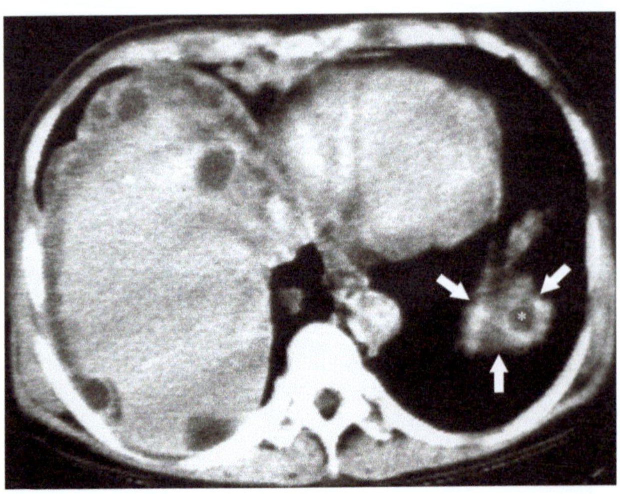

Fig. 3.38 Polycystic echinococcosis (*E. vogeli*). Axial CT scan of the chest (soft tissue window) shows multiple cystic lesions in the liver. There is a pulmonary cyst in the left lower lobe (*asterisk*) with surrounding consolidation (*arrows*) reflecting the inflammatory process

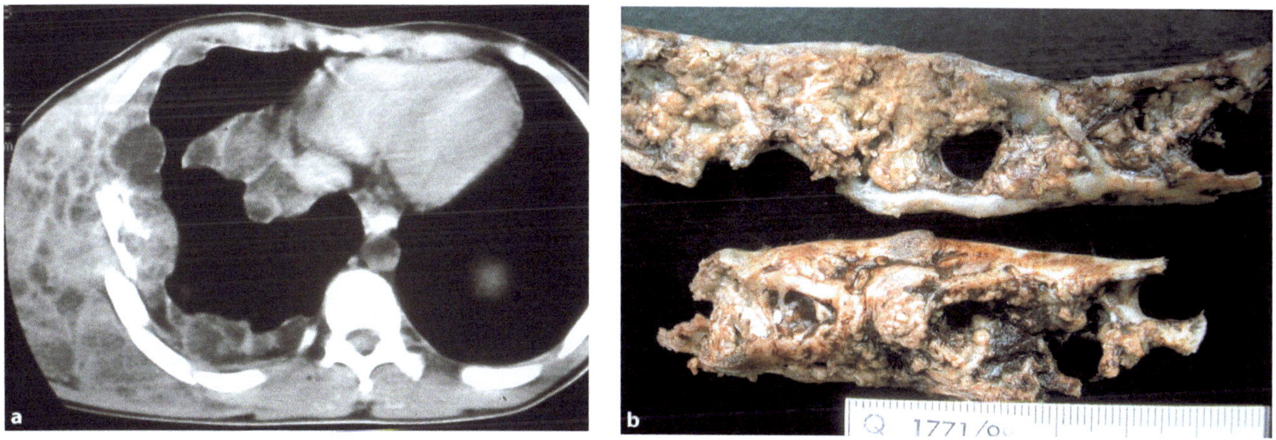

Fig. 3.39 Polycystic echinococcosis *(E. vogeli)* of the chest wall. **a** CT scan of the chest shows cystic thickening of the pleura with chest wall involvement. **b** Photograph of the surgically removed gross specimen demonstrates osseous expansion secondary to rib invasion (Reproduced with permission from Radiographics, Martinez et al. 2005)

fied burned-out lesions can be visualized by plain radiography (Fig. 3.40) in the chest wall muscles.

3.5 Trematodes (Flukes)

3.5.1 Schistosomiasis

Schistosomiasis continues to be a major worldwide public health problem. It is estimated that 200 million people are infected around the world, mostly in Africa. One hundred and twenty million are symptomatic and 20 million have severe disease. Although the infection is endemic in more than 70 countries in all continents, 85% of affected patients live in Africa where Angola, the Central African Republic, Chad, Tunisia, Egypt, Morocco, Ghana, Madagascar, Malawi, Mozambique, Nigeria, Senegal, Sudan, the United Republic of Tanzania, Zambia, Mali, Uganda, and Zimbabwe seem to be the most commonly affected areas. Other affected countries include the Caribbean islands, Japan, Mauritius, Brazil, Cambodia, China, Laos, the Philippines, Botswana, Iran, and Iraq. Although progress has been achieved regarding control of schistosomiasis in the last 2 years, the infection continues to be a devastating and disabling disease, only surpassed by malaria. Mortality is calculated to be near 300,000 deaths per year (Chitsulo et al. 2000; World Health Organization 2006).

There are three important *Schistosoma* species: *S. hematobium*, *S. mansoni*, and *S. japonicum*. Although all three species can cause pulmonary disease (Morris and Knauer 1997), *S. mansoni* and *S. japonicum* are those most frequently observed (Nash et al. 1982). *S. mansoni* is endemic to Africa, Saudi Arabia, Egypt, Sudan, Madagascar, Brazil, Surinam, Venezuela, and Puerto Rico, whereas *S. japonicum* is more frequently seen in East Asia. Infection is acquired through exposure of the skin to water contaminated with cercariae excreted by snails. This parasitic form has the ability to penetrate the skin or the intestinal wall, migrate to the lung and ultimately the liver, where it continues its life cycle (Murray et al. 2005; Botero 2003; Morris and Knauer 1997).

Acute pulmonary schistosomiasis (3–8 weeks after parasitic skin penetration), which results from type 3 immunologic reaction in which eosinophils are sequestered in the lungs, usually resolves within a few weeks. Clinical manifestations often include shortness of breath, wheezing, and dry coughing. The diagnosis is suggested in patients who live in or have traveled to endemic areas and who present with eosinophilia (Morris and Knauer 1997). Patients may have both clinical and radiologic manifestations after the onset of treatment. Katayama fever, more commonly described with *S. mansoni* and *S. japonicum,*

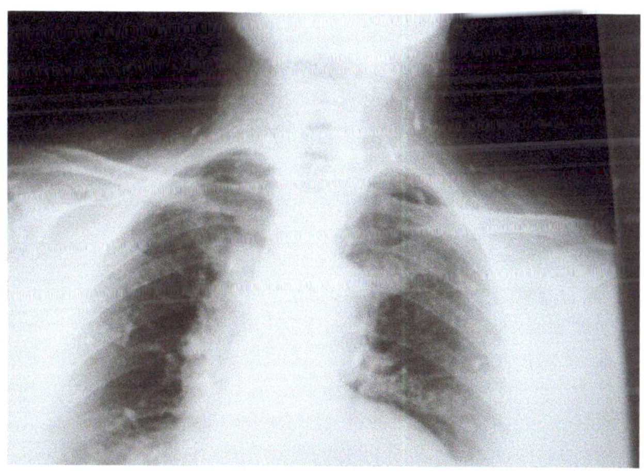

Fig. 3.40 Cysticercosis. Plain radiograph of the chest showing calcified cysticerci of the chest wall and neck muscles

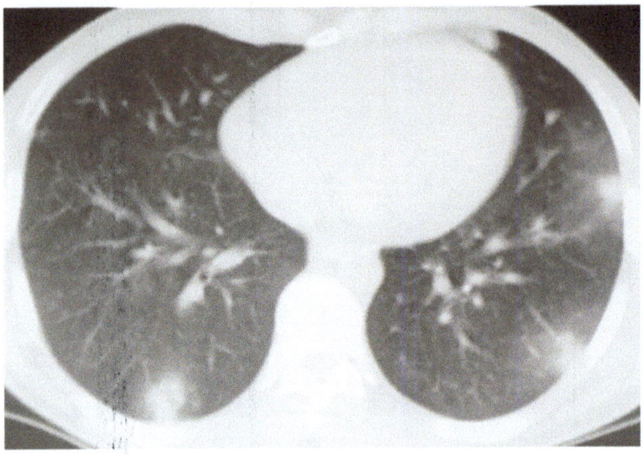

Fig. 3.41 Early pulmonary schistosomiasis. Axial CT scan of the chest shows multiple peripheral subpleural pulmonary nodules surrounded by a halo of ground-glass opacity or attenuation in the lower lobes bilaterally. *S. mansoni* was the proven etiologic factor (Reproduced with permission from Radiographics, Martinez et al. 2005)

refers to pulmonary symptoms that coincide with febrile illness, and is thought to represent an immunologic reaction to the parasite's eggs. Associated symptoms include urticaria, arthralgia, hepatosplenomegaly, hepatitis, eosinophilia, and pulmonary disease. The acute infection is more commonly seen in individuals traveling to endemic regions (Morris and Knauer 1997). Chest radiograph can be normal (Lambertucci et al. 1997, 2005) or show multiple, bilateral, ill-defined, nodular opacities (Lambertucci et al. 1997; Nguyen et al. 2006; Waldman et al. 2001; Cooke et al. 1999; Schwartz 2002; Schwartz et al. 2000) and less frequently, consolidation (Lambertucci et al. 1997; Fatureto et al. 2003) or reticulonodular opacities (Schwartz 2002). These abnormalities are usually transitory and resolve within weeks (Cooke et al. 1999). CT scanning can show solitary (Fatureto et al. 2003) or multiple subpleural soft tissue nodules that may exhibit surrounding ground-glass opacities (the so-called "halo" sign) (Fig. 3.41). Sensitivity is low for the examination of stool and urine for eggs at this stage of infection, although rectal biopsy may help improve the diagnosis. ELISA is a better initial study, but positive results must be confirmed with enzyme-linked immunoelectrotransfer blot. Because serologic tests remain positive for years, even after treatment, they are not helpful for the diagnosis of reinfection or for determining the success of treatment (Schwartz 2002; Schwartz et al. 2000).

Chronic pulmonary disease occurs in patients with hepatosplenic disease in whom portal hypertension and collateral circulation develop. Ultimately, eggs can shunt from the portal system and reach the arterial pulmonary circulation (Schwartz 2002; Andrade and Andrade 1970). A granulomatous reaction to eggs deposited in the pulmonary vasculature leads to intimal fibrosis, pulmonary hypertension, and cor pulmonale. The clinical picture includes dyspnea, chest pain, fatigue, palpitations, coughing, and finally right-sided heart failure. Radiographic and CT findings (Fig. 3.42) include right ventricular enlargement, pulmonary hypertension, dilatation of the azygous vein (due to abundant collaterals draining a hypertensive portal system), and scattered calcified nodules i.e., granulomatas throughout the lungs (Phillips et al. 1975; Pagan Saez 1985). Atypical presentation simulating tuberculosis and neoplasm has been described (El Mallah and Hashem 1953; Schaberg et al. 1991; Tizes et al. 1967). Diagnosis is made by identifying eggs in stool or urine samples or by rectal biopsy; sometimes lung biopsy has been proved effective. Serologic tests are not very helpful because they cannot help differentiate between a former infection and current disease (Richert and Krakaur 1959; Schwartz 2002; Schwartz et al. 2000; Phillips et al. 1975).

3.5.2 Paragonimiasis

Ingestion of raw or partially cooked freshwater crabs or crawfish, containing *Paragonimus westermani* (lung fluke) or other *Paragonimus* species, is the cause of human paragonimiasis. Alternatively, undercooked meat of infected pigs and wild boars are also sources (Nakamura-Uchiyama et al. 2002). The infection is endemic in areas of East Asia, Southeast Asia, Latin America (primarily Peru), and Africa (primarily Nigeria) (Barrett-Connor 1982; Botero 2003; Binford and Connor 1976; Hasleton 1996; Travis et al. 2002; Murray et al. 2002; Fishman et al. 1998). Many cases have been reported in the United States among Indo-Chinese and Latin American immigrants (Nakamura-Uchiyama et al. 2002; Johnson and Johnson 1983; Velez et al. 2002). It is believed that 195 million people are at risk, and 20.7 million are infected in endemic areas (Murray et al. 2002).

After ingestion, the infective larvae of *P. westermani* penetrate the duodenum and migrate to the peritoneal cavity and abdominal wall. Ultimately, parasitic forms travel through the diaphragm to the pleura and lungs (Velez et al. 2002). Although paragonimiasis affects primarily the lungs, skin and central nervous system compromise is also well described. Patients present with fever, chest pain, and respiratory symptoms such as chronic coughing and hemoptysis. Peripheral blood eosinophilia is present in more than 80% of patients (Nakamura-Uchiyama et al. 2002). Diagnosis is confirmed by detecting parasite eggs in the sputum, pleural fluid, or feces; in addition, larvae can often be found at bronchial brushing and washing. Intradermal and serologic tests are also available (Nakamura-Uchiyama et al. 2002).

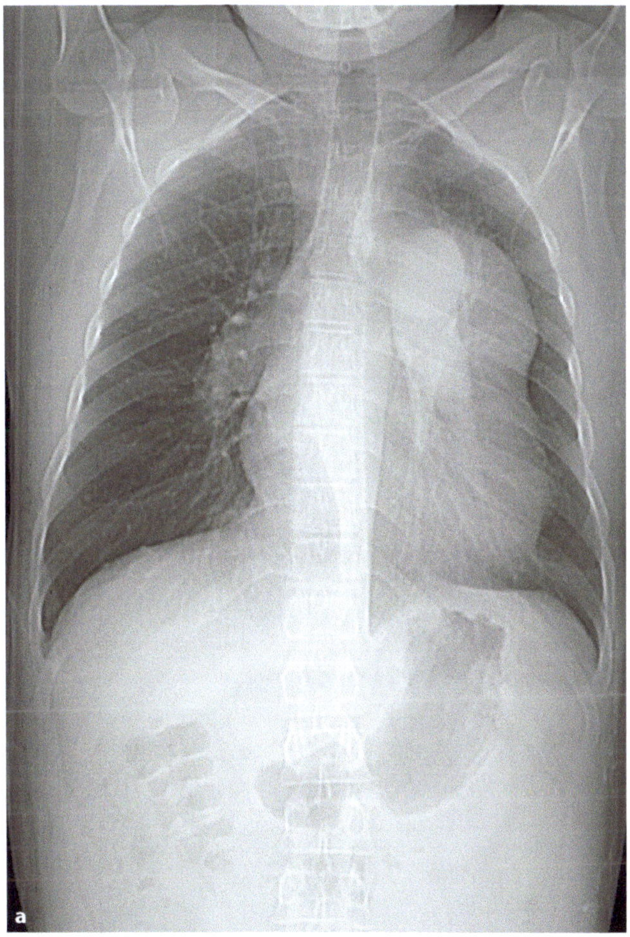

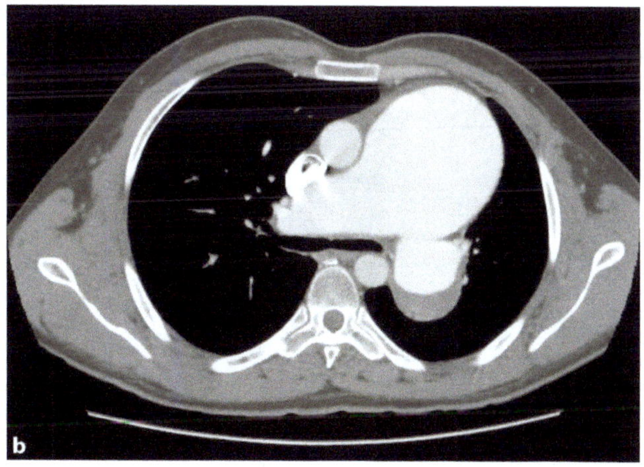

Fig. 3.42 Pulmonary hypertension due to chronic cardiopulmonary schistosomiasis. **a** Scout image of a CT scan of the thorax showing marked enlargement of the main pulmonary trunk, prominent pulmonary arteries demonstrating peripheral pruning, and hypertrophy of the right ventricle. **b** Contrast-enhanced CT scan of the chest showing marked enlargement of the main pulmonary artery trunk and the pulmonary arteries. (Courtesy of Dr. Dany Jasinowodolinski, Fleury-Sao Paolo, Brazil)

Radiologic findings correlate well with the stage of the disease. The penetration of juvenile worms through the diaphragm into the pleural cavity can cause pleural effusion, pneumothorax (Fig. 3.43) and potentially empyema. Migration of worms through the lungs usually manifests as consolidation (Fig. 3.44). Band-like opacities extending from the pleural surface can be identified at this stage, usually representing worm migration tracts (Fig. 3.45). As parasites grow, they tend to settle down. At this time, consolidation resolves and thin-walled cysts appear. When cysts are fluid-filled they manifest on the chest radiograph as round soft tissue nodules (Fig. 3.46), 0.5 to 4 cm in diameter. CT can better identify cysts, even when they are smaller (i.e., 5–15 mm in diameter) (Fig. 3.46) or in the presence of surrounding consolidation due to their hypodense content. If bronchial communication develops, air inside the cyst is better demonstrated on both the plain radiograph and CT (Fig. 3.47). A characteristic appearance at this stage is the ring shadow, which is characterized by a thin-walled cavity with a crescent-shaped opacity inside representing the parasite, usually less than 3 mm thick, and a crescent-shaped area of increased opacity or hyperattenuation within the cyst that represents worms attached to the wall (Fig. 3.48) (Nakamura-Uchiyama et al. 2002; Johnson and Johnson 1983; Velez et al. 2002; Im et al. 1992, 1993, 1997; Mukae et al. 2001; Sharma 1989). Loeffler's-like syndrome with transitory and/or migratory consolidative or ground-glass opacities has also been described (Bahk 1962; Suwanik and Harinsuta 1959). During and after treatment, fibronodular changes can develop in areas previously affected. Calcifications can be present; however, their presence should raise the question of possible coexistent tuberculosis. Fibrosis and cicatricial emphysema, frequent in tuberculosis, are virtually absent in paragonimiasis (Im et al. 1993, 1997).

3.6 Arthropods – Pentastomiasis

Pentastomiasis or porocephalosis is a zoonosis caused by *Armillifer armillatus* that affects snake-eating Africans (Guardia et al. 1991). The parasite penetrates the bowel wall, and migrates into the peritoneum to reach the liver and occasionally the lungs (Fig. 3.49).

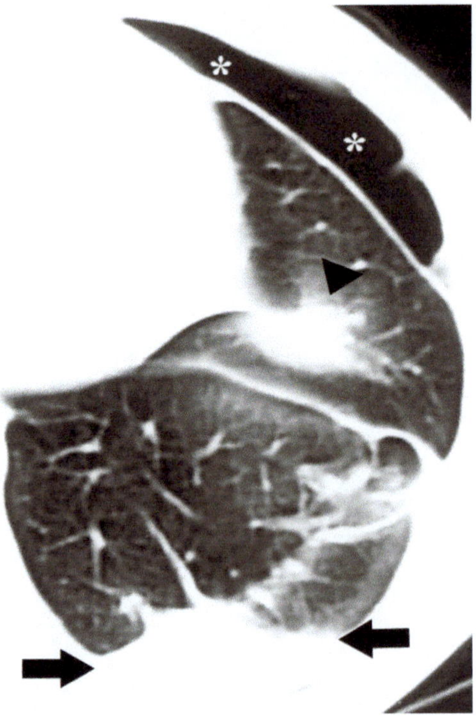

Fig. 3.43 Thoracic paragonimiasis. Axial CT scan of the chest, close-up image, demonstrates left-sided pleural effusion (*arrows*) and pneumothorax (*asterisk*). A small area of consolidation is identified in the lingula (*arrowhead*)

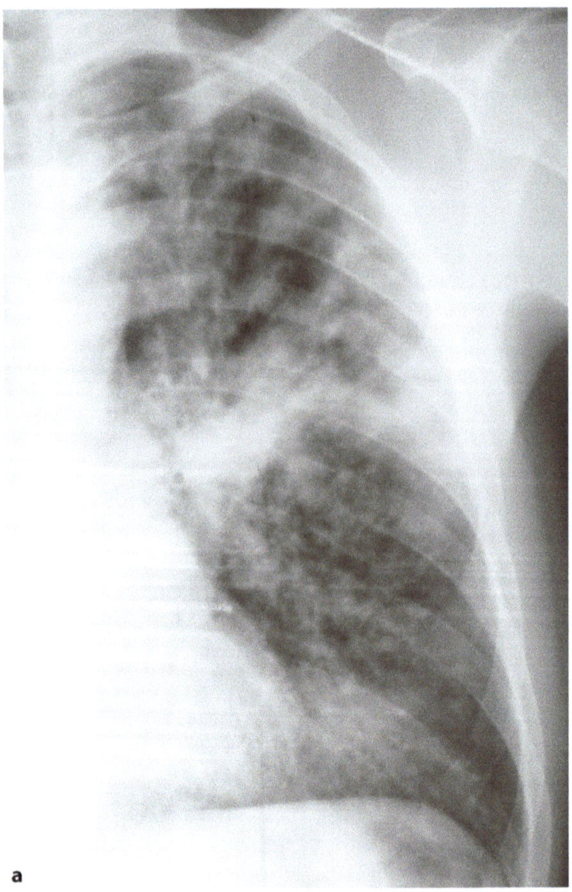

a

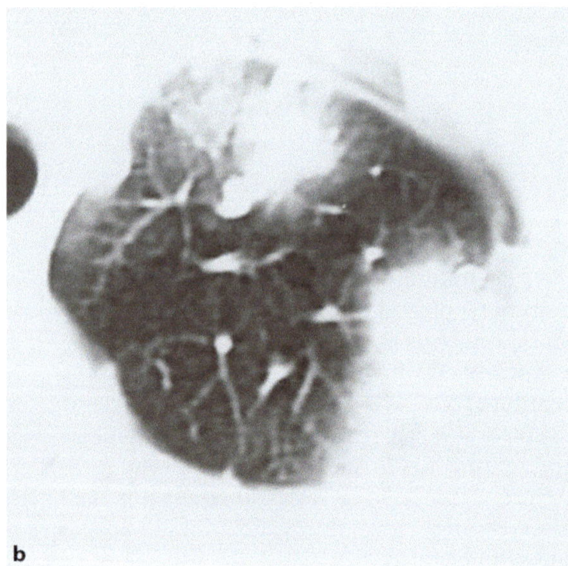

b

Fig. 3.44 Thoracic paragonimiasis. **a** PA chest radiograph, cone view, shows heterogeneous opacities throughout the left hemithorax. **b** Axial CT scan of the chest shows subsegmental areas of consolidation (Reproduced with permission from Radiographics, Martinez et al. 2005)

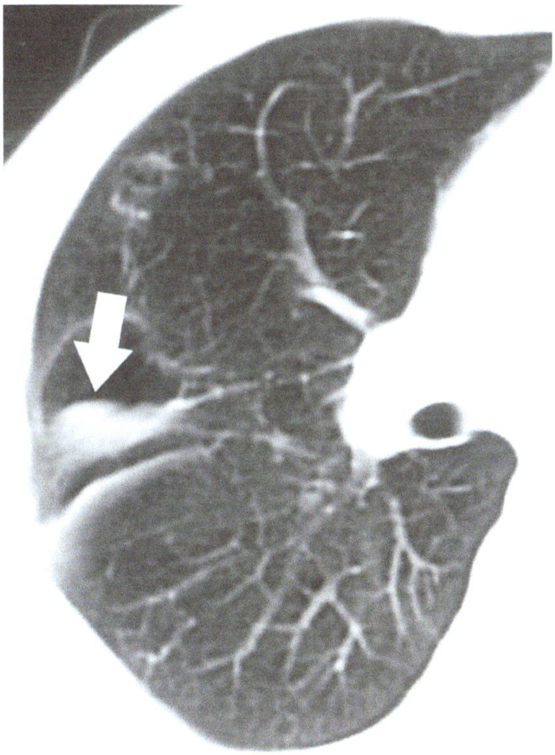

Fig. 3.45 Thoracic paragonimiasis. Axial CT scan of the chest, close-up image, shows band-like opacity in the right middle lobe (*arrow*) that represents worm migration tracts

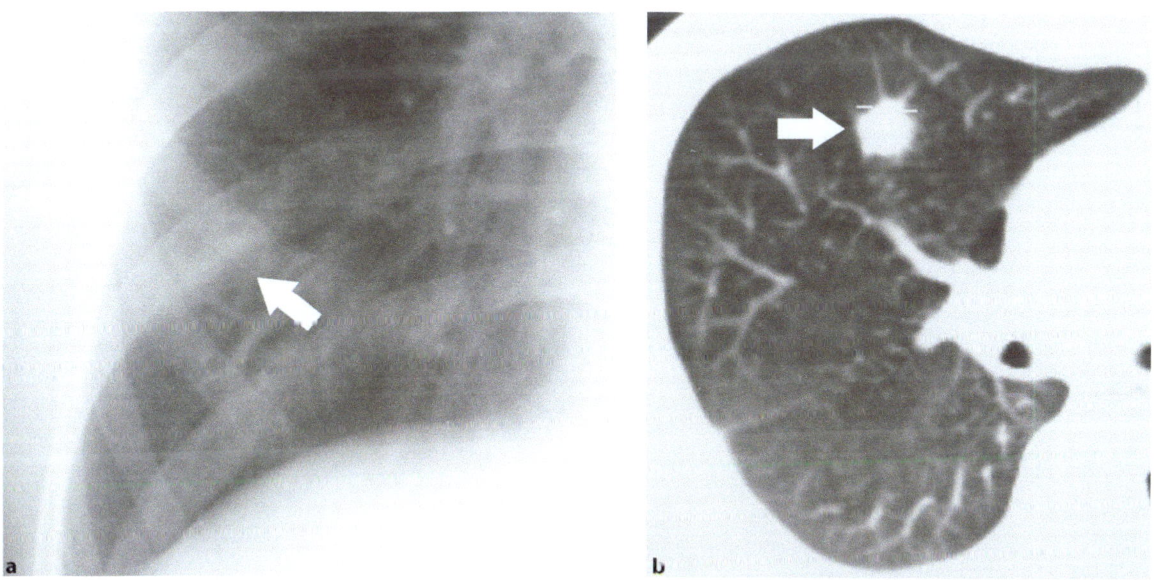

Fig. 3.46 Thoracic paragonimiasis presenting as a solitary pulmonary nodule. **a** PA chest radiograph, cone view, shows an ill-defined opacity (*arrow*) in the right middle lobe. **b** Axial CT scan of the chest, close-up image, shows to better advantage a round soft tissue nodule (*arrow*) in the right middle lobe. Histopathologic analysis performed after surgical resection demonstrated *P. westermani.* (Reproduced with permission from Radiographics, Martinez et al. 2005)

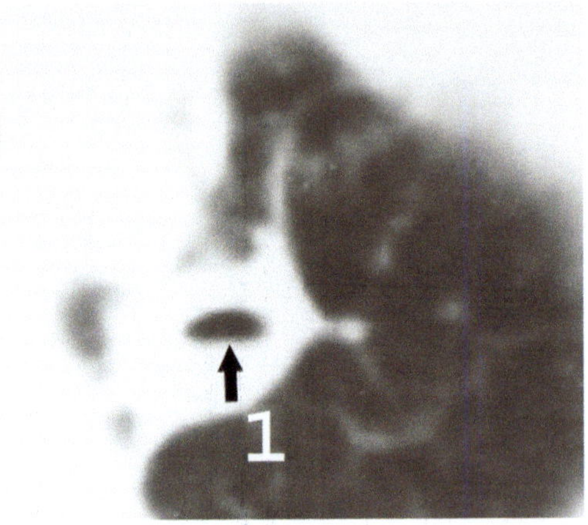

Fig. 3.47 Thoracic paragonimiasis. Axial CT scan of the chest, close-up image, depicts a cavitated nodule in the left upper lobe with thick walls. A small air–fluid level is also identified (*arrow*)

3.7 Eosinophilic Pneumonias/Pulmonary Infiltrates with Eosinophilia/Eosinophilic Lung Diseases

Eosinophilic pneumonias (EP) or lung diseases are rare, and are characterized by the common finding of increased eosinophilia in blood and or tissue, i.e., pulmonary infiltrates, the so-called pulmonary infiltrates with eosinophilia (PIE), a term coined in 1952 which covers a wide spectrum of diseases. It is therefore important to differentiate between parasitic and nonparasitic causes of PIE.

Parasitic EP occurs in almost all metazoan helminthic infections during larval migration of the parasite through the lungs, producing VLM, so-called Loeffler's syndrome described in 1932, and presumably caused by the *Ascaris* larvae. In patients who have not lived in tropical or subtropical regions *Toxocara* and *Ascaris* species should be considered, while for patients who have lived in tropical or subtropical regions *Paragonimus* species, *Strongyloides* species, *Ancylostoma* species, *Schistosoma* species, *Necator americanus*, *Wuchereria bancrofti*, and *Brugia malayi* should be taken into consideration. Tropical pulmonary eosinophilia (TPE) caused by filarial worms *W. bancrofti* and *B. malayi* is the most serious parasitic eosinophilic lung disease, in which cases have typically been reported to masquerade as acute or refractory bronchial asthma. Eosinophils are recruited to the lung to kill the parasite. Despite larval migration through the lungs, there is usually no permanent lung damage (Chitkara and Krishna 2006). Patients present with respiratory symptoms with or without fever. Chest radiographs and CT scans of the chest show migratory peripheral pulmonary infiltrates or consolidation or ground-glass opacities. Blood eosinophilia may or may not be present. The diagnosis is confirmed by the identification of eggs or larvae

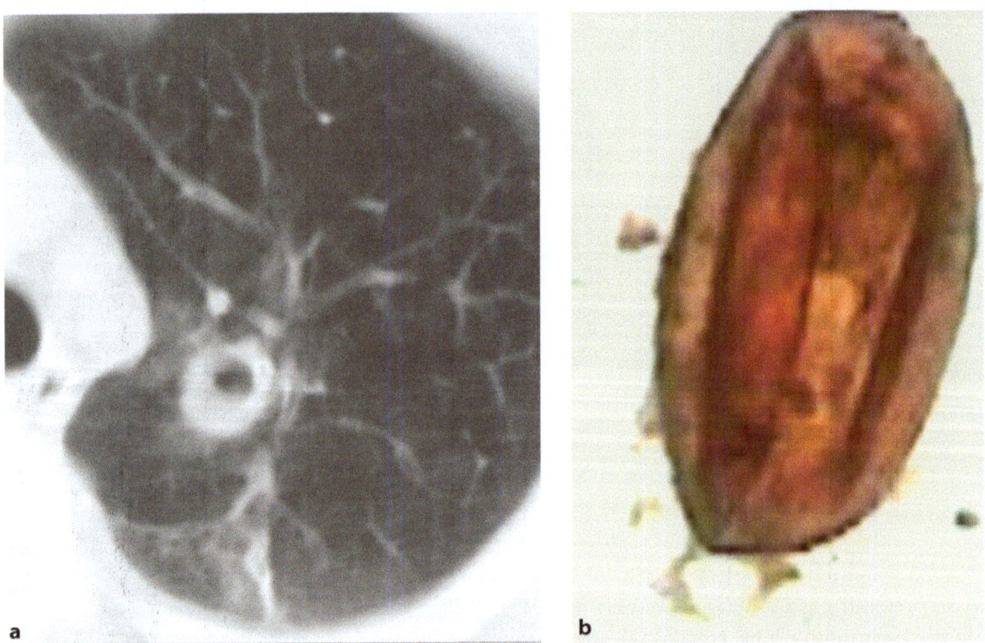

Fig. 3.48 Thoracic paragonimiasis. **a** Axial CT scan of the chest, close-up image, demonstrates a relatively thin-walled cavity with a crescent-dependent opacity representing the actual parasite. **b** Photomicrograph shows an egg of *P. westermani* obtained after the bronchoalveolar lavage

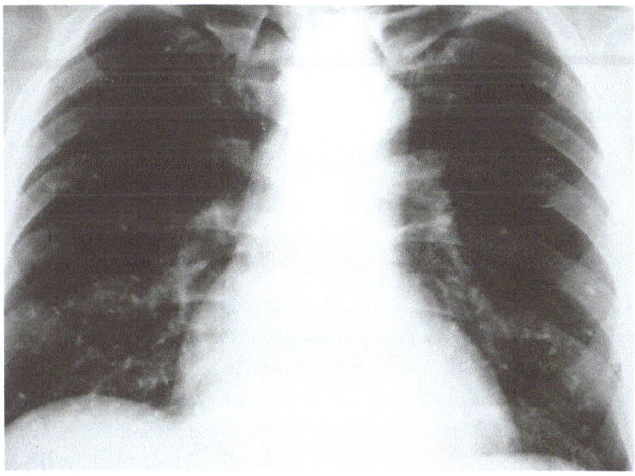

Fig. 3.49 PA chest radiograph showing numerous calcified encysted *Armillifer armillatus* nymphs scattered in the lung fields. (Courtesy of Dr. Gordon Gamsu, Weill-Cornell Medical Center, New York, NY, USA)

in stool, sputum, pleural fluid, bronchoalveolar lavage, or in tissue specimens from transbronchial or thoracoscopic biopsies of the diseased lung segments. Serologic testing is also confirmatory. If all these tests are not diagnostic, empirical treatment with antiparasitic drugs for 2 weeks with resolution of the pulmonary symptoms and radiographic changes is diagnostic.

The nonparasitic causes of PIE include allergic conditions, auto-immune diseases and vasculitides, malignancies, and lastly idiopathic causes. For a detailed description of these pathologies, the reader is referred to the excellent review articles on this subject by Cottin and Alberts (Cottin and Cordier 2005; Alberts 2004).

For clinical understanding, eosinophilic lung diseases (ELD) may be also classified into two groups: intrinsic (primary, cryptogenic, or idiopathic) in which the cause is not known and representing approximately 20% of ELD, and extrinsic (secondary) in which the cause is known. ELD of unknown cause include: simple pulmonary eosinophilia (SPE), acute eosinophilic pneumonia (AEP), chronic eosinophilic pneumonia (CEP), bronchiolitis obstructive obliterans pneumonitis (BOOP) or organizing pneumonia, and idiopathic hypereosinophilic syndrome (IHS). ELD of known cause include:

1. Infectious diseases: fungal infections and hypersensitivity (coccidioidomycosis, histoplasmosis), bacterial and mycobacterial infections (chronic brucellosis, tuberculosis), and parasitic infections (almost all metazoan infestations are accompanied by eosinophilia, mainly during parasitic migration, citing *Strongyloides stercoralis, Ascaris lumbricoides, Schistosoma* and filarial species, *Paragonimus westermani, Ancylostoma duodenale, Toxocara* species, *Clonorchis sinensis, Echinococcus* species).
2. Allergic conditions: allergic bronchopulmonary aspergillosis (ABPA), bronchocentric granulomatosis (BCG), drug reactions or drug-induced pulmonary eosinophilia.
3. Auto-immune diseases and eosinophilic vasculitides: allergic granulomatosis and angiitis (Churg-Strauss syndrome), Wegener's granulomatosis, polyarteritis nodosa (PAN), Langerhan's cell granulomatosis or histiocytosis X, and sarcoidosis.
4. Neoplasm-related eosinophilia: systemic mastocytosis, eosinophilic leukemia, Hodgkin's and B-cell non-Hodgkin's lymphoma, T-cell lymphoblastic leukemia/lymphoma, large cell tumors of the lung, squamous cell carcinomas of the cervix, vagina, penis, skin, and nasopharynx, adenocarcinomas of the stomach, colon, and uterus, and transitional cell bladder carcinoma (Jeong et al.2007; Savani and Sharma 2002).

3.8 Conclusion

Parasite-induced pulmonary diseases result in various imaging patterns that are nonspecific and mimic other inflammatory and neoplastic diseases. The pulmonary parasitic diseases are diagnosed by identification of eggs or larvae in stool, sputum, bronchoalveolar lavage, pleural fluid, tissue specimens from lung biopsy, and serology tests.

References

Ahn PJ, Bertagnolli R, Fraser SL, Freeman JH (2005) Distended thoracic duct and diffuse lymphangiectasia caused by bancroftian filariasis. Am J Roentgenol 185:1011–1014

Akinoglu A, Demiryurek H, Guzel C (1991) Alveolar hydatid disease of the liver: a report on thirty-nine surgical cases in eastern Anatolia, Turkey. Am J Trop Med Hyg 45:182–189

Alberts WM (2004) Eosinophilic interstitial lung disease. Curr Opin Pulm Med 10:419–424

Ali-Munive AR, Torres CA, Lasso JI, Ojeda Leon P, Acosta N (2002) Estrongiloidiasis pulmonar. Presentacion de dos casos. Rev Colomb Neumol 14:33–38

Ammann RW, Eckert J (1996) Cestodes. Echinococcus. Gastroenterol Clin North Am 25:655–689

Ammann RW, Ilitsch N, Marincek B, Freiburghaus AU (1994) Effect of chemotherapy on the larval mass and the long-term course of alveolar echinococcosis. Swiss Echinococcosis Study Group. Hepatology 19:735–742

Andrade ZA, Andrade SG (1970) Pathogenesis of schistosomal pulmonary arteritis. Am J Trop Med Hyg 19:305–310

Asimacopoulos PJ, Katras A, Christie B (1992) Pulmonary dirofilariasis. The largest single-hospital experience. Chest 102:851–855

Bahk Y (1962) Pulmonary paragonimiasis as a cause of Loeffler's syndrome. Radiology 78:598–601

Balikian JP, Mudarris FF (1974) Hydatid disease of the lungs. A roentgenologic study of 50 cases. Am J Roentgenol Radium Ther Nucl Med 122:692–707

Barrett-Connor E (1982) Parasitic pulmonary disease. Am Rev Respir Dis 126:558–563

Bartelink AK, Kortbeek LM, Huidekoper HJ, Meulenbelt J, van Knapen F (1993) Acute respiratory failure due to *Toxocara* infection. Lancet 342:1234

Basset D, Girou C, Nozais IP, et al. (1998) Neotropical echinococcosis in Suriname: *Echinococcus oligarthrus* in the orbit and *Echinococcus vogeli* in the abdomen. Am J Trop Med Hyg 59:787–790

Beaver PC, Snyder CH, Carrera GM, Dent JH, Lafferty JW (1952) Chronic eosinophilia due to visceral larva migrans; report of three cases. Pediatrics 9:7–19

Beggs I (1985) The radiology of hydatid disease. Am J Roentgenol 145:639–648

Berk SL, Verghese A, Alvarez S, Hall K, Smith B (1987) Clinical and epidemiologic features of strongyloidiasis. A prospective study in rural Tennessee. Arch Intern Med 147:1257–1261

Beshear JR, Hendley JO (1973) Severe pulmonary involvement in visceral larva migrans. Am J Dis Child 125:599–600

Bhatia G (1997) Echinococcus. Semin Respir Infect 12:171–186

Binford CH, Connor DH (eds) (1976) Pathology of tropical and extraordinary diseases. Armed Forces Institute of Pathology, Washington, DC

Bloomfield JA (1980) Hydatid disease in children and adolescents. Australas Radiol 24:277–283

Bonakdarpour A (1967) Report of 112 cases from Iran and a review of 611 cases from the United States. Am J Roentgenol 99:660–667

Bonilla CA, Rosa UW (1994) *Toxoplasma gondii* pneumonia in patients with the acquired immunodeficiency syndrome: diagnosis by bronchoalveolar lavage. South Med J 87:659–663

Botero D (2003) RMPhteM, Colombia: corporación para investigaciones biológicas

Bruno P, McAllister K, Matthews JI (1982) Pulmonary strongyloidiasis. South Med J 75:363–365

Camara EJ, Lima JA, Oliveira GB, Machado AS (1993) Pulmonary findings in patients with chagasic megaesophagus. Study of autopsied cases. Chest 83:87–91

Cantoni S, Frola C, Gatto R, Loria F, Terzi MI, Vallebona A (1993) Hydatid cyst of the interventricular septum of the heart: MR findings. Am J Roentgenol 161:753–754

Carlini ME, White AC Jr, Atmar RL (1999) Vivax malaria complicated by adult respiratory distress syndrome. Clin Infect Dis 28:1182–1183

Cayea PD, Rubin E, Teixidor HS (1981) Atypical pulmonary malaria. Am J Roentgenol 137:51–55

Charoenratanakul S (1997) Tropical infection and the lung. Monaldi Arch Chest Dis 52(4):376–379

Chitkara RK, Krishna G (2006) Parasitic pulmonary eosinophilia. Semin Respir Crit Care Med 27(2):171–184

Chitkara RK, Sarinas PS (1997) Dirofilaria, visceral larva migrans, and tropical pulmonary eosinophilia. Semin Respir Infect 12:138–148

Chitsulo L, Engels D, Montresor A, Savioli L (2000) The global status of schistosomiasis and its control. Acta Trop 77:41–51

Chu E, Whitlock WL, Dietrich RA (1990) Pulmonary hyperinfection syndrome with *Strongyloides stercoralis*. Chest 97:1475–1477

Cook GA, Rodriguez H, Silva H, Rodriguez-Iturbe B, Bohorquez de Rodriguez H (1987) Adult respiratory distress secondary to strongyloidiasis. Chest 92:1115–1116

Cooke GS, Lalvani A, Gleeson FV, Conlon CP (1999) Acute pulmonary schistosomiasis in travelers returning from Lake Malawi, sub-Saharan Africa. Clin Infect Dis 29:836–839

Cosgriff TM (1990) Pulmonary edema in falciparum malaria. Slaying the dragon of volume overload. Chest 98:10–12

Cottin V, Cordier J-F (2005) Eosinophilic pneumonias. Allergy 60:841–857

Crompton DW (2001) Ascaris and ascariasis. Adv Parasitol 48:285–375

Crowe SM, Carlin JB, Stewart KI, Lucas CR, Hoy JF (1991) Predictive value of CD4 lymphocyte numbers for the development of opportunistic infections and malignancies in HIV-infected persons. J Acquir Immune Defic Syndr 4:770–776

Curlin ME, Barat LM, Walsh DK, Granger DL (1999) Noncardiogenic pulmonary edema during vivax malaria. Clin Infect Dis 28:1166–1167

Dahniya MH, Hanna RM, Ashebu S, et al. (2001) The imaging appearances of hydatid disease at some unusual sites. Br J Radiol 74:283–289

D'Alessandro A (1997) Polycystic echinococcosis in tropical America: Echinococcus vogeli and E. oligarthrus. Acta Trop 67:43–65

D'Alessandro A, Rausch RL, Cuello C, Aristizabal N (1979) Echinococcus vogeli in man, with a review of polycystic hydatid disease in Colombia and neighboring countries. Am J Trop Med Hyg 28:303–317

D'Alessandro A, Ramirez LE, Chapadeiro E, Lopes ER, de Mesquita PM (1995) Second recorded case of human infection by Echinococcus oligarthrus. Am J Trop Med Hyg 52:29–33

Davidson AC, Bateman C, Shovlin C, Marrinan M, Burton GH, Cameron IR (1988) Pulmonary toxicity of malaria prophylaxis. BMJ 297:1240–1241

Davidson RA (1992) Infection due to Strongyloides stercoralis in patients with pulmonary disease. South Med J 85:28–31

Dent JH, Nichols RL, Beaver PC, Carrera GM, Staggers RJ (1956) Visceral larva migrans; with a case report. Am J Pathol 32:777–803

Duffield JS, Jacob AJ, Miller HC (1996) Recurrent, life-threatening atrioventricular dissociation associated with toxoplasma myocarditis. Heart 76:453–454

El Mallah SH, Hashem M (1953) Localized bilharzial granuloma of the lung simulating a tumour. Thorax 8:148–151

Etievent JP, Vuitton D, Allemand H, Weill F, Gandjbakhch I, Miguet JP (1986) Pulmonary embolism from a parasitic cardiac clot secondary to hepatic alveolar echinococcosis. J Cardiovasc Surg (Torino) 27:671–674

Fatureto MC, Correia D, Silva MB, et al. (2003) [Pulmonary schistosoma nodule simulating neoplasia: case report]. Rev Soc Bras Med Trop 36:735–737

Feldman GJ, Parker HW (1992) Visceral larva migrans associated with the hypereosinophilic syndrome and the onset of severe asthma. Ann Intern Med 116:838–840

Fishman AP (1998) Fishman's pulmonary diseases and disorders. McGraw-Hill, New York

Fishman AP, Elias JA, Fishman JA, Grippi MA, Kaiser LR, Senior MR (1998) Fishman's pulmonary diseases and disorders, 3rd edn. McGraw-Hill, New York

Ford J, Reiss-Levy E, Clark E, Dyson AJ, Schonell M (1981) Pulmonary strongyloidiasis and lung abscess. Chest 79:239–240

Franquet T, Plaza V, Llauger J, Gimenez A, Bordes R (1999) Hydatid pulmonary embolism from a ruptured mediastinal cyst: high-resolution computed tomography, angiographic, and pathologic findings. J Thorac Imaging 14:138–141

Froes HP (1930) Identification of a nematode larvae in the exudate of a sero-haemorrhagic pleural effusion. J Trop Med Hyg 33:18–19

Gachot B, Wolff M, Nissack G, Veber B, Vachon F (1995) Acute lung injury complicating imported *Plasmodium falciparum* malaria. Chest 108:746–749

Goodman PC, Schnapp LM (1992) Pulmonary toxoplasmosis in AIDS. Radiology 184:791–793

Gottstein B, Reichen J (2002) Hydatid lung disease (echinococcosis/hydatidosis). Clin Chest Med 23:397–408, ix

Gouliamos AD, Kalovidouris A, Papailiou J, Vlahos L, Papavasiliou C (1991) CT appearance of pulmonary hydatid disease. Chest 100:1578–1581

Guardia SN, Sepp H, Scholten M, Morava-Protzner I (1991) Pentastomiasis in Canada. Arch Pathol Lab Med 115(5):515–517

Hagar JM, Rahimtoola SH (1991) Chagas' heart disease in the United States. N Engl J Med 325:763–768

Hasleton PS (ed) (1996) Spencer's pathology of the lung. Mc Graw-Hill, New York

Hofman P, Bernard E, Michiels JF, Thyss A, Le Fichoux Y, Loubiere R (1993a) Extracerebral toxoplasmosis in the acquired immunodeficiency syndrome (AIDS). Pathol Res Pract 189:894–901

Hofman P, Drici MD, Gibelin P, Michiels JF, Thyss A (1993b) Prevalence of toxoplasma myocarditis in patients with the acquired immunodeficiency syndrome. Br Heart J 70:376–381

Holliman RE (1988) Toxoplasmosis and the acquired immune deficiency syndrome. J Infect 16:121–128

Horton RJ (1989) Chemotherapy of *Echinococcus* infection in man with albendazole. Trans R Soc Trop Med Hyg 83:97–102

Hotez PJ, Pritchard DI (1995) Hookworm infection. Sci Am 272:68–74

Ibarra-Perez C et al. (1981) Thoracic complications of amebic abscess of the liver: report of 501 cases. Chest 79:672–677

Im JG, Whang HY, Kim WS, Han MC, Shim YS, Cho SY (1992) Pleuropulmonary paragonimiasis: radiologic findings in 71 patients. Am J Roentgenol 159:39–43

Im JG, Kong Y, Shin YM, et al. (1993) Pulmonary paragonimiasis: clinical and experimental studies. Radiographics 13:575–586

Im JG, Chang KH, Reeder MM (1997) Current diagnostic imaging of pulmonary and cerebral paragonimiasis, with pathological correlation. Semin Roentgenol 32:301–324

Inoue K, Inoue Y, Arai T, et al. (2002) Chronic eosinophilic pneumonia due to visceral larva migrans. Intern Med 41:478–482

Ishi H, Mukae H, Inone Y, Kadota J, Kohno S, Vchiyama F, Nawa Y (2001) A rare case of eosinophilic pleuritis due to sparganosis. Intern Med 40(8):783–785

Iwatani K, Kubota I, Hirotsu Y, Wakimoto J, Yoshioka M, Mori T, Ito T, Namori H (2006) Sparganum mansoni parasitic infection in the lung showing a nodule. Pathol Int 56:674–677

Jeong YJ, Kim KI, Seo IJ, et al. (2007) Eosinophilic lung disease: a clinical, radiological, and pathologic overwiew. Radiographics 27:617–639

Jiang C (2002) Two cases of liver alveolar echinococcosis associated with simultaneous lung and brain metastases. Chin Med J (Engl) 115:1898–1901

Johnson RJ, Johnson JR (1983) Paragonimiasis in Indochinese refugees. Roentgenographic findings with clinical correlations. Am Rev Respir Dis 128:534–538

Kabiri EH, El Maslout A, Benosman A (2001) Thoracic rupture of hepatic hydatidosis (123 cases). Ann Thorac Surg 72:1883–1886

Kern P, Bardonnet K, Renner E, et al. (2003) European Echinococcosis Registry: human alveolar echinococcosis, Europe, 1982–2000. Emerg Infect Dis 9:343–349

Kilic D, Tercan F, Sahin E, Bilen A, Hatipoglu A (2006) Unusual radiologic manifestations of the echinococcus infection in the thorax. J Thorac Imaging 21:32–36

Kirchhoff LV, Neva FA (1985) Chagas' disease in Latin American immigrants. JAMA 254:3058–3060

Kochar AS (1985) Human pulmonary dirofilariasis. Report of three cases and brief review of the literature. Am J Clin Pathol 84:19–23

Koul PA, Koul AN, Wahid A, Mir FA (2000) CT in pulmonary hydatid disease: unusual appearances. Chest 118:1645–1647

Kremery V Jr, Gould I, Sobota K, Spanik S (1992) Two cases of disseminated toxocariasis in compromised hosts successfully treated with mebendazole. Chemotherapy 38:367–368

Krysl J, Muller NL, Miller RR, Champion P (1991) Patient with miliary nodules and diarrhea. Can Assoc Radiol J 42:363–366

Kurkcuoglu IC, Eroglu A, Karaoglanoglu N, Polat P (2002a) Tension pneumothorax associated with hydatid cyst rupture. J Thorac Imaging 17:78–80

Kurkcuoglu IC, Eroglu A, Karaoglanoglu N, Polat P (2002b) Complications of albendazole treatment in hydatid disease of lung. Eur J Cardiothorac Surg 22:649–650

Kuznen A (2006) Parasitic diseases of the respiratory tract. Curr Opin Pulm Med 12:212–221

Kuzucu A, Soysal O, Ozgel M, Yologlu S (2004) Complicated hydatid cysts of the lung: clinical and therapeutic issues. Ann Thorac Surg 77:1200–1204

Lahiri K (1993) Parasitic infections of the respiratory tract (diagnosis and management). J Postgrad Med 39:144–148

Lambertucci JR, Rayes AA, Barata CH, Teixeira R, Gerspacher-Lara R (1997) Acute schistosomiasis: report on five singular cases. Mem Inst Oswaldo Cruz 92:631–635

Lambertucci JR, Moreira RF, Barbosa AJ (2005) Solitary pulmonary nodule caused by *Schistosoma mansoni* in a patient with medullary thyroid carcinoma. Rev Soc Bras Med Trop 38:536–537

Landay MJ, Setiawan H, Hirsch G, Christensen EE, Conrad MR (1980) Hepatic and thoracic amoebiasis. Am J Roentgenol 135:449–454

Lavrard I, Chouaid C, Roux P, et al. (1995) Pulmonary toxoplasmosis in HIV-infected patients: usefulness of polymerase chain reaction and cell culture. Eur Respir J 8:697–700

Lee EY, Maguire JH (1999) Acute pulmonary edema complicating ovale malaria. Clin Infect Dis 29:697–698

Lemle A (1999) Chagas' disease. Chest 115:906

Le Roux BT (1969) Pleuro-pulmonary amoebiasis. Thorax 24:91–101

Levinson ED, Ziter FM Jr, Westcott JL (1979) Pulmonary lesions due to *Dirofilaria immitis* (dog heartworm). Report of four cases with radiologic findings. Radiology 131:305–307

Libanore M, Bicocchi R, Sighinolfi L, Ghinelli F (1991) Pneumothorax during pulmonary toxoplasmosis in an AIDS patient. Chest 100:1184

Lopera RD, Melendez RD, Fernandez I, Sirit J, Perera MP (1989) Orbital hydatid cyst of *Echinococcus oligarthrus* in a human in Venezuela. J Parasitol 75:467–470

MacPherson CN, Romig T, Zeyhle E, Rees PH, Were JB (1987) Portable ultrasound scanner versus serology in screening for hydatid cysts in a nomadic population. Lancet 2:259–261

Mahrholdt H, Wagner A, Judd RM, Sechtem U, Kim RJ (2005) Delayed enhancement cardiovascular magnetic resonance assessment of non-ischaemic cardiomyopathies. Eur Heart J 26:1461–1474

Makris AN, Sher S, Bertoli C, Latour MG (1993) Pulmonary strongyloidiasis: an unusual opportunistic pneumonia in a patient with AIDS. Am J Roentgenol 161:545–547

Malouf J, Saksouk FA, Alam S, Rizk GK, Dagher I (1985) Hydatid cyst of the heart: diagnosis by two-dimensional echocardiography and computed tomography. Am Heart J 109:605–607

Mamere AE, Muglia VF, Simao GN, Belucci AD, dos Santos AC, Trad CS, Takayanagui OM (2004) Disseminated cysticercosis with pulmonary involvement. J Thorac Imaging 19(2):109–111

Mandell GL, Bennett JE, Dolin R (2005) Principles and practice of infectious diseases. Elsevier/Churchill Livingstone, Philadelphia

Marcos FG, Popovsky S, Osorio ML (1969) Hydatid cyst of the mediastinum. Dis Chest 56:160–162

Mariani M, Pagani M, Inserra C, De Servi S (2006) Complete atrioventricular block associated with toxoplasma myocarditis. Europace 8:221–223

Mariuz P, Bosler EM, Luft BJ (1997) Toxoplasma pneumonia. Semin Respir Infect 12:40–43

Martinez S, Restrepo CS, Carrillo JA, et al. (2005) Thoracic manifestations of tropical parasitic infections: a pictorial review. Radiographics 25:135–155

Maruyama H, Nawa Y, Noda S, Mimori T, Choi WY (1996) An outbreak of visceral larva migrans due to *Ascaris suum* in Kyushu, Japan. Lancet 347:1766–1767

Mendelson MH, Finkel LJ, Meyers BR, Lieberman JP, Hirschman SZ (1987) Pulmonary toxoplasmosis in AIDS. Scand J Infect Dis 19:703–706

Meneghelli UG, Barbo ML, Magro JE, Bellucci AD, Llorach Velludo MA (1986) Polycystic hydatid disease (*Echinococcus vogeli*): clinical and radiological manifestations and treatment with albendazole of a patient from the Brazilian Amazon region. Arq Gastroenterol 23:177–183

Meneghelli UG, Martinelli AL, Llorach Velludo MA, Bellucci AD, Magro JE, Barbo ML (1992a) Polycystic hydatid disease (*Echinococcus vogeli*). Clinical, laboratory and morphological findings in nine Brazilian patients. J Hepatol 14:203–210

Meneghelli UG, Martinelli AL, Bellucci AD, Villanova MG, Velludo MA, Magro JE (1992b) Polycystic hydatid disease (*Echinococcus vogeli*). Treatment with albendazole. Ann Trop Med Parasitol 86:151–156

Miralles A, Bracamonte L, Pavie A, et al. (1994) Cardiac echinococcosis. Surgical treatment and results. J Thorac Cardiovasc Surg 107:184–190

Moore W, Franceschi D (2005) PET findings in pulmonary dirofilariasis. J Thorac Imaging 20(4):305–306

Morar R, Feldman C (2003) Pulmonary echinococcosis. Eur Respir J 21:1069–1077

Morris DL, Dykes PW, Marriner S, et al. (1985) Albendazole – objective evidence of response in human hydatid disease. JAMA 253:2053–2057

Morris W, Knauer CM (1997) Cardiopulmonary manifestations of schistosomiasis. Semin Respir Infect 12:159–170

Mukae H, Taniguchi H, Matsumoto N, et al. (2001) Clinicoradiologic features of pleuropulmonary Paragonimus westermani on Kyushu Island, Japan. Chest 120:514–520

Munteis E, Mellibovsky L, Marquez MA, Minguez S, Vazquez E, Diez A (1997) Pulmonary involvement in a case of *Plasmodium vivax* malaria. Chest 111:834–835

Murray PR, Rosenthal KS, Kobayashi GS, Pfaller M (2002) Medical microbiology,4 th edn. Mosby, St. Louis, MO

Murray PR, Rosenthal KS, Pfaller M (2005) Medical microbiology. St. Louis, MO

Nadir A, Kaptanoglu M, Cosar D, Sahin E (2005) Pulmonary hydatid cysts: report of six uncommon cases. Turk Respir J 6:109–112

Nakamura-Uchiyama F, Mukae H, Nawa Y (2002) Paragonimiasis: a Japanese perspective. Clin Chest Med 23:409–420

Nash TE, Cheever AW, Ottesen EA, Cook JA (1982) Schistosome infections in humans: perspectives and recent findings. NIH conference. Ann Intern Med 97:740–754

Nawa Y, Maruyama H, Ogata K (1997) Current status of gnasthostomiasis doloresi in Miyazaki Prefecture, Japan. Southeast Asian J Trap Med Public Health 28 [Suppl 1]:11–13

Nguyen LQ, Estrella J, Jett EA, Grunvald EL, Nicholson L, Levin DL (2006) Acute schistosomiasis in nonimmune travelers: chest CT findings in 10 patients. Am J Roentgenol 186:1300–1303

Odev K, Acikgozoglu S, Gormus N, Aribas OK, Kiresi DA, Solak H (2002) Pulmonary embolism due to cardiac hydatid disease: imaging findings of unusual complication of hydatid cyst. Eur Radiol 12:627–633

Oguzkaya F, Akcali Y, Kahraman C, Emirogullari N, Bilgin M, Sahin A (1997) Unusually located hydatid cysts: intrathoracic but extrapulmonary. Ann Thorac Surg 64:334–337

Oksenhendler E, Cadranel J, Sarfati C, et al. (1990) *Toxoplasma gondii* pneumonia in patients with the acquired immunodeficiency syndrome. Am J Med 88:18N–21N

Ozdemir N, Akal M, Kutlay H, Yavuzer S (1994) Chest wall echinococcosis. Chest 105:1277–1279

Pagan Saez H (1985) Schistosoma mansoni: its radiographic manifestations. Presented at the International Congress of Radiology, Brussels 1981. Bol Asoc Med P R 77:195–201

Pedrosa I, Saiz A, Arrazola J, Ferreiros J, Pedrosa CS (2000) Hydatid disease: radiologic and pathologic features and complications. Radiographics 20:795–817

Phillips JF, Cockrill H, Jorge E, Steiner R (1975) Radiographic evaluation of patients with schistosomiasis. Radiology 114:31–37

Phills JA, Harrold AJ, Whiteman GV, Perelmutter L (1972) Pulmonary infiltrates, asthma and eosinophilia due to *Ascaris suum* infestation in man. N Engl J Med 286:965–970

Polat P, Kantarci M, Alper F, Suma S, Koruyucu MB, Okur A (2003) Hydatid disease from head to toe. Radiographics 23:475–494; quiz 536–477

Pomeroy C, Filice GA (1992) Pulmonary toxoplasmosis: a review. Clin Infect Dis 14:863–870

Prata A (1994) Chagas' disease. Infect Dis Clin North Am 8:61–76

Prijyanonda B, Pradatsundarasar A, Viranuvatti V (1955) Pulmonary gnathostomiasis: a case report. Ann Trop Med Parasitol 49(2):121–122

Proffitt RD, Walton BC (1962) *Ascaris* pneumonia in a two-year-old girl. Diagnosis by gastric aspirate. N Engl J Med 266:931–934

Qian ZX (1988) Thoracic hydatid cysts: a report of 842 cases treated over a thirty-year period. Ann Thorac Surg 46:342–346

Rabaud C, May T, Lucet JC, Leport C, Ambroise-Thomas P, Canton P (1996) Pulmonary toxoplasmosis in patients infected with human immunodeficiency virus: a French National Survey. Clin Infect Dis 23:1249–1254

Ramos L, Hernandez-Mora M, Illanas M, Llorente MT, Marcos J (1975) Radiological characteristics of perforated pulmonary hydatid cysts. Radiology 116:539–542

Ravdin JI (1988) Amebiasis: human infection by *Entamoeba histolytica*. Wiley, New York

Reeder MM, Palmer PE (1980) Acute tropical pneumonias. Semin Roentgenol 15:35–49

Reittner P, Szolar DH, Schmid M (1996) Case report. Systemic manifestation of *Echinococcus alveolaris* infection. J Comput Assist Tomogr 20:1030–1032

Reuter S, Seitz HM, Kern P, Junghanss T (2000) Extrahepatic alveolar echinococcosis without liver involvement: a rare manifestation. Infection 28:187–192

Reuter S, Jensen B, Buttenschoen K, Kratzer W, Kern P (2000) Benzimidazoles in the treatment of alveolar echinococcosis: a comparative study and review of the literature. J Antimicrob Chemother 46:451–456

Richert JH, Krakaur RB (1959) Diffuse pulmonary schistosomiasis; report of two cases proved by lung biopsy. J Am Med Assoc 169:1302–1306

Rochitte CE, Oliveira PF, Andrade JM, et al. (2005) Myocardial delayed enhancement by magnetic resonance imaging in patients with Chagas' disease: a marker of disease severity. J Am Coll Cardiol 46:1553–1558

Rodrigues-Silva R, Peixoto JR, de Oliveira RM, MagalhaesPinto R, Gomes DC (2002) An autochthonous case of *Echinococcus vogeli* Rausch & Bernstein, 1972 polycystic echinococcosis in the state of Rondonia, Brazil. Mem Inst Oswaldo Cruz 97:123–126

Roig J, Romeu J, Riera C, Texido A, Domingo C, Morera J (1992) Acute eosinophilic pneumonia due to toxocariasis with bronchoalveolar lavage findings. Chest 102:294–296

Roldan EO, Moskowitz L, Hensley GT (1987) Pathology of the heart in acquired immunodeficiency syndrome. Arch Pathol Lab Med 111:943–946

Roy BT, Chirurgi VA, Theis JH (1993) Pulmonary dirofilariasis in California. West J Med 158:74–76

Sahasrabudhe NS, Jadhav MV, Deshmukh SD, Holla VV (2003) Pathology of Toxoplasma myocarditis in acquired immunodeficiency syndrome. Indian J Pathol Microbiol 46:649–651

Sahin E, Kaptanoglu M, Nadir A, Ceran C (2006) [Traumatic rupture of a pulmonary hydatid cyst: a case report]. Ulus Travma Acil Cerrahi Derg 12:71–75

Sakai S, Shida Y, Takahashi N, et al. (2006) Pulmonary lesions associated with visceral larva migrans due to *Ascaris suum* or *Toxocara canis*: imaging of six cases. Am J Roentgenol 186:1697–1702

Sakakibara A, Baba K, Niwa S, et al. (2002) Visceral larva migrans due to *Ascaris suum* which presented with eosinophilic pneumonia and multiple intra-hepatic lesions with severe eosinophil infiltration – outbreak in a Japanese area other than Kyushu. Intern Med 41:574–579

Saksouk FA, Fahl MH, Rizk GK (1986) Computed tomography of pulmonary hydatid disease. J Comput Assist Tomogr 10:226–232

Salinas-Lopez N, Jimenez-Guzman F, Cruz-Reyes A (1996) Presence of Echinococcus oligarthrus (Diesing, 1863) Luhe, 1910 in Lynx rufus texensis Allen, 1895 from San Fernando, Tamaulipas state, in north-east Mexico. Int J Parasitol 26:793–796

Sane AC, Barber BA (1997) Pulmonary nodules due to *Toxocara canis* infection in an immunocompetent adult. South Med J 90:78–79

Sarinas PS, Chitkara RK (1997) Ascariasis and hookworm. Semin Respir Infect 12:130–137

Savani DM, Sharna OP (2002) Eosinophilic lung disease in the tropics. Clin Chest Med 23:377–396

Schaberg T, Rahn W, Racz P, Lode H (1991) Pulmonary schistosomiasis resembling acute pulmonary tuberculosis. Eur Respir J 4:1023–1026

Schnapp LM, Geaghan SM, Campagna A, et al. (1992) *Toxoplasma gondii* pneumonitis in patients infected with the human immunodeficiency virus. Arch Intern Med 152:1073–1077

Schwartz E (2002) Pulmonary schistosomiasis. Clin Chest Med 23:433–443

Schwartz E, Rozenman J, Perelman M (2000) Pulmonary manifestations of early schistosome infection among nonimmune travelers. Am J Med 109:718–722

Senturk H, Mert A, Ersavasti G, Tabak F, Akdogan M, Ulualp K (1998) Bronchobiliary fistula due to alveolar hydatid disease: report of three cases. Am J Gastroenterol 93:2248–2253

Shah MK (1999) Human pulmonary dirofilariasis: review of the literature. South Med J 92:276–279

Shambesh MA, Craig PS, Macpherson CN, Rogan MT, Gusbi AM, Echtuish EF (1999) An extensive ultrasound and serologic study to investigate the prevalence of human cystic echinococcosis in northern Libya. Am J Trop Med Hyg 60:462–468

Shamsuzzaman SM, Hashiguchi Y (2002) Thoracic amebiasis. Clin Chest Med 23:479–492

Sharma OP (1989) The man who loved drunken crabs. A case of pulmonary paragonimiasis. Chest 95:670–672

Simpson WG, Gerhardstein DC, Thompson JR (1993) Disseminated *Strongyloides stercoralis* infection. South Med J 86:821–825

Slim MS, Khayat G, Nasr AT, Jidejian YD (1971) Hydatid disease in childhood. J Pediatr Surg 6:440–448

Snyder CH (1961) Visceral larva migrans. Ten years' experience. Pediatrics 23:85–91

Society for Cardiovascular Magnetic Resonance (2003) Abstracts of the Society for Cardiovascular Magnetic Resonance 6th Annual Scientific Sessions. Lake Buena Vista, Florida, USA. February 7–9, 2003. J Cardiovasc Magn Reson 5:1–313

Spillmann R (1975) Pulmonary ascariasis in tropical communities. Am J Trop Med Hyg 24:791–800

Suwanik R, Harinsuta C (1959) Pulmonary paragonimiasis; an evaluation of roentgen findings in 38 positive sputum patients in an endemic area in Thailand. Am J Roentgenol Radium Ther Nucl Med 81:236–244

Tanios MA, Kogelman L, McGovern B, Hassoun PM (2001) Acute respiratory distress syndrome complicating *Plasmodium vivax* malaria. Crit Care Med 29:665–667

Tawney S, Masci J, Berger HW, Subietas A (1986) Pulmonary toxoplasmosis: an unusual nodular radiographic pattern in a patient with AIDS. Mt Sinai J Med 53:683–685

Taylor DH, Morris DL, Reffin D, Richards KS (1989) Comparison of albendazole, mebendazole and praziquantel chemotherapy of *Echinococcus multilocularis* in a gerbil model. Gut 30:1401–1405

Taylor WR, White NJ (2002) Malaria and the lung. Clin Chest Med 23:457–468

Teggi A, Lastilla MG, De Rosa F (1993) Therapy of human hydatid disease with mebendazole and albendazole. Antimicrob Agents Chemother 37:1679–1684

Tercan F, Kacar N, Kilic D, Oguzkurt L, Turkoz R, Habesoglu MA (2005) Hydatid cysts of the bilateral pulmonary arteries and left ventricle wall: computed tomography and magnetic resonance imaging findings. J Comput Assist Tomogr 29:31–33

Tizes R, Zaki MH, Minkowitz S (1967) Pulmonary schistosomiasis. Report of a case found with a solitary lesion. Am J Trop Med Hyg 16:595–598

Torres JR, Perez H, Postigo MM, Silva JR (1997) Acute noncardiogenic lung injury in benign tertian malaria. Lancet 350:31–32

Travis WD, Colby TV, Koss MN, Rosado-de-Christenson ML, Müller NL, King TE Jr (2002) Non-neoplastic disorders of the lower respiratory tract. Armed Forces Institute of Pathology, Washington, DC

Treugut H, Schulze K, Hubener KH, Andrasch R (1980) Pulmonary involvement by *Echinococcus alveolaris*. Radiology 137:37–41

Tuzun M, Hekimoglu B (2001) Pictorial essay. Various locations of cystic and alveolar hydatid disease: CT appearances. J Comput Assist Tomogr 25:81–87

Umezawa ES, Stolf AM, Corbett CE, Shikanai-Yasuda MA (2001) Chagas' disease. Lancet 357:797–799

Van Knapen F, Buijs J, Kortbeek LM, Ljungstrom I (1992) Larva migrans syndrome: *toxocara, ascaris*, or both? Lancet 340:550–551

Velez ID, Ortega JE, Velasquez LE (2002) Paragonimiasis: a view from Columbia. Clin Chest Med 23:421–431, ix–x

Von Sinner W (1990a) Pleural complications of hydatid disease (*Echinococcus granulosus*). Rofo 152:718–722

Von Sinner W (1990b) Successful treatment of disseminated hydatid disease using albendazole monitored by CT. Eur J Radiol 11:232–233

Von Sinner W, te Strake L, Clark D, Sharif H (1991) MR imaging in hydatid disease. Am J Roentgenol 157:741–745

Von Sinner WN, Rifai A, te Strake L, Sieck J (1990) Magnetic resonance imaging of thoracic hydatid disease. Correlation with clinical findings, radiography, ultrasonography, CT and pathology. Acta Radiol 31:59–62

Vuitton DA, Zhou H, Bresson-Hadni S, et al. (2003) Epidemiology of alveolar echinococcosis with particular reference to China and Europe. Parasitology 127 [Suppl]:S87–S107

Waldman AD, Day JH, Shaw P, Bryceson AD (2001) Subacute pulmonary granulomatous schistosomiasis: high resolution CT appearances – another cause of the halo sign. Br J Radiol 74:1052–1055

Wallace GD (1973) The role of the cat in the natural history of *Toxoplasma gondii*. Am J Trop Med Hyg 22:313–322

Wilson JF, Rausch RL, McMahon BJ, Schantz PM (1992) Parasiticidal effect of chemotherapy in alveolar hydatid disease: review of experience with mebendazole and albendazole in Alaskan Eskimos. Clin Infect Dis 15:234–249

Wilson JF, Rausch RL, Wilson FR (1995) Alveolar hydatid disease. Review of the surgical experience in 42 cases of active disease among Alaskan Eskimos. Ann Surg 221:315–323

Wolach B, Sinnreich Z, Uziel Y, Gotesman G, Pomerantz A (1995) Toxocariasis: a diagnostic dilemma. Isr J Med Sci 31:689–692

Woodring JH, Halfhill H 2nd, Reed JC (1994) Pulmonary strongyloidiasis: clinical and imaging features. Am J Roentgenol 162:537–542

World Health Organization (1997) Amoebiasis. Wkly Epidemiol Rec 72:97–99

World Health Organization (1999) Chagas disease, Venezuela, 1999. Wkly Epidemiol Rec 74:290–292

World Health Organization (2000a) Management of severe malaria: a practical handbook. World Health Organization, Geneva

World Health Organization (2000b) Chagas disease, Chile. Wkly Epidemiol Rec 75:10–12

World Health Organization (2000c) Chagas disease, Brazil. Wkly Epidemiol Rec 75:153–155

World Health Organization (2002) Prevention and control of schistosomiasis and soil-transmitted helminthiasis. World Health Organ Tech Rep Ser 912:i–vi, 1–57, back cover

World Health Organization (2005) World Malaria Report 2005. World Health Organization

World Health Organization (2006) Schistosomiasis and soil-transmitted helminth infections – preliminary estimates of the number of children treated with albendazole or mebendazole. Wkly Epidemiol Rec 81:145–163

Yassin MA, Errayes MM, Khan FY, Elbozon EA, Ellahi AY (2007) Can worms cause chest pain? Saudi Med J 28(1):142–143

Zidi A, Zannad-Hantous S, Mestiri I, Ghrairi H, Baccouche I, Djilani H, Ben Miled Mrad K (2006) Hydatid cyst of the mediastinum: a report of 14 cases. J Radiol 87:1869–1874

Zumla AI, James DG (2002) Immunologic aspects of tropical lung disease. Clin Chest Med 23:283–308, vii

Chapter

Imaging of Parasitic Diseases of the Gastrointestinal Tract

4

Mohamed E. Abd El Bagi

Contents

4.1 Introduction

There is increasing public concern (Gittleman 2001) and an increase in the worldwide prevalence of gastrointestinal parasites (GIP) due to bidirectional transcontinental traveling. Some may harbor parasites within their bodies and thereby spread the disease to new habitats. Others may acquire parasitic disease when they visit endemic areas for the first time. GIP are the most prevalent of all parasites. They cause significant morbidity and mortality leading to a high global impact of disability-adjusted life years. The objective of this chapter is to summarize the main epidemiological, clinical and radiological features of the commonest GIP.

Human parasites are not a thing of the past. In addition to the factors described above, the importation of GIP with refugees (Barnett 2004), their world wide re-emergence (Macpherson 2005), and the question of their association with malignancy (Robinson and Ketongole-Mbidde 2006) are also matters of concern. As transcontinental travel becomes excessive, it is feared that organisms of lower evolutionary potential may gain greater evolutionary advantages from migration and the subsequent change in habitat and climate (Morgan 2007).

The gastrointestinal tract (GIT) has a triple relation with parasites that may affect man. It is the entrance gate into the body for most human parasites. Thereafter, it becomes the reservoir for transformation, growth, and multiplication of the vast majority of parasites. Finally, the GIT is the factory outlet for expulsion of ova, trophozoites, cysts, and adult worms and their offspring into the environment to become a source of contamination through water, food stuffs or direct human contact (Box 4.1).

Like all organisms, parasites are classified by the international code of Zoological Nomenclature according to their morphology and genetic structure (Zaman and Keong 1990). Each parasite is thereby binomial, with the name of the genus beginning with an upper case letter and the name of the species in starting with a lower case letter, e.g., *Entamoeba histolytica*.

Reproduction of GIP is variable. Most cestodes (tapeworms) are hermaphrodites with each segment of the parasite containing a set of male and female reproductive organs. The group of unicellular protozoa, like amoeba and malaria, may reproduce asexually by simple binary fission (amoeba), schizogony where the nucleus divides into multiple daughters (malaria), or endodyogeny by internal budding from the nucleus (toxoplasmosis). Sexual reproduction occurs where there is conjugation with or without an increase in number (Zaman and Keong 1990).

One interesting feature of human parasites is their adaptation to undergo profound morphologic changes. This is seen more frequently in obligate parasites that live only in the host. Moreover, some facultative parasites that can live either in the host or independently are on the road to obligate parasitism (Markell et al. 1992). The simultaneous transcontinental migration of parasites within a human host from one habitat to another can dramatically affect the host interaction (Poulin 2006).

The lifecycle of parasites may be simple, involving a single host or complex involving two or more hosts (primary host, secondary host, and intermediate host). The objective of learning about the lifecycle is to find out which is the invasive stage that causes morbidity and at which stage can the diagnosis be made using available clinical, laboratory or imaging techniques (Box 4.2).

Box 4.1 What is the relation between GIT and human parasites?

1. Main entrance gate
2. Multiplication reservoir
3. Factory outlet for spread

Box 4.2 What should you learn from the lifecycle?

1. The infective stage
2. The stage amenable to diagnosis

The routes of transmission of parasites into the human body include:

1. Ingestion
2. Skin penetration
3. Mucus membrane penetration
4. Venereal transmission
5. Congenital transmission
6. Blood transfusion
7. Organ transplantation

Parasites that can infect the human GIT are innumerable. Medical schools' curricula are under an ever-increasing pressure of time constraints. Allocated time to study GIP is limited, particularly in Western countries.

This chapter is not an exhaustive census, but a representation of the imaging features of common GIP. The main objective of this text is to highlight how radiology and imaging can contribute to the diagnosis and management of GIP (Martinez et al. 2005; Abd El Bagi et al. 2004; Sammak et al. 1999).

4.2 History of GIP

Gastrointestinal parasites have been known since ancient Egyptian civilization (3000–400BC) and are particularly documented in the papyri of Thebes (1500BC). They were also documented by the Greek's Aristotle (384–322BC), Hippocrates (460–375BC), and Galen (129–200AD), and in the Chinese writings of the second and third century.

The best historical summary was provided by Abu Bakr Rhazes (850–923) and thereafter by Avicenna (981–1037). Patrick Manson (1898) coined the term Tropical Medicine and incriminated vectors in parasite transmission (Reeder and Palmer 1994). Proper helminthology took off in the 17th and 18th century after the germ theory of Louis Pasteur, who demolished the concept of spontaneous generation. Robert Koch, as early as those times, introduced methods of preventing disease caused by microorganisms.

At this moment in time, parasitology was not left out of the recent information explosion that has characterized all sciences. It is now possible to identify subspecies of various protozoa by recombinant DNA analysis of materials taken from their vectors (Markell et al. 1992).

4.3 Prevalence of GIP

A quarter of the world's population is at risk of harboring parasites (Table 4.1) (Reeder and Palmer 1994). GIP are the commonest parasites that affect human beings. The prevalence of GIP is an index for collective ill health (Table. 4.2) (World Bank 1993). It is inversely proportional to the level of local sanitation and personal hygiene. GIP are common in the tropics and rural areas, but are not exclusive to them. Parasites are not restricted to the tropics or to the poor. Certain parasites are endemic in the temperate climates of Northern Europe. Peculiarly, parasites are rare in nomadics due to interrupted contact with contaminated soil (World Health Organization 1981).

Western travelers are at risk proportional to their length of stay in the tropics (Nettleman 1996), particularly Western soldiers deployed to under-prescribed communities (Leutscher and Bagley 2003). High-risk sexual practices, and thereby AIDS, have increased the prevalence and severity of GIP (Heyworth 1996; Phillips 1981). Refugees and adoption of foreign children from developing countries into the USA bring along a variety of GIP (Chen et al. 2003a). Global warming can affect the world's biodata and the functioning ecosystems to produce temperature-mediated proliferation and wider distribution of parasites (Poulin 2006). Recent studies have demonstrated that infective cercarial output from snails can dramatically increase with global temperature rise (Poulin and Mouritsen 2006). The overall behavior of human beings has a pivotal role to play in the macro- and microepidemiology of emerging and re-emerging parasitic zoonoses. Changing demographics and the concomitant alterations to the environment converge to favor parasitic spread. Proclivity for eating meat, undercooked fish or pickled food is a contributing factor (Macpherson 2005).

The increasing world population and urbanization are not matched by adequate sanitation. Ironically, certain economic projects intended to promote regional development have brought about disastrous parasitic proliferation (Markell et al. 1992). The best examples are the high dam in Egypt and the Sinnar dam in the Sudan, constant irrigation sources for cotton growing, have led to proliferation of bilharziasis with high mortality and morbidity. Building highways in Brazil was associated with the proliferation of Chagas' disease. There are thus worries about the effect of the new Chinese super dam on the environment.

Eradication of parasites is dependent on the economic and educational status of the community. The question is whether total eradication would disturb the ecology and the natural equilibrium on earth and whether parasites have preceded or succeeded man's descent to earth? The United Nations Millennium Project Quick Impact Initiative, endorsed in 2005, is committed to the control of malaria and neglected tropical diseases, including GIP, in developing countries.

Table 4.1 Prevalence of parasites (WHO 1995)

Parasite		Prevalence
Ascaris	roundworm	>1,000 millions
Plasmodia	malaria	>500
Trichuris	whipworm	>500
Amebiasis	dysentery	250–500
Enterobius vermicularis	pinworm	400
Ancylostoma	hookworm	400
Giardiasis	dysentery	200
Schistosomiasis	bilharzia	200
Filariasis	threadworms	90
Strongyloides	hookworm	80
Taenia	tapeworm	78
Echinococcosis	hydatid	Unknown
Dracunculus	guinea worm	3

Table 4.2 Reported relative incidence of gastrointestinal parasites (GIP)

Group	Percentage	Reference
Ethiopian immigrants	93	Berger et al. (1989)
Hyper endemic areas	Up to 98	Walsh (1986)
Adopted children	9–67	Chen et al. (2003a)
Kampuchean refugees	64	Barnett (2004)
Foreign Corps in Madagascar	42	Leutscher and Bagley (2003)
Immunocompromised patients	32.4	Botero et al. (2003)
World at large	25	Reeder (1998)

4.4 Impact of GIP

Parasites can occur in those who look well. Fortunately, only a few parasites give rise to mortality while the majority would cause a high degree of morbidity, e.g., chronic ill health. Malaria affects 500 million people and kills about 2.3 million annually (Facer and Tanner 1997). Parasites can live for a long time within the human body, e.g., *Ascaris* (1–16 years), *Schistosoma* (up to 30 years), and *Strongyloides* (up to 35 years) (Markell et al. 1992). Commonly, patients present with chronic fatigue syndrome, which leads to high loss of workers' productivity. This is expressed as disability-adjusted life years (DALY; Table 4.3) (World Bank 1993). Recently, the global impact of malaria alone has reached 35 million DALYs (Facer and Tanner1997).

Gastrointestinal parasites are the commonest worldwide cause of GIT blood loss. They can present with massive GIT bleeding (Sangkhathat et al. 2003). The damage caused by parasites has been previously classified as follows (Thomas 1986):

1. Action of the parasite:
   a) Mechanical injury
   b) Production of toxins
   c) Deprivation of nutrients and metabolites
   d) Introduction of pathogenic organisms

2. Reaction of the host:
   a) Tissue reaction, inflammation, granulomas, or fibrosis
   b) Immunologic response
   c) Eosinophilia

The worst scenario is the carcinogenic nature of some parasites (Box 4.3). A recent alarming study reported an incidence of GIP of as much as 28% in proven cancer patients in Uganda (Robinson and Katongole-Mbidde 2006).

Box 4.3 What are the precancerous parasites?

Chagas' disease	Esophageal carcinoma
S. japonicum	Gastric and liver carcinoma
Clonorchiasis	Cholangiocarcinoma
Opisthorchiasis	Cholangiocarcinoma
S. hematobium	Bladder cancer

Table 4.3 Disability-adjusted life years (DALY)

	Market economy countries (%)	Developing countries (%)
Injuries	12.7	14.7
Infections and parasites	4.6	37.7

4.5 Clinical Presentation

There are common symptoms and signs among nearly all GIP including:

Vague symptoms
1. Obscure abdominal pain
2. Loss of appetite
3. Fatiguability and malaise
4. Nausea
5. Vomiting
6. Colics

Childhood symptoms
7. Deterioration at school
8. Disturbed sleep
9. Teeth grinding at night
10. Body or perianal itch
11. Diarrhea and malabsorption
12. Anemia, eosinophilia

High parasite burden
13. Melaena
14. Hematemesis
15. Parasite-orrhea
16. Parasite-emesis

Complications
17. Abscesses
18. Intestinal obstruction/perforation complications
19. Gastric outlet obstruction
20. Hepatitis, cholangitis, jaundice, gallstones
21. Pancreatitis
22. Ectopic manifestations in the chest, brain or musculoskeletal system

A high index of clinical suspicion is necessary to select patients for confirmatory tests for GIP. High-risk groups are now well identified, which makes patient selection for further tests easier (Table 4.4).

Table 4.4 Detection of GIP

Feature	Detection
Vague symptoms	To be picked up by the family physician
Childhood symptoms	To be noticed by parents and school teachers
Complications	Hospital-based diagnosis
Refugees and adopted children	Assumed to harbor GIP, start empirical therapy

4.6 Diagnosis of GIP

Traditionally, microscopic stools examination was the gold standard for diagnosis of GIP (Fig. 4.1). Repetition of the tests over a few days may be necessary. The patient and his family may catch a live worm or proglottids in the stools (Fig. 4.2a–d). At times patient may cough it out, e.g., in the case of ascariasis. The electron microscope has superbly elaborated on the morphology of tiny parasites, particularly the intracellular obligates.

Recently, endoscopy coupled with biopsy has contributed greatly to the diagnosis of parasites and the management of their complications (Fig. 4.3) (El Sheikh 1991).

The frequently encountered radiologic manifestations of common GIP are summarized in (Table 4.5) (Sammak et al. 1999).

4.7 Protozoa

4.7.1 Amebiasis

Four species of amoeba occur in the human being. Some are commensals.

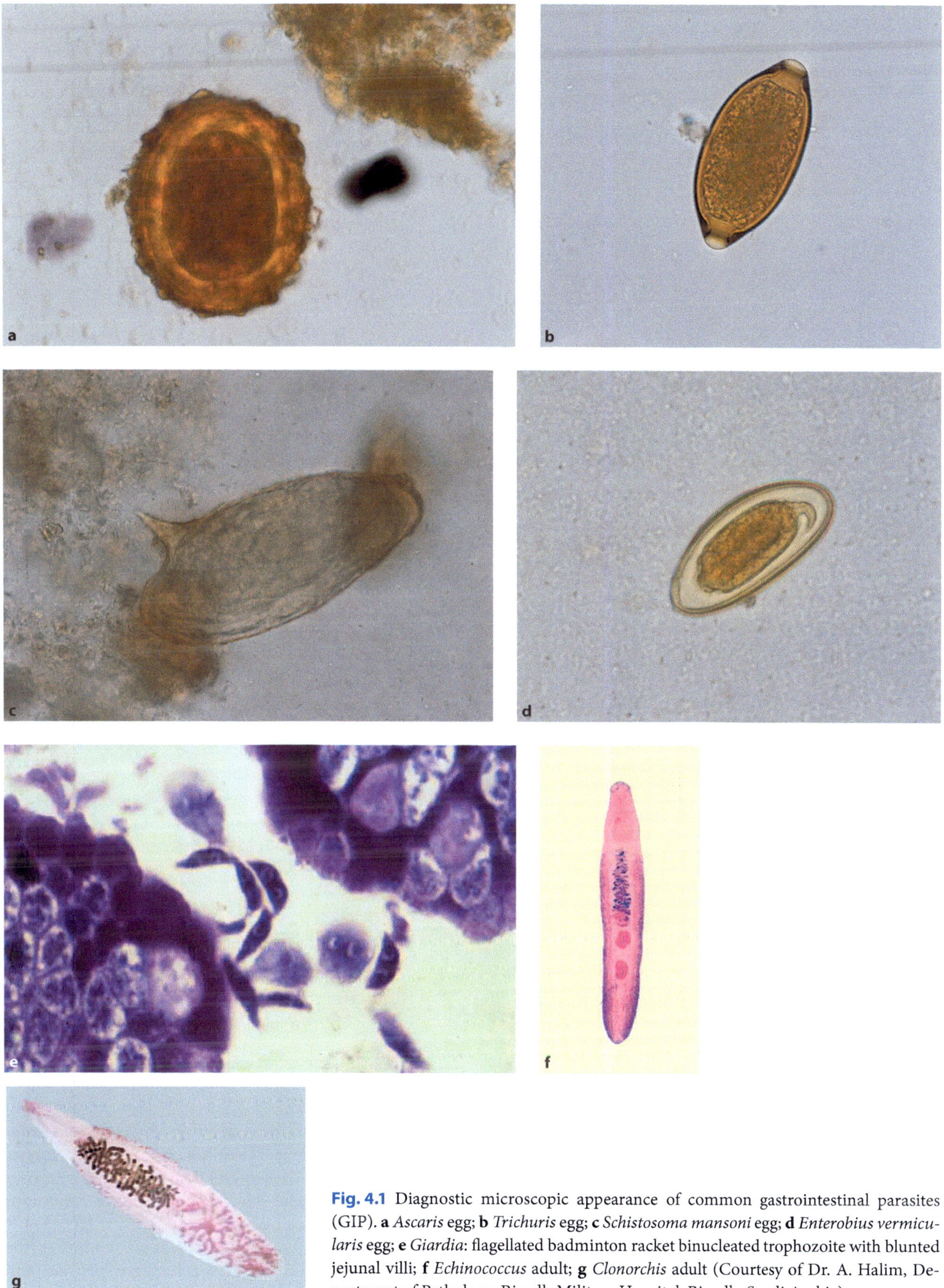

Fig. 4.1 Diagnostic microscopic appearance of common gastrointestinal parasites (GIP). **a** *Ascaris* egg; **b** *Trichuris* egg; **c** *Schistosoma mansoni* egg; **d** *Enterobius vermicularis* egg; **e** *Giardia*: flagellated badminton racket binucleated trophozoite with blunted jejunal villi; **f** *Echinococcus* adult; **g** *Clonorchis* adult (Courtesy of Dr. A. Halim, Department of Pathology, Riyadh Military Hospital, Riyadh, Saudi Arabia)

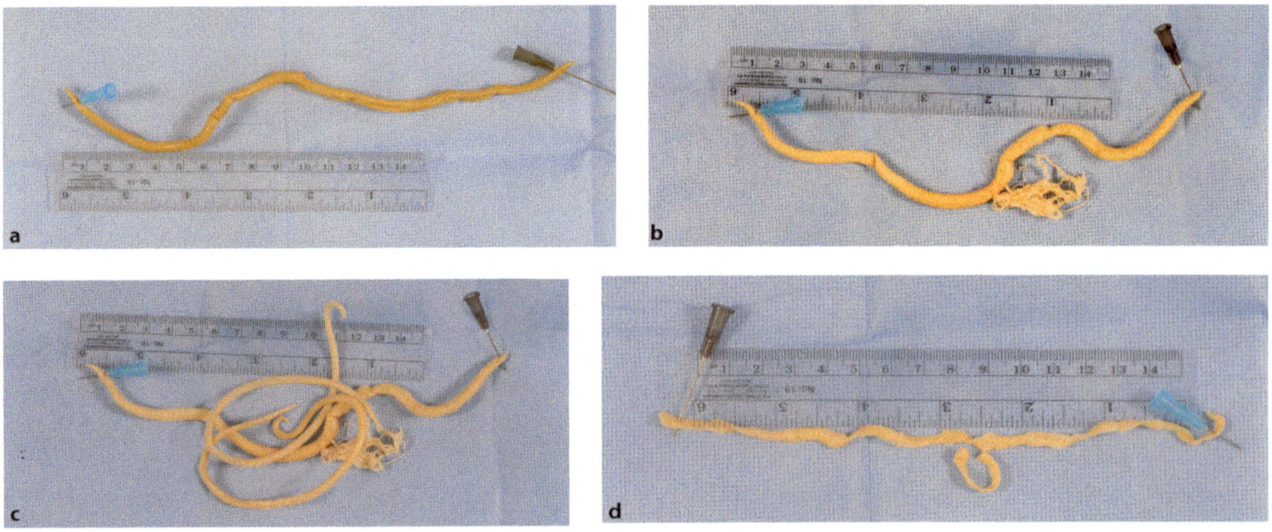

Fig. 4.2 Adult worms caught in stools. **a** Male *Ascaris*; **b** female *Ascaris*; **c** *Ascaris* bolus; **d** part of *Taenia* worm (Courtesy of Dr. A. Saeed, Department of Pathology, Riyadh Military Hospital, Riyadh, Saudi Arabia)

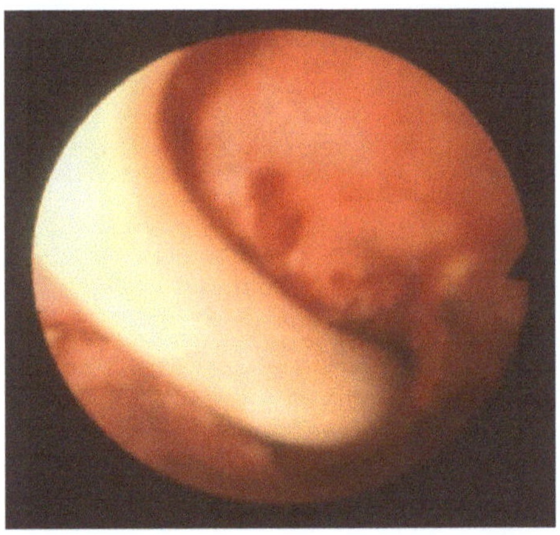

Fig. 4.3 Endoscopic view of *Ascaris lumbricoides* worm sticking out of the duodenal papilla, causing obstruction of the common bile duct and jaundice. This was removed endoscopically (Courtesy of Dr. M. Al Karawi, Department of Gastroenterology, Riyadh Military Hospital, Riyadh, Saudi Arabia)

Table 4.5 Common radiological manifestations of GIP

Manifestation	GIP
Megaesophagus, megacolon	*Trypanosoma cruzi*
Thick duodenojejunal mucosa and nodularity	*Giardia lamblia, Ancylostoma duodenale, Necator Americanus, Capillaria philippinensis, Strongyloides stercoralis*
Stomach strictures	*Anisakis marina*
Terminal ileum edema	*Capillaria philippinensis, Anisakis marina, Angiostrongylus costaricensis*
Ulcerative colitis	Amebiasis, *Strongyloides stercoralis, Trichuris trichiura*
Bowel ischemia	*Angiostrongylus costaricensis*
Linear filling defects	*Ascaris lumbricoides, Taenia saginata, Clonorchis sinensis, Fasciola hepatica, Opisthorchis viverrini*

Entamoeba histolytica is the pathogenic genus that causes colitis and liver abscess in the tropics, while *Entamoeba dispar* may cause infections in men engaging in high-risk sexual practices in developed countries (Katz and Taylor 2001; Li and Stanley 1996). Actually, amebiasis was found to be commoner in homosexuals than tuberculosis or hepatitis (Sargeaunt et al. 1983). Amebiasis is spread widely from pole to pole (Box 4.4). It is the second commonest cause of death from parasite disease after malaria (Kimura et al. 1997). Incidence may reach 50–80% in hyperendemic tropical countries like Mexico and India due to poor housing conditions and personal hygiene (Walsh 1986). In West Africa 60% of the victims are children. In Western countries the disease is rarely seen outside orphanages, prisons, and asylums.

Box 4.4 Amebiasis

1. *E. Histolytica* is the commonest cosmopolitan parasite
2. Causes colitis and liver abscess in the tropics
3. *E. dispar* occurs where there are high-risk sexual practices
4. Active trophozoites erode the intestinal wall
5. Cysts are responsible for transmission

4.7.1.1 Clinical Presentation

1. Asymptomatic with accidental discovery of cysts in stools (80–90%).
2. Symptomatic
   a) Acute dysentery
   b) Fulminant colitis or toxic megacolon
   c) Chronic colitis, appendicitis (the friable appendix)
   d) Colonic mass
   e) Bowel perforation
3. Extraintestinal
   a) Hepatitis
   b) Liver, lung or brain abscess

The characteristic presentation of amoebic dysentery is the very frequent passage of small stools or mucous associated with tenesmus leading to patient exhaustion.

4.7.1.2 Pathogenesis

Trophozoites of the virulent strains of the organism are capable of breaking through the immunological barriers of the intestine to the mucosa by producing necrotizing proteolytic enzymes. The amoeba then settles in the submucosa and erodes the blood vessels to feed on red blood corpuscles, producing flask-shaped ulcers.

The parasite is resistant to ordinary concentrations of chlorine in water. It is recommended that people use calcium hypochlorite or iodine derivatives to purify polluted water.

4.7.1.3 Radiologic Manifestations

1. Bowel distention and bowel wall thickening (Fig. 4.4), and thumb printing
2. Pneumatosis intestinalis (Fig. 4.4c)
3. Toxic megacolon
4. Bowel perforation
5. Chronic ulcers, linear, aphthous or flask-shaped
6. Thickened or conical cecum (Fig. 4.5.e)
7. Normal terminal ileum. This helps to differentiate amoebic colitis from Crohn's disease (Fig. 4.5)
8. Pseudotumor (ameboma) or apple core lesions (Fig. 4.6)
9. Napkin ring appearance
10. Diffuse colitis

Essentially these are either signs of inflammatory bowel disease or of a colonic mass mimicking a tumor or granuloma, particularly in the cecum. Extraintestinal signs and complications are discussed in the relevant chapters. Intestinal infection usually precedes ectopic complications.

The differential diagnosis of intestinal amebiasis includes other causes of inflammatory bowel disease like ulcerative colitis, Crohn's disease, tuberculosis, ischemic colitis or pseudomembranous colitis (Juniper 1962). CT is now replacing conventional techniques for diagnosis of the disease and the detection of extraintestinal complications. Diagnosis of liver abscess is relatively easy with ultrasound. In the acute presuppurative phase it may not be so obvious and can be missed, because it may be slightly hyperechoic or even isoechoic with liver parenchyma; however, in the suppurative phase it becomes hypoechoic and easily detectable (Dairymple 1982). We prefer to drain amoebic abscesses to remove the toxic effect of the denatured liver cells, which dramatically relieves the patient's symptoms (Saraswat et al. 1992). Metronidazole is the treatment of choice, which can serve as a therapeutic test.

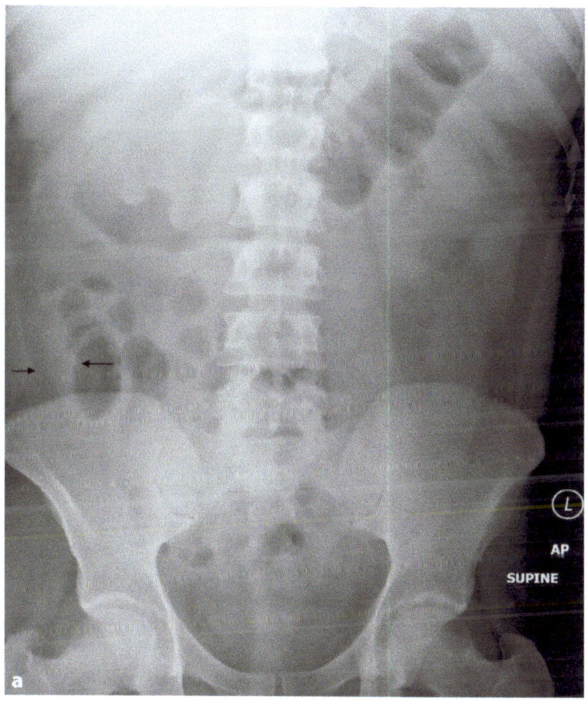

Fig. 4.4 Colonic amebiasis. **a** Plain radiograph of an adult patient with right iliac fossa pain and diarrhea. There is wall thickening (*arrows*) and slight distention of the cecum. **b,c** *see next page*

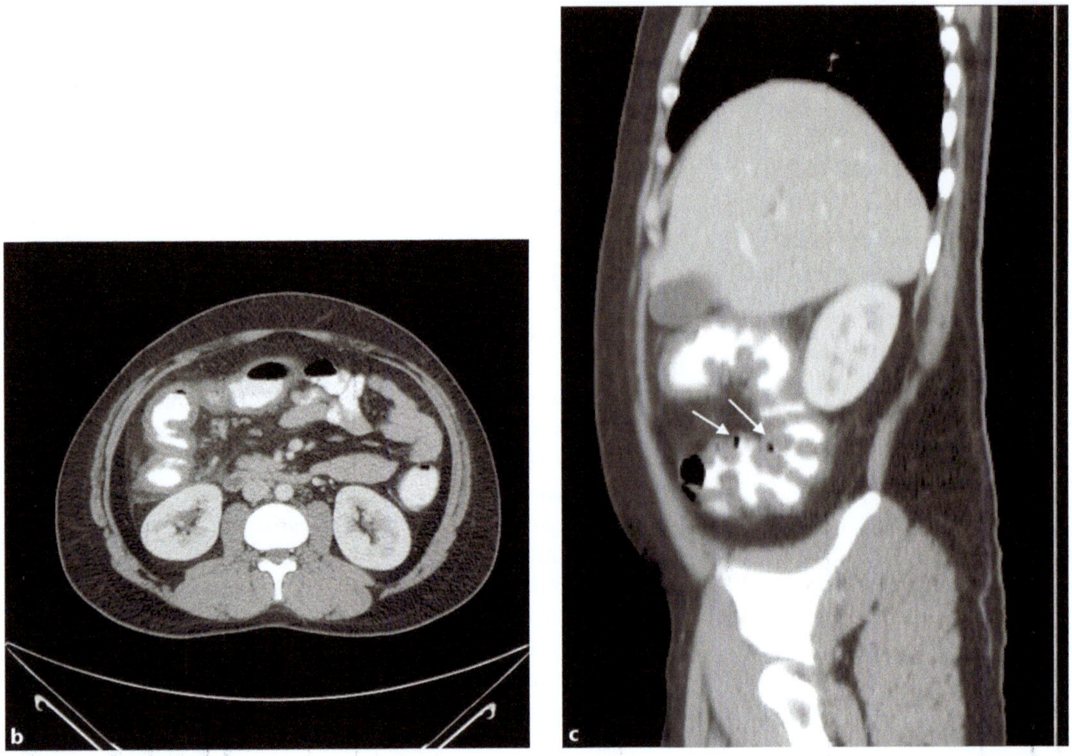

Fig. 4.4 (*continued*) Colonic amebiasis. **b** Axial CT scan of the abdomen confirmed extensive wall thickening of the cecum and hepatic flexure. **c** Parasagittal reconstructed CT scan image showing evidence of pneumatosis coli (*arrows*)

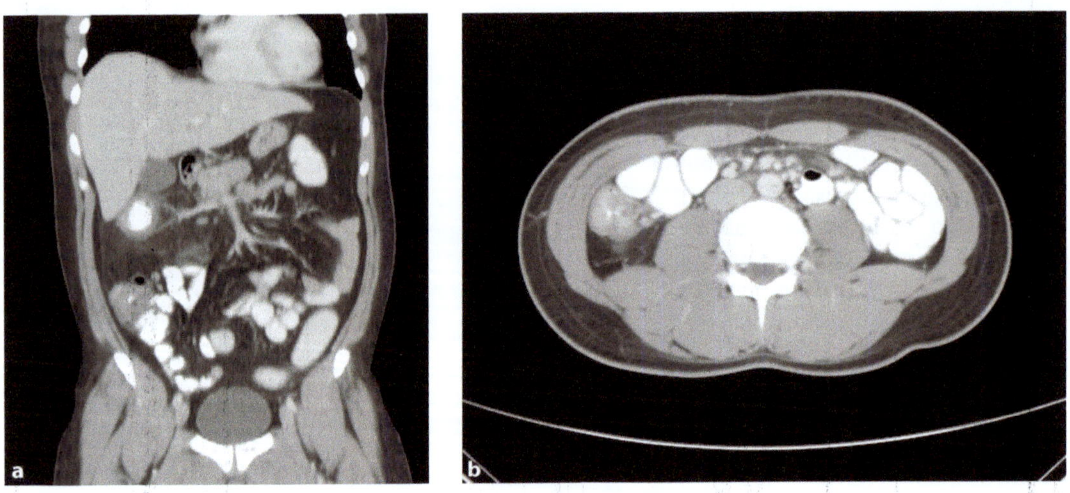

Fig. 4.5 Differentiation between amebiasis and Crohn's disease. **a** Coronal reconstruction of a CT scan showing contracted cecum with normal terminal ileum due to amebiasis. **b** Axial CT scan of the abdomen showing a thickened and contracted cecum due to Crohn's disease. **c**–e *see next page*

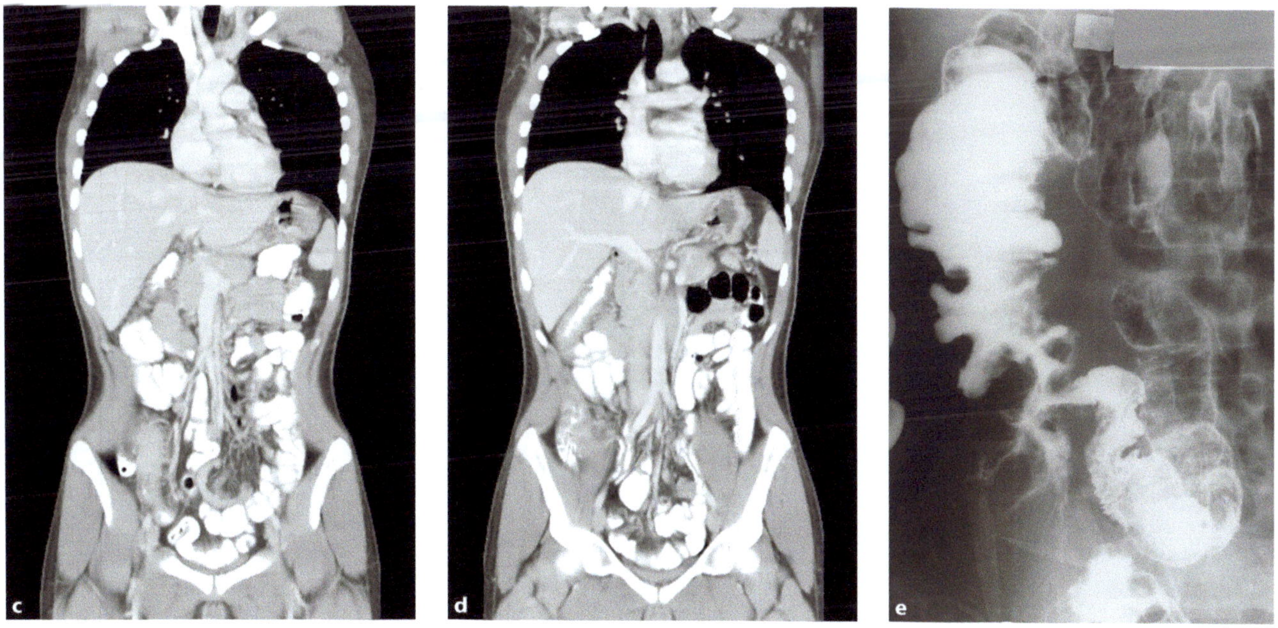

Fig. 4.5 (*continued*) Differentiation between amebiasis and Crohn's disease. **c**,**d** The coronal reconstruction CT scan images of the abdomen of the same patient in (**b**) showed markedly thickened terminal ileum with irregular outline due to Crohn's disease. **e** Barium enema showing contracted irregular cecum due to amebiasis with normal terminal ileum

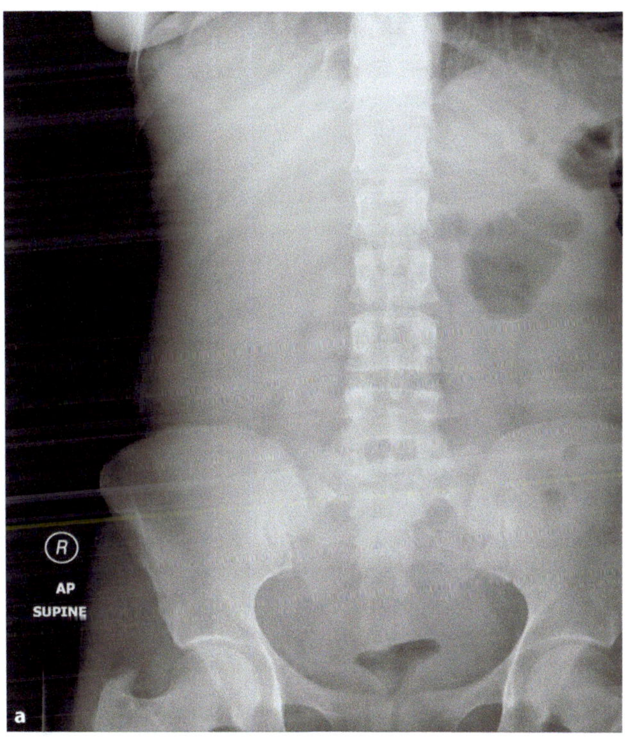

Fig. 4.6 Amebiasis presenting as a palpable mass in the right iliac fossa. **a** Plain radiograph of an adult patient who presented with a right iliac fossa mass and dysentery, showing the paucity of intestinal gas in the right iliac fossa. **b**,**c** *see next page*

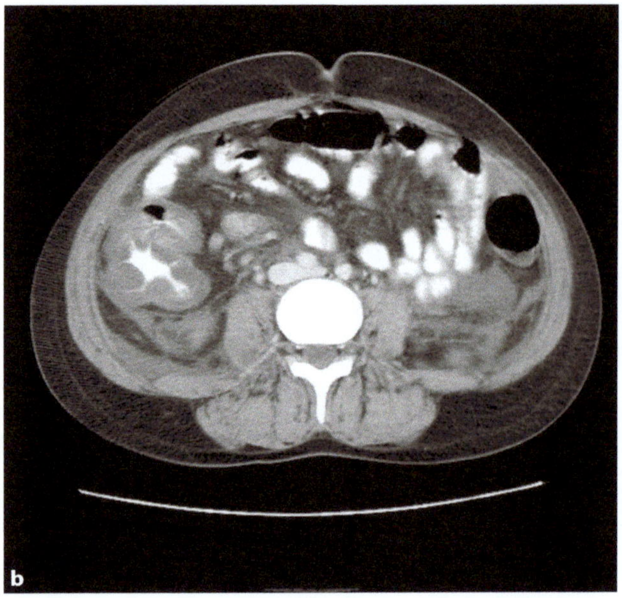

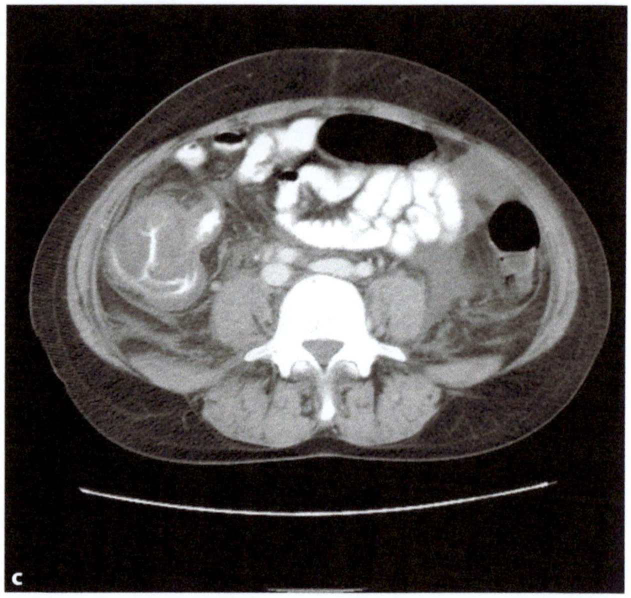

Fig. 4.6 (*continued*) Amebiasis presenting as a palpable mass in the right iliac fossa. **b,c** Axial CT scans of the cecum showing a markedly thickened cecum due to amebiasis (Courtesy of Dr. Mona Al Shahed, Department of Radiology, Riyadh Military Hospital, Riyadh, Saudi Arabia)

4.7.2 Flagellates

There are three types of flagellates that can affect man:

1. Intestinal flagellates, e.g., *Giardia lamblia*
2. Genital flagellates, e.g., *Trichomonas* (*T. vaginalis*, *T. hominis*)
3. Hemoflagellates:
   a) Leishmaniasis including visceral type (kala-azar) due to *L. donovani*, mucocutaneous type due to *L. brasiliensis*, or ulcers due to *L. tropica* (Oriental sores)
   b) Trypanosomiasis (African sleeping sickness) is due to *T. gambiense*, while the South American form (Chagas' disease) is due to *T. cruzi*

The resurgence of kala-azar in Europe is linked to HIV (Wilson and Streil 1996). Visceral leishmaniasis was also reported in American veterans of the Desert Storm war (Magill et al. 1993).

4.7.2.1 Giardiasis

4.7.2.1.1 Prevalence of Giardiasis

Giardiasis was found in 47% of Columbian children and 3–20% of children in some parts of the United States (Reeder 1997). In the tropics 4–16% of the population may harbor *Giardia*. In the USA, "gay bowel syndrome" was described in patients practicing oro-anal sex (Laughon 1988).

4.7.2.1.2 Pathogenesis

The parasite can live as a human commensal. Trophozoites adhere their suckers to the mucosa of the jejunum leading to mucosal inflammatory changes and may reflux into the duodenum and the biliary tree. They may exist as a characteristically active flagellate or as a cyst. Endoscopy may reveal inflammation, erosions, and nodularity of the mucosa (El Sheikh Mohammed et al. 1991). Jejunal biopsy may demonstrate shortening and blunting of the intestinal villi due to a reduction in the height of the columnar epithelium associated with hypercellularity of the lamina propria (Fig. 4.1e).

4.7.2.1.3 Clinical Presentation

Presentation could be acute or chronic including abdominal discomfort, diarrhea, dyspepsia, malabsorption, steatorrhea, anorexia, and even weight loss (Hartonget al. 1979). Reflux into the biliary tree may present as jaundice. There is a strong association between giardiasis and dysgammaglobulinemia (Reeder 1997). Macrocytic anemia and lactase deficiency can occur (Farthing 1996).

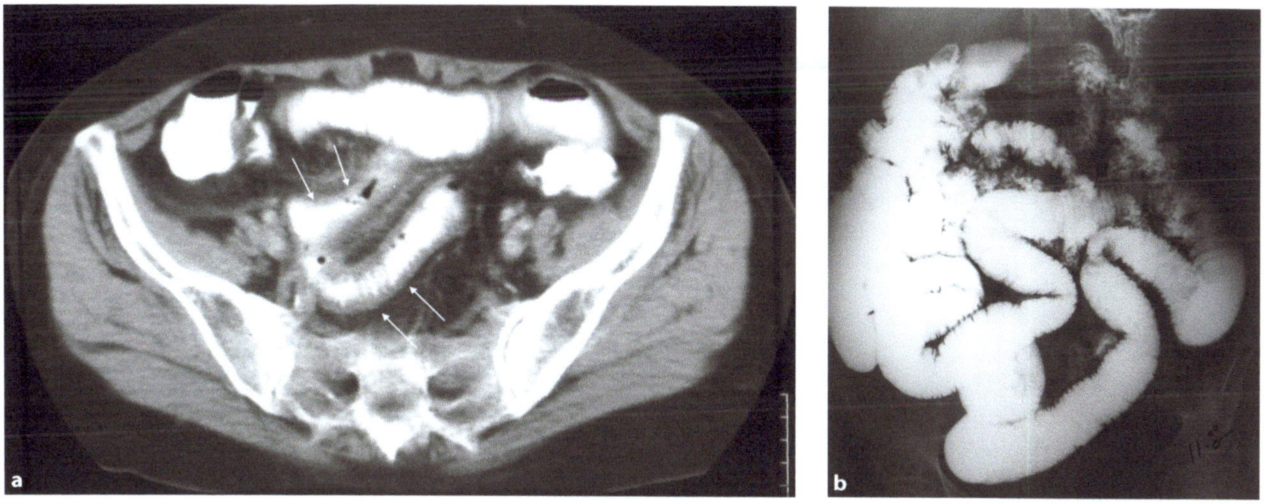

Fig. 4.7 Intestinal giardiasis. **a** Contrast-enhanced CT scan of the abdomen showing a fixed jejunal loop (*arrows*) with a thickened wall. **b** Barium follow-through demonstrating thickening of the jejunal mucosal folds

4.7.2.1.4 Radiological Features

The majority of those harboring *Giardia* may show no clinical or radiologic signs. Barium follow-through examination (Fig. 4.7) may show thickened mucosal folds and signs of malabsorption. These include rapid transit, intestinal dilatation, segmentation of the barium column, and coarsening and poor coating of the mucosal folds due to excess secretions (Reeder 1998). Spastic areas may be seen. Compensatory lymphoid hyperplasia is an attempt to produce more gammaglobulin, it manifests as fine nodularity distorting the normal feathery jejunal pattern. The radiological changes are nonspecific and the differential diagnosis of this appearance includes lymphangiectasia, Whipple's disease, lymphoma, amyloidosis, and hookworm infestation. Jejunal biopsy is essential for confirmation.

4.7.2.2 American Trypanosomiasis

Chagas' disease due to *T. cruzi* is endemic in Brazil, affecting 18 million people and causing the death of 50,000 annually (WHO 1991). This parasite is peculiarly restricted to one continent, so far.

In the acute phase of the disease the patient may present with myocarditis or meningoencephalitis. This is commoner in children. Unilateral eye swelling is an early sign (Romana's sign) (Marsden 1995). In the sub-acute phase hepatosplenomegaly and lymphadenopathy are apparent.

Megaesophagus (Chagasic achalasia; Fig. 4.8) and megacolon represent the chronic phase due to destruction of the Meissner and Auerbach's nerve plexuses. Lesions are pre cancerous in 7% (Mattoso and Reeder1998).

4.7.3 Cryptosporidiasis

This is a parasite that does not usually infect man. *Cryptosporidium parvum* is a minute rare parasite, but is of worldwide distribution. The first case was reported in a child in 1976 (Markell et al. 1992). Thereafter, it was reported in AIDS patients in association with diarrhea. It affects primarily the epithelial cells of the GIT, including the small and large bowel, causing diarrhea and occasionally pneumatosis intestinalis (Fig. 4.9) (Collins 1992). The diagnosis is made by stool examination and bowel biopsy for identification of the organism.

4.7.4 Rare Protozoa

Balantidium coli (balantidiasis) is a protozoan that is not usually pathogenic in man, but has been occasionally reported in mental hospitals. It mainly affects the colon and clinical presentation varies from asymptomatic forms to severe dysenteric syndromes. Diagnosis is by colonic endoscopy and biopsy (Gonzales de Canales Simon 2000).

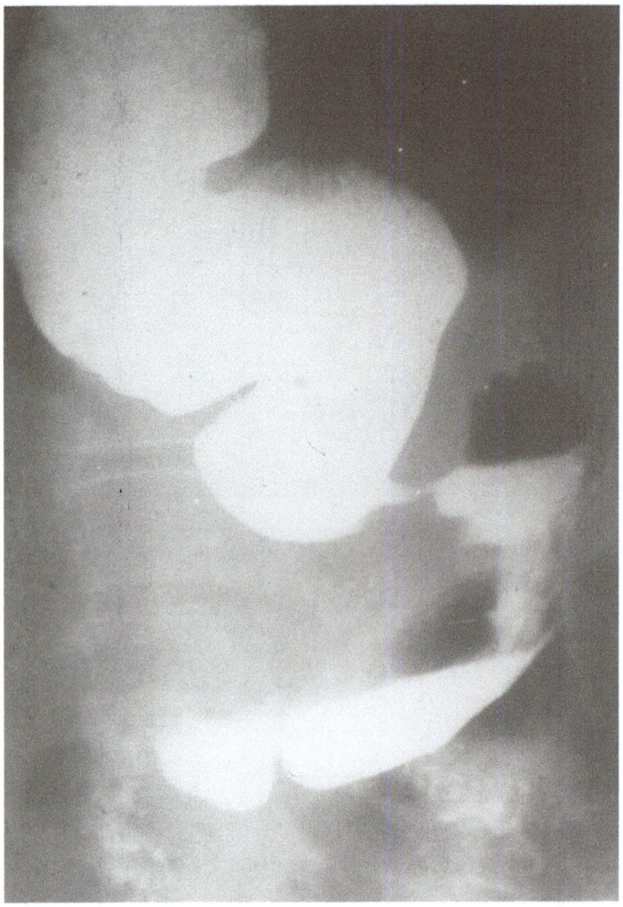

Fig. 4.8 Megaesophagus due to destruction of the submucosal and myenteric nerve plexuses

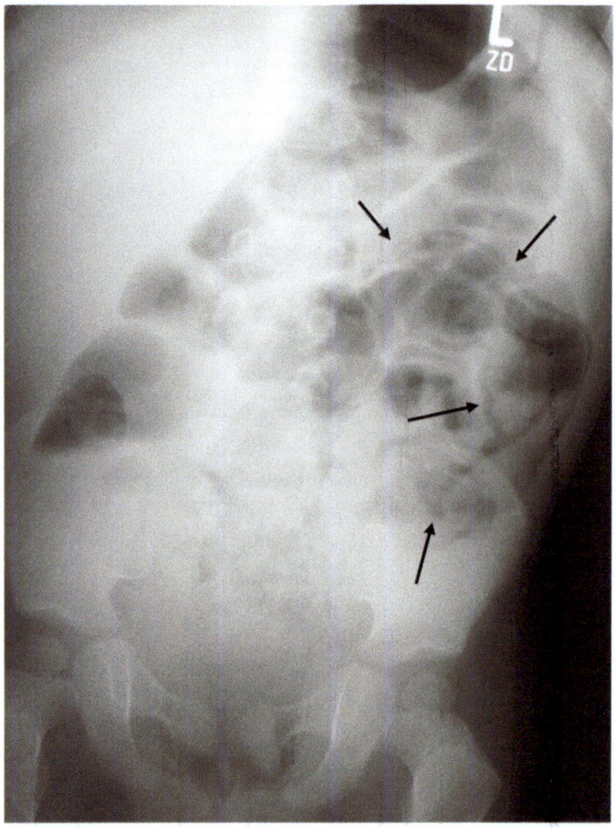

Fig. 4.9 Plain abdominal radiograph showing pneumatosis intestinalis (*arrows*) in a child with cryptosporidiasis

4.8 Nematodes (Helminths – "Roundworms")

These are the commonest GIT parasites.

4.8.1 Ascariasis

Ascaris lumbricoides affects over 1.4 billion people with a heavy infestation in 2 million people, killing 20,000 of them annually. In certain tropical countries up to 93% of the population are infected (Khuroo 1996). The worm may reach 16–40 cm, with the male a little slenderer than the female (Fig. 4.2a,b). Worm burden within the patient may reach 1,000 worms per capita due to continuous reproduction (Fig. 4.2.c).

4.8.1.1 Clinical Presentation

1. Incidental finding
2. Passage of worms with vomitus or stools
3. Abdominal symptoms
4. Intestinal obstruction
5. Jaundice, biliary colic, cholangitis
6. Pancreatitis
7. Chest symptoms

4.8.1.2 Radiological Findings

Linear filling defects may be seen on barium follow-through (Fig. 4.10a–c) or barium enema (Fig 4.11). Barium may be seen within the GIT of the parasite itself (Fig. 4.10c). The worm may rarely be seen by plain abdominal radiograph in patients with a high worm load (Fig. 4.10d) or on ultrasound and abdominal CT scan (Mahmood et al. 2001; Sauvage et al. 2006). Worm clumps may cause intestinal obstruction (Schulze et al. 2005). Endoscopic retrieval of worms obstructing the biliary tree was reported (Fig. 4.3) (Karawi et al. 1989).

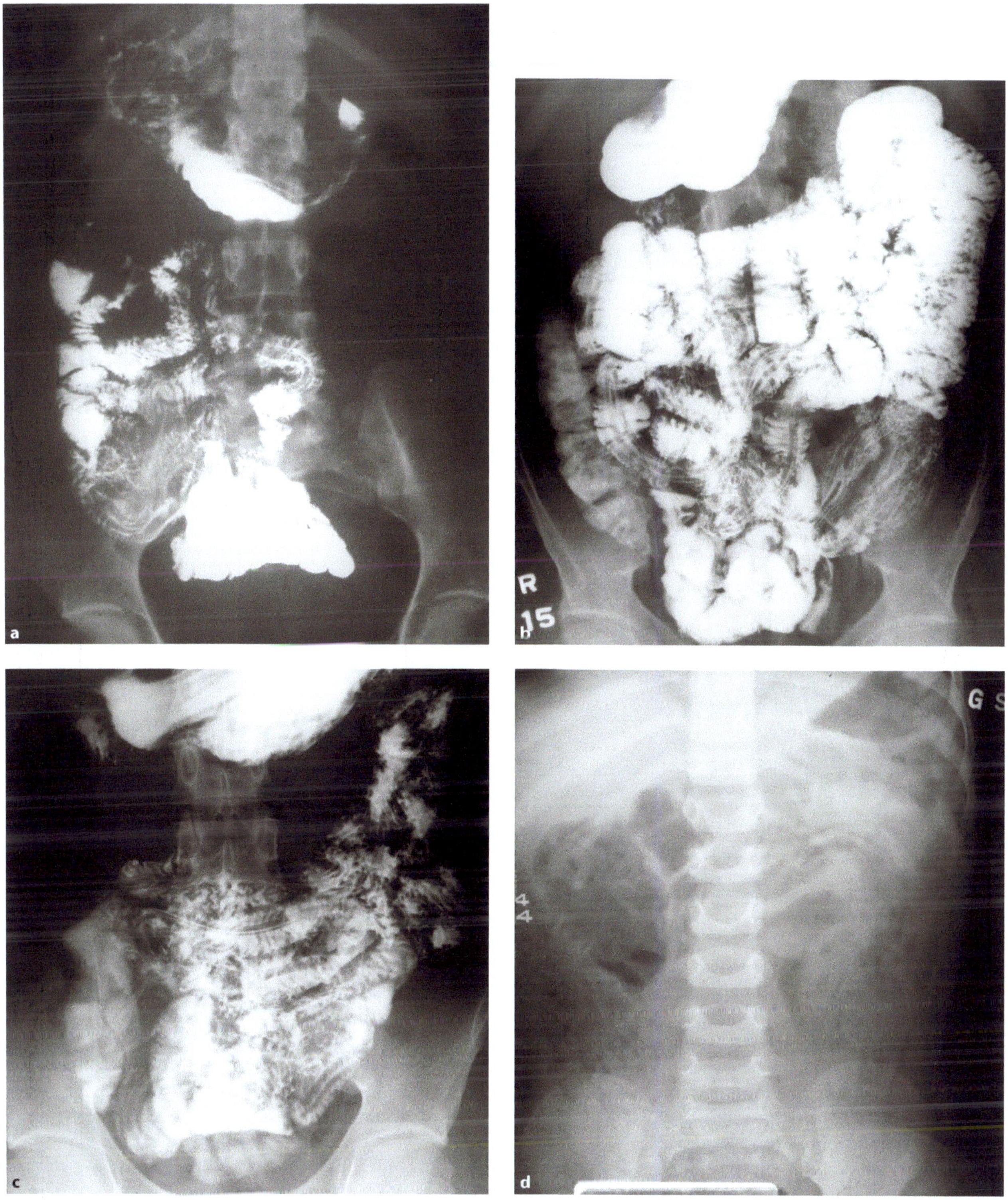

Fig. 4.10 Intestinal ascariasis. **a,b** Barium follow-through examinations showing elongated filling defects due to *Ascaris*. **c** Opacification of the *Ascaris* digestive tract by barium sulphate. **d** Plain abdominal radiograph demonstrating abnormal bowel gas pattern due to the presence of *Ascaris* in the small bowel

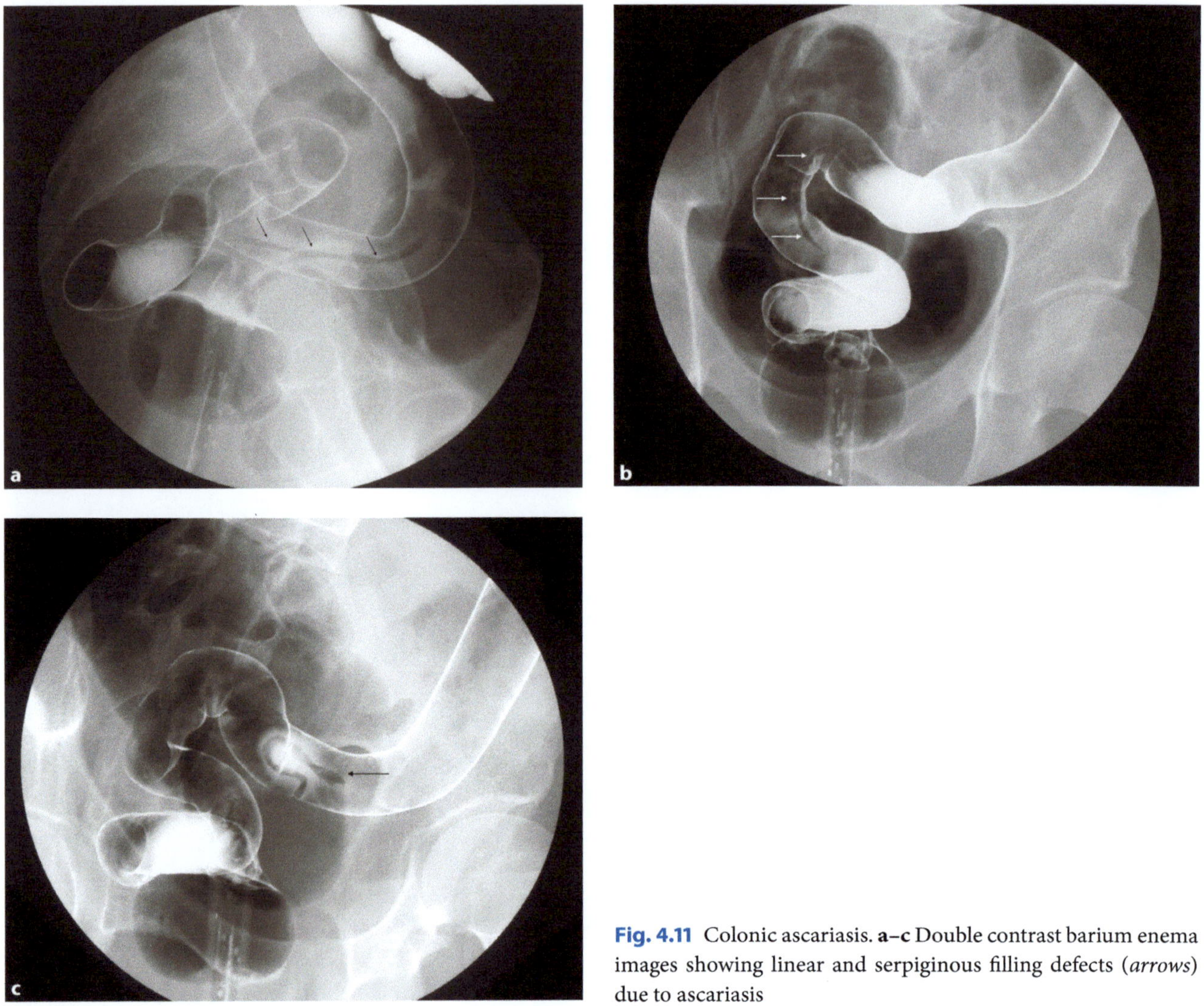

Fig. 4.11 Colonic ascariasis. **a–c** Double contrast barium enema images showing linear and serpiginous filling defects (*arrows*) due to ascariasis

4.8.2 Strongyloidiasis

The larva penetrates the skin to reach the lungs and the intestine via the bloodstream. The disease is endemic in the Caribbean, West Africa, and Southeast Asia. This nematode, *S. stercoralis*, was noted to proliferate in immunocompromised patients (Armignacco et al. 1989). The most dangerous and peculiar aspect of this parasite is that it can undergo a complete life cycle within the patient (autoinfection or hyperinfection) leading to endless proliferation and a fatal hyperinfection syndrome by transformation of rhabditiform larva into the filiform stage within the patient (Hakim and Genta 1986). Moreover, it can complete a life cycle in the external environment (free-living cycle). Apparently, male forms of this parasite do not exist (Polenakovik and Polenakovik 2006). I am afraid that this worm may be a time bomb for the next century if global warming escalates. Strongyloidiasis is prevalent worldwide; *S. stercoralis* affects the submucosa and lamina propria of the duodenum and upper jejunum, and rarely the large bowel. Plain films may show distended bowel. Barium studies show loss of mucosal pattern, rigidity, and tubular narrowing of the intestinal walls (Fig. 4.12). Acute hyperinfections may involve the lungs and central nervous system.

► **Fig. 4.12** Intestinal and colonic strongyloidiasis. **a** Barium follow-through showing thickened mucosal folds of the small intestine. **b** Delayed images showing loss of mucosal pattern in the terminal ileum, and in the transverse and descending colon segments. **c** Photomicrograph from a colonic biopsy showing crypt infestation by several *Strongyloides stercoralis* parasites (*arrows*; H&E, ×40). *Insets*: *A* two adult worms, one seen in longitudinal section and one in cross-section (H&E, ×200), *B* Higher magnification of the latter showing the intestine and two reproductive tubes (H&E, ×400) (Courtesy of Dr. Fadi Mrad, Department of Internal Medicine and Drs. Ayman Tawil and Zaher Chakhachiro, Department of Pathology, American University of Beirut Medical Center, Beirut, Lebanon)

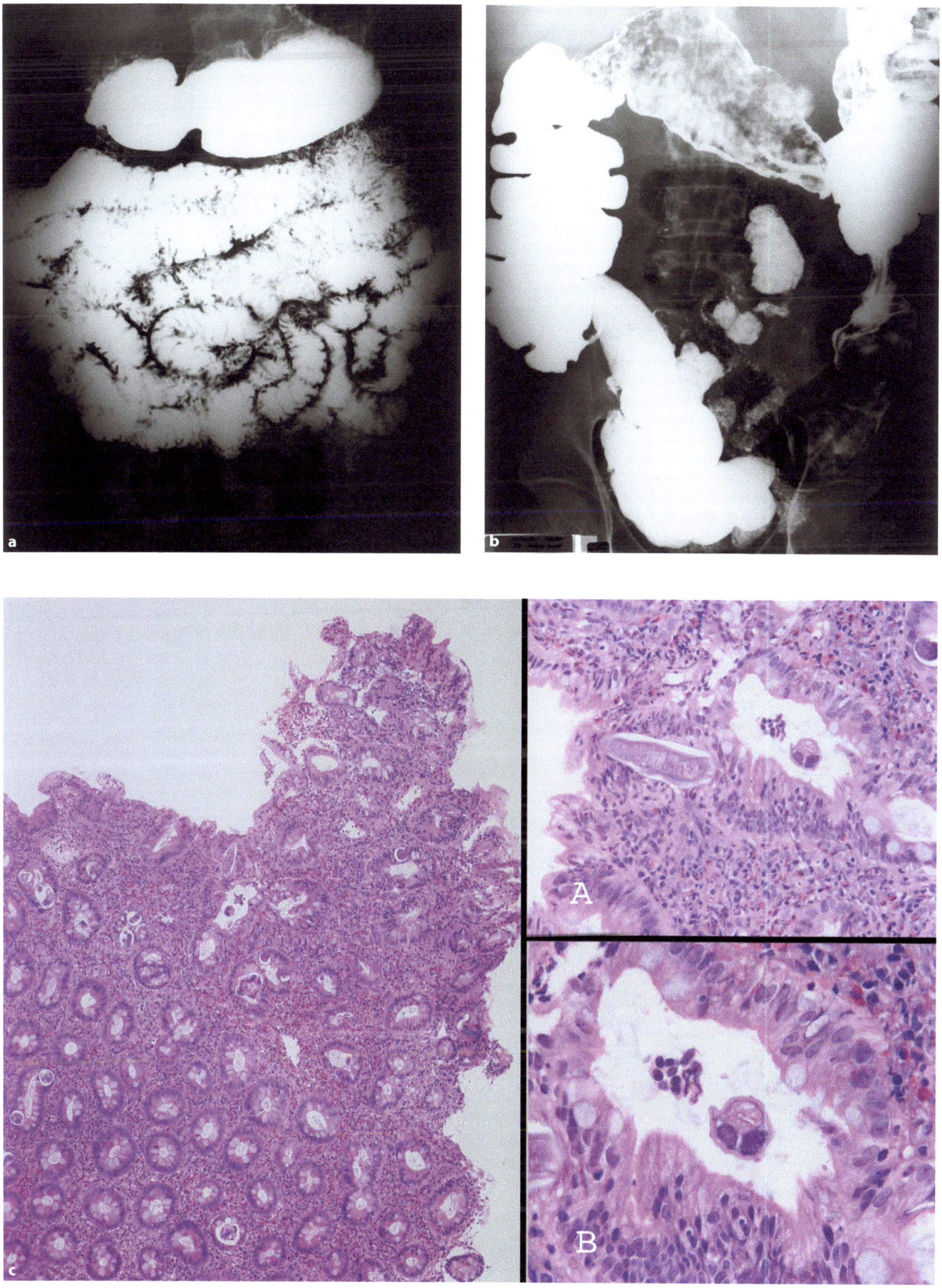
a
b
c
A
B

4.8.3 Rare Nematodes

4.8.3.1 *Enterobius vermicularis* (Enterobiasis, Oxyuriasis)

This peculiar small "pinworm" lives in the cecum. The worm migrates at night to lay eggs in the perianal region and subsequently dies (Lewis et al. 1975). It may cause perianal itching, which can be severe, disturbing sleep. *E. vermicularis* is the commonest helminthic parasite in the temperate countries (Goldsmid et al. 1992). Reinfection by hand contamination or via the fecal–oral route is common (Markell et al. 1992). Patients may present with appendicitis (Abu-Rumman 2001) or eosinophilic ileocolitis (Macedo and MacCarty 2000).

4.8.3.2 *Ancylostoma duodenale* and *Necator americanus*

The *A. duodenale* "hookworm" is common around the Mediterranean and Africa while the *N. americanus* "hookworm" is common in the New World and America. These parasites attach themselves to the bowel wall of the small intestine by their chitinous teeth to suck the blood. Patients usually present with anemia. Barium studies may be unrevealing or show nonspecific changes including spasm and thickened mucosal folds (Thomas 1986). The diagnosis of hookworm can be made by capsule endoscopy (Chao and Ray 2006).

4.8.3.3 *Trichuris trichiura* (Trichuriasis)

The *T. trichiura* "whipworm" is very common, but fortunately usually harmless. It lives in the cecum and rectum causing mild dysentery and anemia. In severe cases it may lead to rectal prolapse (Gilles 1995) and colonic trichuriasis (Tokmak et al. 2006).

4.8.3.4 *Anisakis marina* (Anisakiasis)

This is a parasite of marine mammals like seals and dolphins. It is transported to humans when they eat squid or fish. The parasites cause upper GIT symptoms with wall thickening and even strictures. The terminal ileum may be involved and appendicitis was seen in 80% of cases (Repiso Ortega et al. 2003).

4.8.3.5 *Capillaria philippinensis* (Intestinal Capillariasis)

Intestinal capillariasis is a severe protein-losing enteropathy caused by the small nematode *Capillaria philippinensis*. Infection in man occurs as a result of eating raw or inadequately cooked small freshwater fish harboring the infective larvae of the parasite in their intestine. Intestinal capillariasis is endemic in Southeast Asia. The disease was also reported in the Middle East (Iran and Egypt). The first Egyptian case was reported in 1989 (Youssef et al. 1989), but it appears to be an emerging infection in that country (Mansour et al. 1990; Austin et al. 1999; Anis et al. 1998; El-Dib and Doss 2002; Ahmad et al. 1999). The diagnosis is usually made by the detection of eggs and larvae in stool samples.

4.8.3.6 *Angiostrongylus costaricensis* (Angiostrongyliasis)

Abdominal angiostrongyliasis is acquired by ingesting infected mollusks or contaminated vegetables by their secretions containing larvae. The disease affects the terminal ileum, appendix, cecum, and ascending colon causing abdominal pain, recurrent gastrointestinal hemorrhage, or intestinal perforation. Pathologically, there is an eosinophilic inflammatory reaction leading to bowel ischemia or necrosis. Radiologically, there is evidence of bowel wall-thickening and edema with ulcerations. The clinical and radiological changes are nonspecific, and the differential diagnosis includes acute appendicitis, Crohn's disease, and other pathologies. Stool examinations are nondiagnostic. Positive diagnosis is established by serology, endoscopic biopsy or at surgery, which is the treatment of choice (Loria-Cortes and Lobo-Sanahuja 1980).

4.9 Cestodes (Helminths – "Tapeworms")

These are long ribbon-like parasites acquired by eating raw meat containing live cysticerci (Box 4.5). *Taenia saginata* is common in beef-eating communities, while *T. solium* is commoner in pork-eating communities. *Diphyllobothrium latum* is relatively common in Scandinavia, leading to anemia and selective vitamin B12 deficiency. Sparganosis caused by *Spirometra mansoni* can be transmitted to man through the practice of eating or using snakes and frogs in medicines (Rha et al. 1999).

Cestodes do not have a digestive system and rely on sucking their food from the human intestine. This is why they do not ingest barium like *Ascaris*. All tapeworms are hermaphrodites. For the *Taenia* species, humans are the definitive hosts. A recent report described the reflective, ribbon-like appearance of *Taenia saginata* on ultrasound (Fabijanic et al. 2001). CT is useful to demonstrate gut wall and peritoneal involvement with tapeworms and flukes (Rha et al. 1999). Cysticercosis is the larval stage of *Taenia solium*. It causes more harm than the worm itself when deposited in the brain or the orbits. In may also deposit in muscles and can calcify in all sites (Markell et al. 1992).

Box 4.5 What are the types of tapeworms?

Diphyllobothrium latum	Fish tapeworm	10 m
Taenia saginata	Beef tapeworm	5 m
Taenia solium	Pork tapeworm	3 m
Cysticercosis	Larva of tapeworm	0.5 – 5 cm
Hymenolepis nana	Dwarf tapeworm	2 – 4 cm
Echinococcus	Dog tapeworm	0.6 cm

4.9.1 *Echinococcosis* (Hydatid Disease)

This parasite is common in countries where animal husbandry is popular. Hydatid is not principally a tropical disease (Lewall 1998). No country is really exempt, although it is peculiarly rare on the West African coastline and in the South Pacific islands, except Australia where it is endemic. Its exact prevalence, however, is unknown. *Echinococcus granulosus* is widespread (von Sinner 1997) and *E. multilocularis* is restricted to the subarctic region. The tiny adult worm (Fig. 4.1f) lives in the intestine of dogs or foxes (Amman and Eckert 1996). It releases eggs into the environment, which are ingested by the intermediate host of sheep or cattle. Humans are accidental hosts. There are two methods of acquiring the disease. Either by eating improperly disinfected vegetables or by close contact with dogs. Peculiarly, hydatid disease practices favorite host specificity in the primary host. Although domestic cats are canines, they do not act as a primary host (Lewall 1998). Swallowed eggs hatch in the stomach. Hatched embryos migrate to lodge in the liver (60–90%), lungs, kidneys, and bones. The majority are asymptomatic and are discovered accidentally as cyst calcifications or as a mass on conventional plain abdominal radiographs (Fig. 4.13) (Beggs 1983). Like liver cysts, extrahepatic abdominal cysts exhibit calcifications (Fig. 4.13). Ultrasound is the favorite diagnostic test. Symptoms depend on the site of involvement. GIT involvement by hydatid cysts is by extrinsic compression. Peritoneal cysts follow previous liver surgery. They were seen in 3.8% of one study (Polat 2003). Cyst rupture causes anaphylactic shock and peritoneal seeding (von Sinner 1997). Silent or chronic leakage may fill the whole abdomen, compatible with peritoneal dissemination (Fig. 4.14). CT scanning is an accurate test for the diagnosis and classification of the disease. If available, MRI demonstrates cyst contents, size, and multiplanar relations (Fig. 4.15). Spontaneous rupture into the GIT is extremely rare, occurring only in 0.5%, manifesting itself as hydatidemesis or hydatidorrhea (Pedrosa et al. 2000). Hydatid cysts can be effectively treated by image-guided drainage (Khuroo et al. 1991). Even solid-appearing hydatid cysts can be drained percutaneously (Haddad et al. 2000). Endoscopic transpapillary drainage is an effective therapy when there is endobiliary rupture (Fig. 4.16) (Al Karawi et al. 1987).

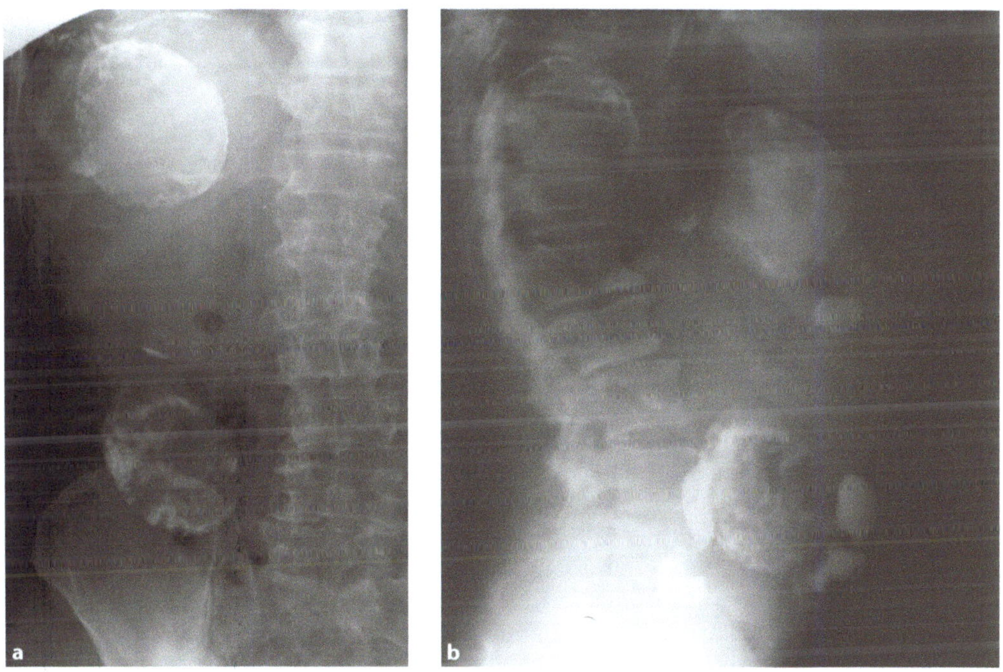

Fig. 4.13 Calcified hepatic and peritoneal hydatid cysts on plain radiography. **a** Anteroposterior and **b** lateral projections showing multiple calcified hepatic and peritoneal echinococcal cysts

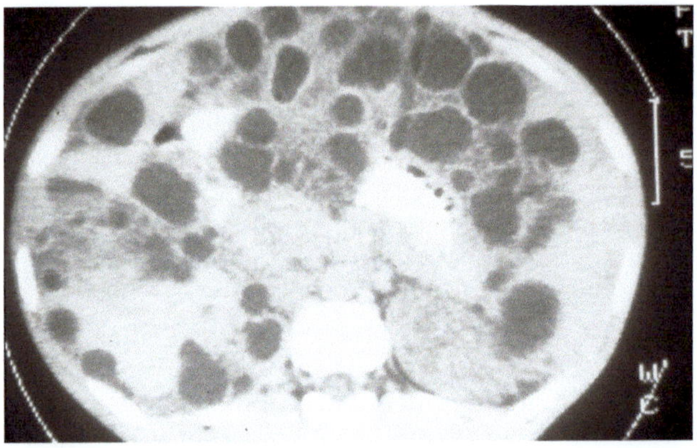

Fig. 4.14 Computed tomography scan of the abdomen showing disseminated abdominal hydatidosis

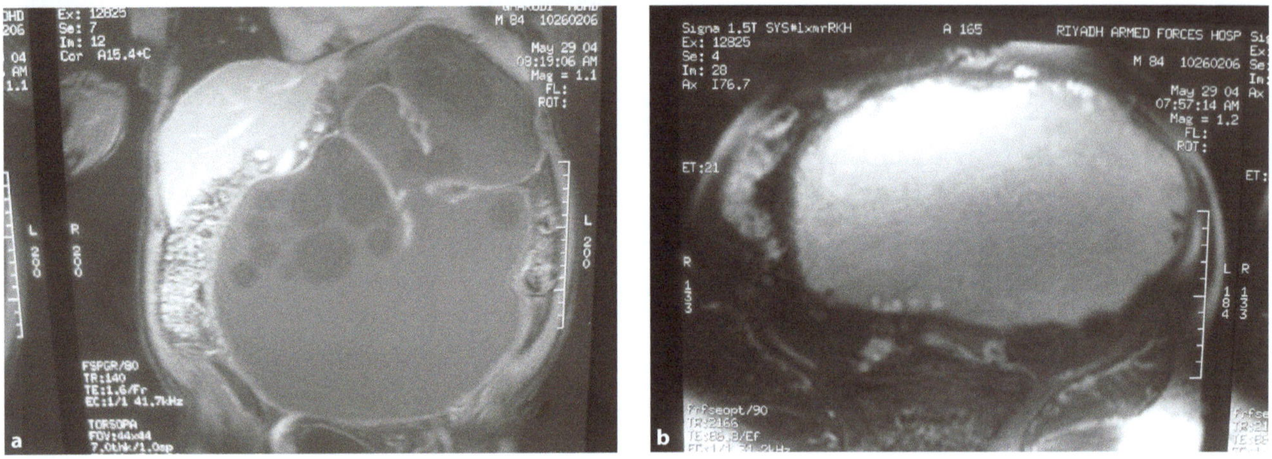

Fig. 4.15 Magnetic resonance imaging of a giant intra-abdominal hydatid cyst. **a** T1-weighted coronal MR image showing a hypointense large hydatid cyst with internal septations and small daughter cysts. **b** Axial T2-weighted MR image showing a hyperintense hydatid cyst occupying the abdominal cavity

4.9.2 Taeniasis and Cysticercosis

Taenia solium is the pork tapeworm and is common in Mexico, Africa, and China. Infection occurs if incompletely cooked pork meat is consumed. *Taenia saginata* infection occurs from poorly cooked beef and this worm may reach a length of 25 m. Cysticercosis represents the larval stage of *Taenia solium* tapeworms. In humans they are most commonly lodged in the muscles or central nervous system, and in swine they are found in muscles. Eye infection in humans leads to blindness. This should not be confused with the river blindness due to microfilaria of *Onchocerca volvulus* especially prevalent around the river Jur in southern Sudan. Subcutaneous calcified small cysts can be demonstrated by plain radiographs or ultrasound and CT scanning. The disease is common in Africa, South America and the Far East (Abd El Bagi et al. 2004). Barium studies are capable of demonstrating intestinal *Taenia saginata*, and the sonographic appearance of colon taeniasis consists of a double-reflective, ribbon-like structure in the lumen of the bowel (Fabijanic et al. 2001). MR enterography potentially plays a role in the diagnosis of taeniasis *(Taenia saginata)* too (Paolantonio et al. 2006).

4.9.3 Rare Cestodes

4.9.3.1 *Diphyllobothrium latum* (Diphyllobothriasis)

The fish tapeworm of humans, *Diphyllobothrium latum*, is common in northern temperate areas of the world (e.g., Scandinavia and Canada) where pickled or insufficiently cooked fresh water fish is prominent in the diet. The adult worm is several meters in length and does not cause many symptoms. Anemia is a presenting feature and vitamin B12 deficiency is a rare but serious complication (Abd El Bagi et al. 2004). The first case of diphyllobothriasis from Saudi Arabia was recently reported in a Saudi patient who had traveled to Southeast Asia (Al-khalife et al. 2006).

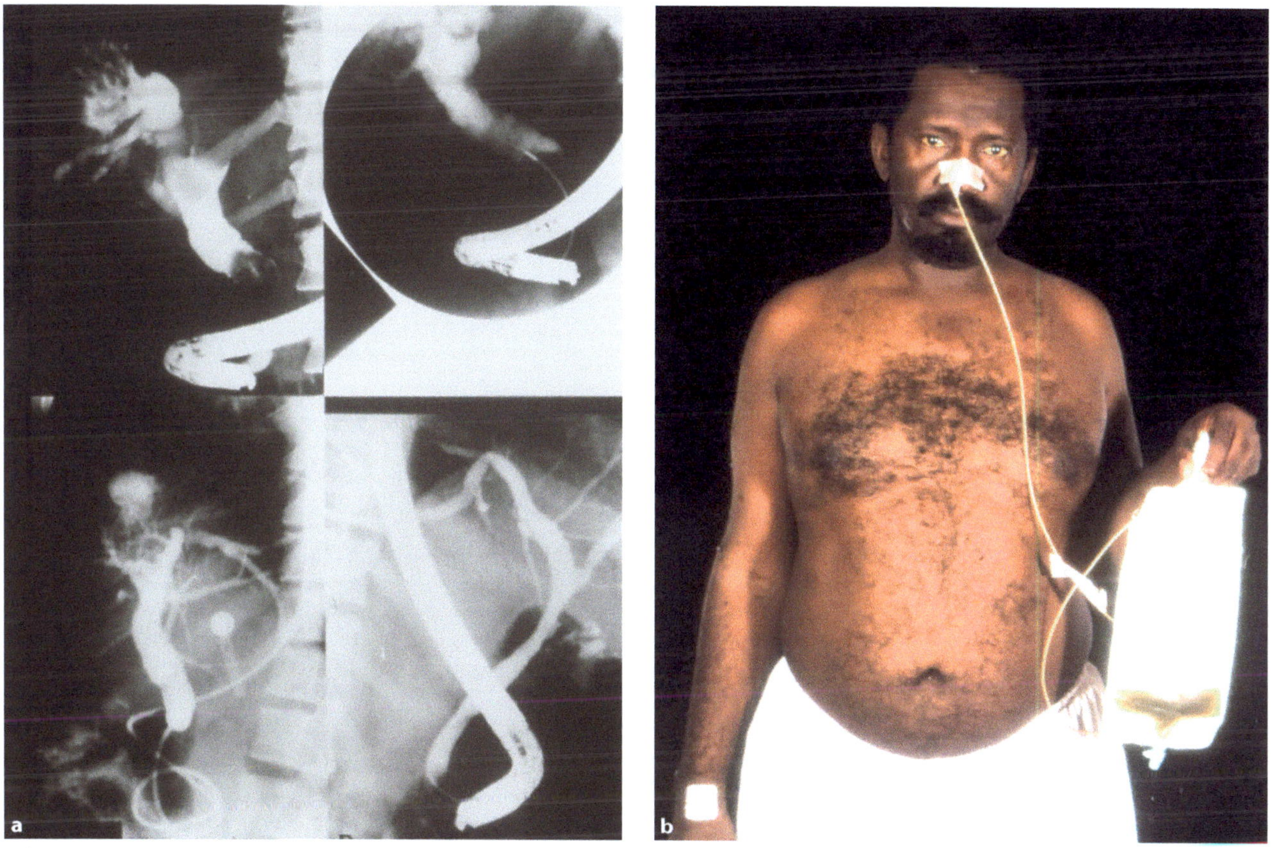

Fig. 4.16 Endobiliary rupture of hepatic hydatid cyst causing obstructive jaundice. **a** Endoscopic retrograde cholangiopancreatography followed by daughter cyst extraction. **b** Transpapillary nasobiliary drainage for irrigation and flushing of membranes and small daughter cysts causing obstructive jaundice with yellowish eye sclera (Courtesy of Dr. M. Al Karawi, Department of Gastroenterology, Riyadh Military Hospital, Riyadh, Saudi Arabia)

4.9.3.2 *Hymenolepis nana* (Hymenolepiasis)

Hymenolepis nana is a dwarf tapeworm in humans, but it is a common parasite of the house mouse. It is most prevalent in children in Central Europe and Latin America. It is estimated that 20 million people are infected. The adult worm is a few centimeters long and lives in the small intestines of humans. *H. diminuta* is a larger tapeworm than *H. nana*, measuring 1 m in length (Abd El Bagi et al. 2004).

4.9.3.3 *Spirometra mansoni* (Sparganosis)

Sparganosis affects primarily the central nervous system, subcutaneous tissues, and muscles. When accidentally ingested by humans, bowel perforation and peritonitis may occur (Dunn and Palmer 1998), or even intestinal obstruction due to intramural sparganosis (Cho et al. 1987).

4.10 Trematodes (Helminths – "Flukes")

Trematodes are leaf-like worms except schistosomes, which are elongated. They all pass through asexual development in a snail host. They are all hermaphrodites except schistosomes, which are dioecious. Classification of flukes depends on the organ infected.

1. Intestinal flukes: the large fluke *Fasciolopsis buski*, measuring 2–7 cm in length, is prevalent in China. It lives in the intestine and may cause ulceration or hemorrhage (Zaman 1984). The minute fluke *Heterophyes heterophyes* occurs in the Far East and Egypt where people eat pickled fresh water fish (Markell et al. 1992). Other intestinal flukes include *Metagonimus yokogawai* and *Echinostoma ilocanum.*
2. Liver flukes: opisthorchiasis and clonorchiasis are prevalent in the Far East and immigrants from those countries. Clonorchiasis is famous for causing cholangiocarcinoma (Choi et al. 2004). *Fasciola hepatica* is prevalent in the Far East and Egypt. It is ac-

quired by eating cyst-laden water plants (Pulpeiro et al. 1991).
3. Lung fluke: paragonimiasis is a disease of the Far East related to eating raw cray fish and the delicacy of eating live "drunken crab" immersed in wine (Markell et al. 1992). The parasite settles in the lungs, but may reach the peritoneum or brain (Martinez et al. 2005).
4. Blood fluke: schistosomiasis.

4.10.1 Schistosomiasis

There are five species of schistosoma that affect humans. Eggs of *Schistosoma mansoni*, *S. japonicum* and *S. intercalatum* are passed in stools. *S. mansoni* is prevalent in Egypt, in the Sudanese cotton-growing fields, and in the West Indies, affecting the GIT (Box 4.6). Schistosomas are dioecious with the two sexes dissimilar in appearance. Females are longer than the males. The female has a gynecophoral canal in which the male reposes. Unlike other trematodes, which are ingested, *Schistosoma* enters the body through the skin. Humans are the definitive hosts. Soft water snails are intermediate hosts.

Schistosoma japonicum is confined to the Far East. Unlike *S. mansoni* it can infect other mammals. It is small and tends to lodge in the branches of the superior mesenteric vein. *S. mekongi* is prevalent in Cambodia, while *S. intercalatum* is prevalent in Western Africa causing mild disease. *S. japonicum* is prevalent in China and not in Japan. *S. japonicum* is precancerous for hepatoma and adenocarcinoma of the stomach. *S. mansoni* is not precancerous (Elliot 1996; Palmer 1998). Intestinal schistosomiasis is prevalent in 53 countries, affecting 60 million people. It causes 200,000 deaths annually.

Box 4.6 Gastrointestinal schistosomiasis

- Widespread, caused by man-made lakes
- An occupational hazard to farmers
- The egg is the main cause of disease
- Liver failure is late
- Cirrhosis is nutrition-related
- *S. japonicum* is precancerous
- *S. mansoni* is not precancerous
- Fibrosis causes portal hypertension
- Portosystemic shunts open
- Bleeding varices cause death
- Praziquantel is the drug of choice

4.10.1.1 Pathogenesis

The parasite entry through the skin causes dermatitis and petechial hemorrhage. *S. mansoni* females depart from the male to deposit their laterally spined eggs into small venules of the inferior mesenteric territory (Fig. 4.1c). The eggs cannot pass through capillaries because of their larger size. The eggs of *S. mansoni* provoke periluminal chronic inflammation, polyposis, ulceration or strictures of the colon. Reflux into the portal system leads to Symmer's periportal fibrosis (Symmer 1904). This causes portal hypertension. Periportal fibrosis can be assessed and classified by ultrasound. Even simple portable handheld ultrasound machines can provide accurate diagnosis (Homeida et al. 1988). The issue of periportal fibrosis received a lot of worldwide attention and the original classification was revised twice to become more elaborate. It is divided into seven subtypes varying from starry sky to bird's claw appearance (WHO 1996). Portosystemic shunts may lead to variceal bleeding episodes. *S. hematobium* lodges in the urinary system. Mixed infection of *S. mansoni* and *S. hematobium* can occur in hyperendemic areas.

4.10.1.2 Clinical Presentations

These are summarized in (Table 4.6). The "swimmer's itch" represents cutaneous itching or schistosomal der-

Table 4.6 Clinical presentation of intestinal bilharziasis

	Symptom	Timing
1.	Swimmer's itch	Within 24 h
2.	Katayama syndrome (toxemic hypersensitivity)	After a month
3.	Dysentery	After 2 months
4.	Hepatomegaly	May regress
5.	Splenomegaly	After a year
6.	Periportal fibrosis	Detected by US
7.	Portal hypertension	About 2 years
8.	Ascites, varices, and congestive enteropathy	Late stages
9.	Pulmonary hypertension	Late
10.	Liver failure	Not an early feature
11.	Acute variceal bleeding	May be fatal

matitis at the skin entry of the cercaria into the human body after swimming in infected ponds. The "Katayama syndrome" is a severe febrile illness accompanied by abdominal pain, diarrhea, cough, hepatosplenomegaly, acute bilharzial colitis, and eosinophilia, which may occur 4–6 weeks following exposure (Yasawy 2004).

4.10.1.3 Radiological Manifestations

Portal hypertension leads to the opening of portosystemic shunts (Mohamed et al. 1990). Serpiginous filling defects can be seen in barium studies of the esophagus or stomach (Fig. 4.17a). Water enhanced transcutaneous ultrasound (WETCUS) can detect and classify congestive gastropathy secondary to portal hypertension (Fig. 4.17b,c) (Abd El Bagi et al. 1998). Varices and collateral veins can be demonstrated on contrast – enhanced CT scan and color Doppler ultrasound (Figs. 4.18, 4.19b). Endoscopy can demonstrate esophageal and perigastric varices with the potential for sclerotherapy (Mohamed et al. 1990).

Endoscopic ultrasound is a useful adjunct to endoscopy, but makes the procedure more invasive and lengthy (Fig. 4.19a).

Gastric and duodenal erosions are present in 50% of cases. The small bowel may show thickening due to congestive enteropathy. Ischemic changes may become evident as thumb printing. Mesenteric or portal vein thrombosis can occur due to perivascular fibrosis and granulomas (Fig. 4.18c). Ascites are a late complication. Colonic polyposis or strictures may be seen. Pericolonic granulomas may calcify (Fig. 4.20) (Sammak et al. 1999).

In later stages, the spleen may reach a visibly enormous size (Fig. 4.21a). Splenomegaly can be demonstrated by ultrasound (Fig. 4.21.b) or CT (Fig. 4.21c). Up to 13 cm in length is considered the normal size of the spleen in malaria homelands.

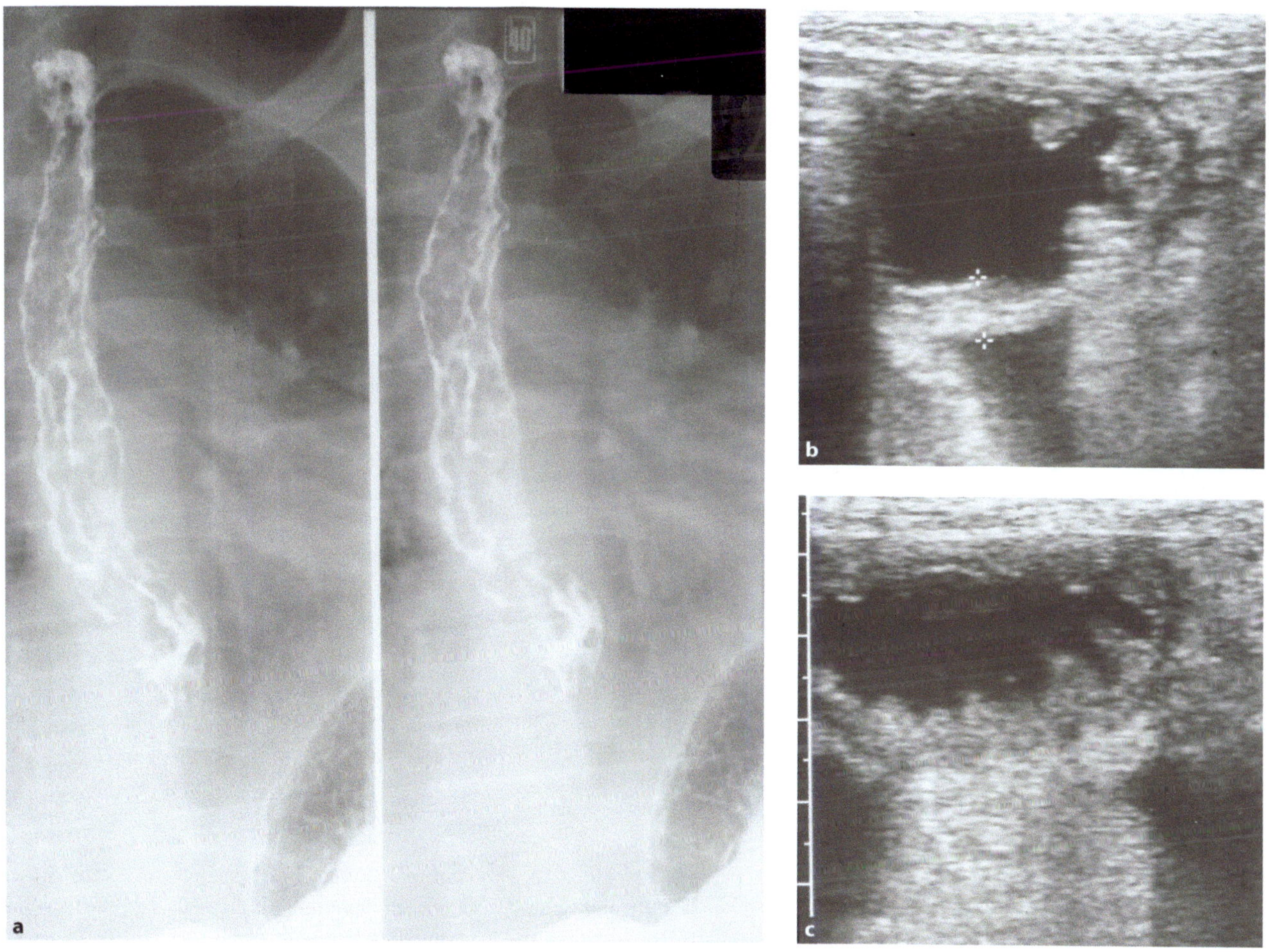

Fig. 4.17 **a** Barium swallow showing serpiginous filling defects in the lower half of the esophagus and gastric fundus due to varices. **b** Water enhanced transcutaneous ultrasound of the stomach showing thickening of the gastric wall (*cursors*) and ascites. **c** "Shark teeth" polypoid mucosal thickening due to portal hypertensive gastropathy

4.10.2 Rare Intestinal Flukes

Fasciolopsis buski (fasciolopsiasis), *Metagonimus yokogawai* (metagonimiasis), *Echinostoma ilocanum*, and *E. lindoense* (echinostomiasis), and *Heterophyes heterophyes* (heterophyiasis) are intestinal flukes endemic in Southeast Asia, the Middle East (Egypt and Iran), and North Africa.

Humans are accidentally infected by consuming infected raw or undercooked fish or crustaceans, or contaminated vegetables. The intestinal flukes attach to the mucosa of the proximal bowel with oral and ventral suckers, causing ulcerations, necrosis, granulomas, and fibrosis. The diagnosis is usually made by identification of characteristic eggs on stool examination (Liu and Harinasuta 1996).

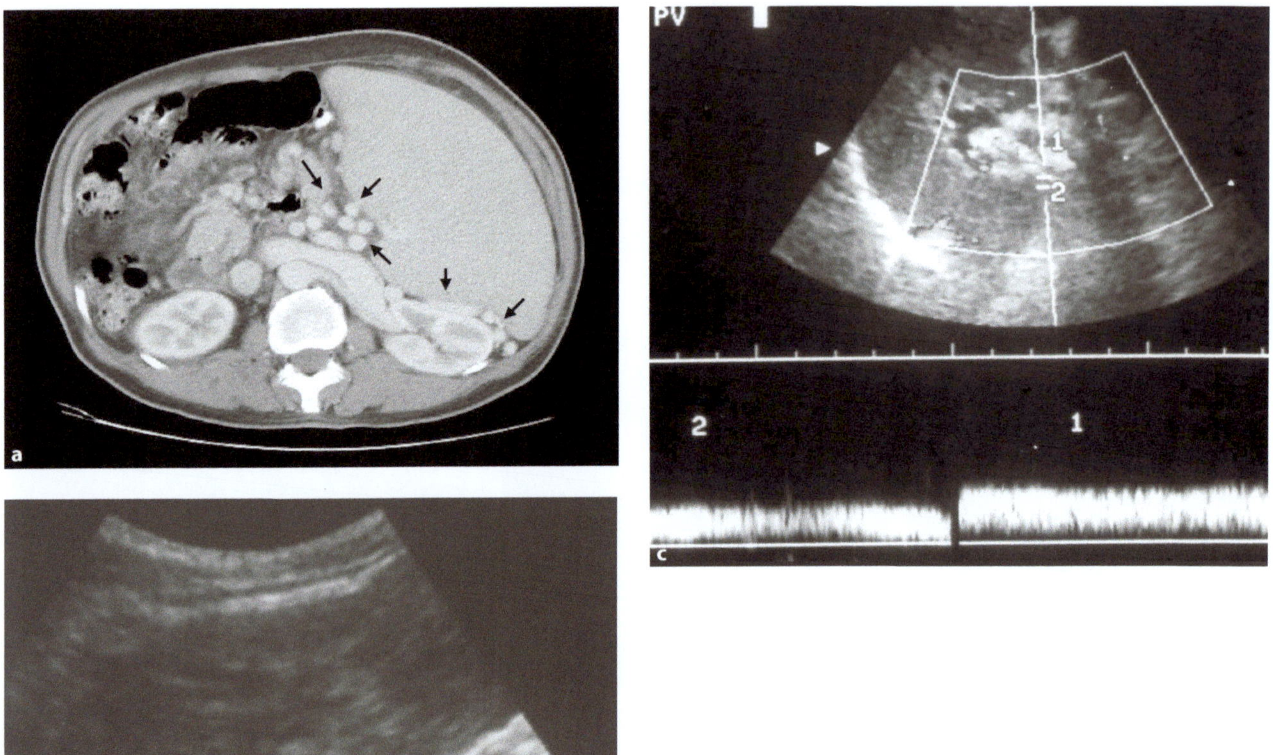

Fig. 4.18 Schistosomal portal hypertension. **a** CT scan showing splenomegaly with lienorenal collaterals (*arrows*). **b** US scan of the liver showing grade III periportal fibrosis (*arrows*) (Homeida et al. 1988) or class C rings and pipes (WHO 1996). **c** Split-second Doppler ultrasound image and spectral waveforms of cavernous transformation of the portal vein due to thrombosis caused by periportal fibrosis

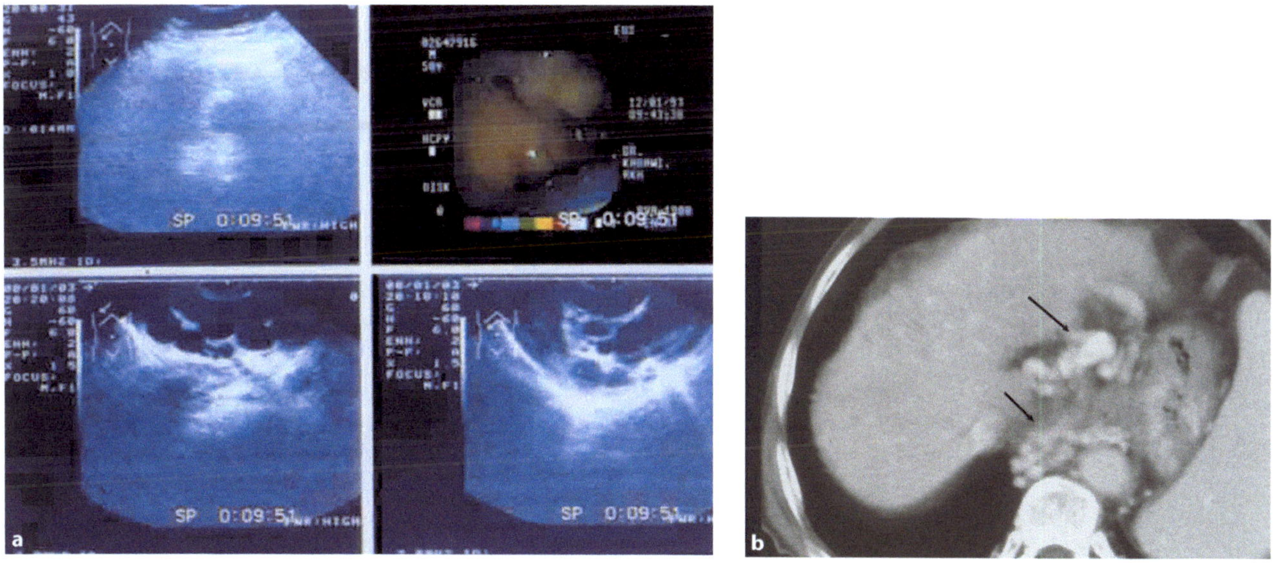

Fig. 4.19 Gastric varices. **a** Endoscopic view and endoscopic ultrasound demonstrating giant perigastric varices. **b** Contrast-enhanced CT scan image in the same patient showing the perigastric varices (*arrows*) and splenomegaly (Courtesy of Dr. Mohamed El Sheikh, Department of Gastroenterology, Riyadh Military Hospital, Riyadh, Saudi Arabia)

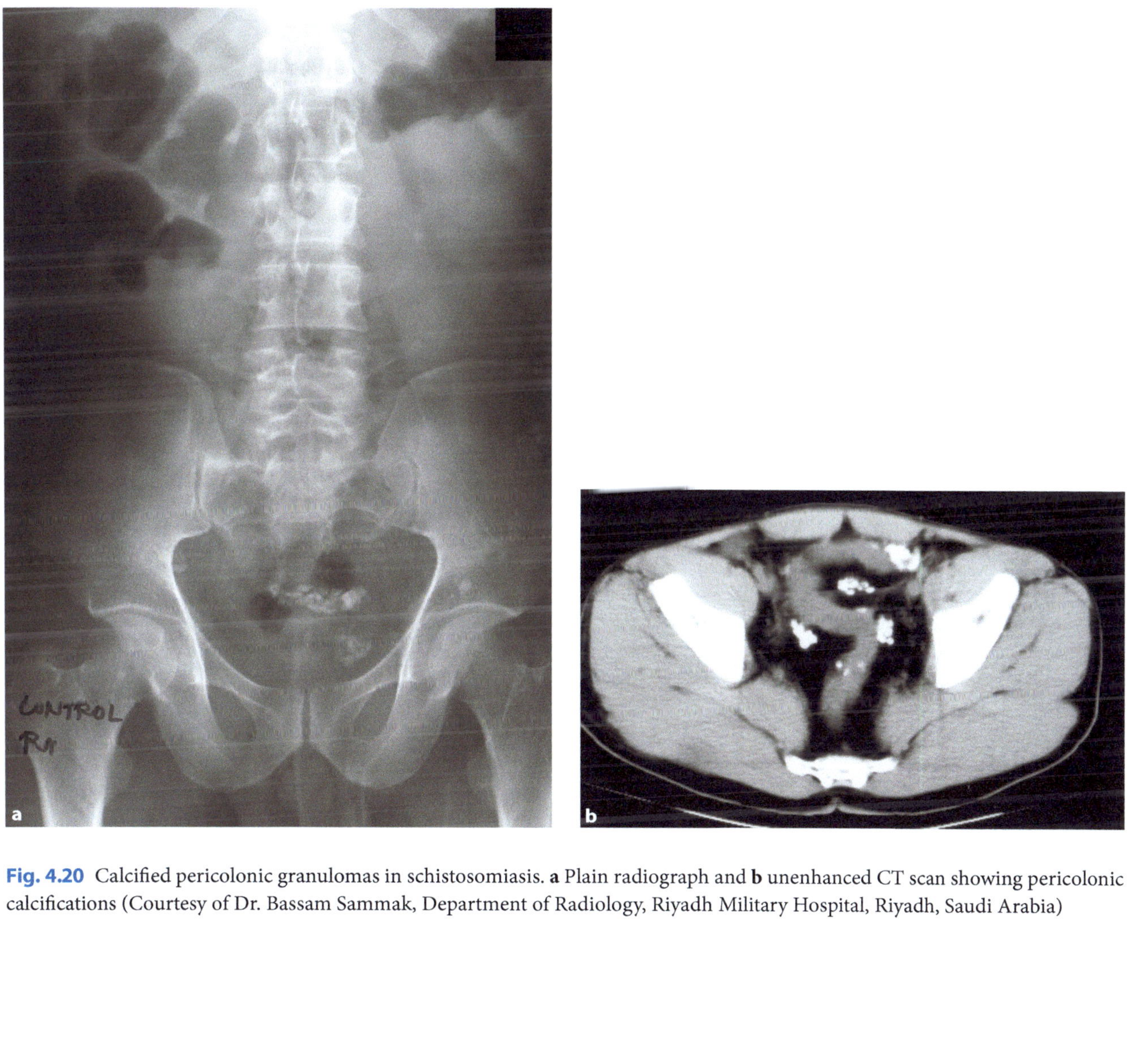

Fig. 4.20 Calcified pericolonic granulomas in schistosomiasis. **a** Plain radiograph and **b** unenhanced CT scan showing pericolonic calcifications (Courtesy of Dr. Bassam Sammak, Department of Radiology, Riyadh Military Hospital, Riyadh, Saudi Arabia)

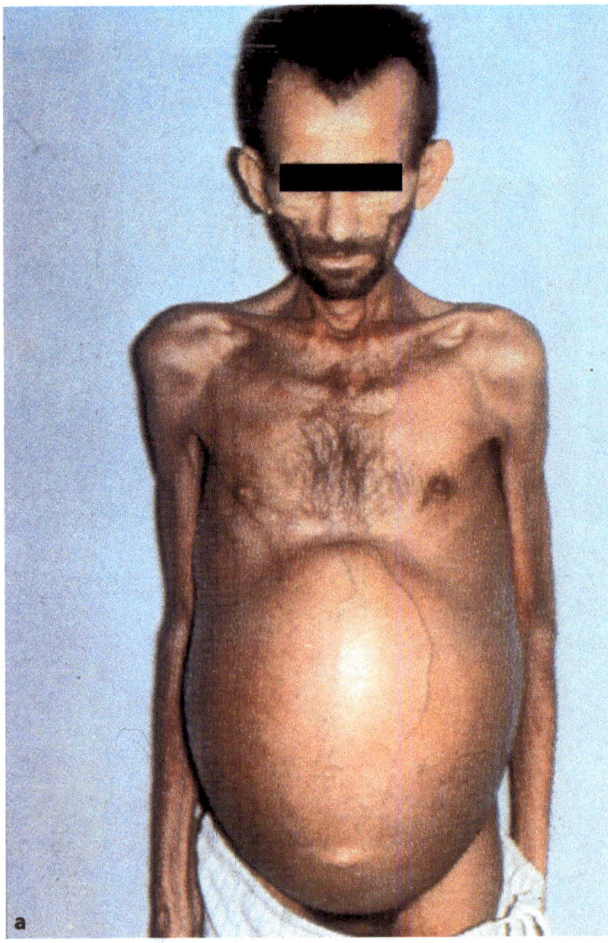

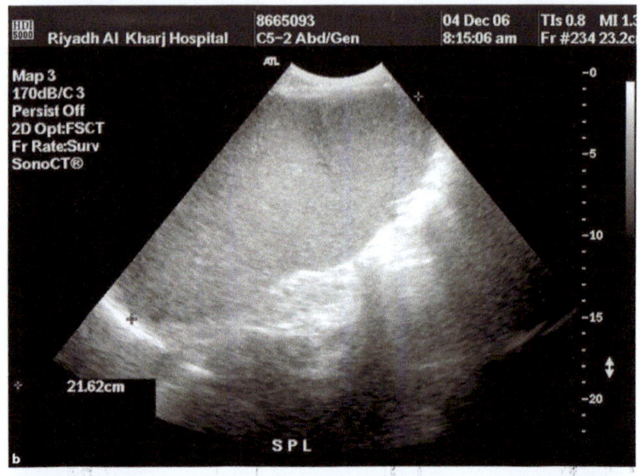

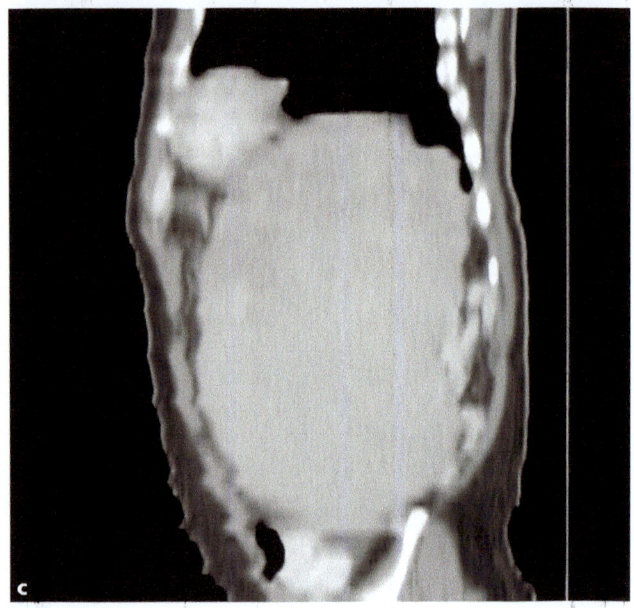

Fig. 4.21 Huge splenomegaly in schistosomiasis. **a** An adult cachectic peasant with ascites and huge splenomegaly. **b** Splenomegaly by ultrasound. **c** Parasagittal reconstructed CT scan image showing marked splenomegaly

4.11 Arthropods

4.11.1 Pentastomiasis

lives in the respiratory tract of snakes. Humans are infected by eating raw snakes or contaminated food. Patients are usually asymptomatic. Parasites cause typical calcifications (Fig. 4.22) in the body and trunk, not involving the limbs, unlike cysticerci (Thomas 1986).

4.11.2 Linguatulosis

Human ingestion of encysted nymphs in viscera, especially the raw liver of infected sheep or goats with *Linguatula serrata*, results in their liberation into the stomach and then migration upward up to the nasal passages, producing nasopharyngeal linguatulosis or "halzoun," first described from Lebanon (Khoury 1905), and has no radiological significance. Symptoms subside in a few days.

In previously endemic areas of Lebanon, the locals and physicians are familiar with this entity, where it is locally treated by the intake and gargling with a traditional alcoholic drink called "Arak." *L. serrata* infections are also known to occur in other countries of the Middle East, especially Sudan and Egypt (Morsy et al. 1999), where the ingestion of raw or undercooked infected viscera can result in a very similar entity called "Marrara."

4.12 Parasite-induced Acute Abdomen

Acute abdomen caused by parasites is infrequent, representing 3.9% of acute abdominal surgeries in a large series reported by Essomba et al. from Cameroon (2006).

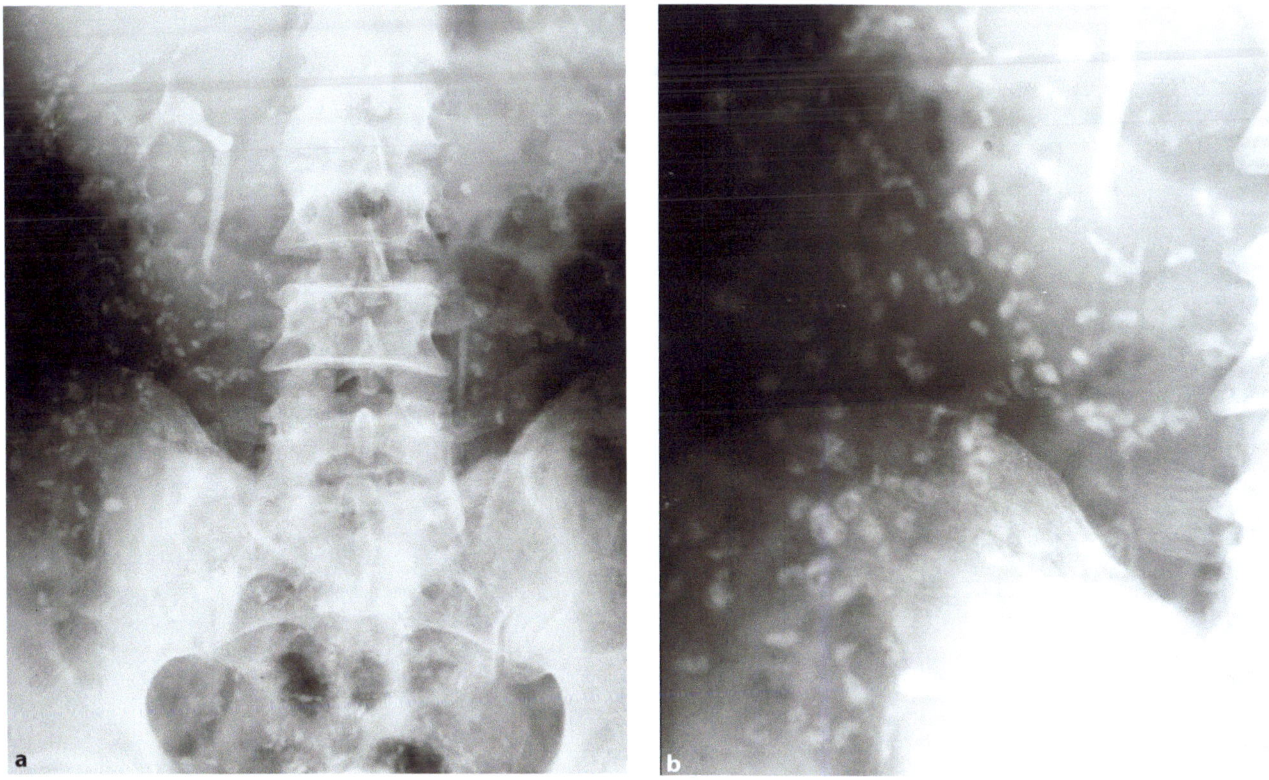

Fig. 4.22 Pentastomiasis of the peritoneum. **a** Intravenous urography film showing numerous scattered peritoneal calcifications due to burned-out pentastomiasis. **b** Close-up or magnified view demonstrating typical comma-shaped calcifications of pentastomiasis

The etiologies were: peritonitis secondary to the intraperitoneal rupture of amebic liver abscesses (47%), intestinal obstruction due to intestinal parasitism by *Ascaris lumbricoides* (18%) (Fig. 4.23), appendicitis of parasitic origin (15%), amebic typhlitis (11%), pancreatitis and angiocholitis secondary to ampulla of Vater obstruction by an adult *Ascaris* worm (3%), intestinal perforation by *Ascaris* (3%), and intestinal intussusception (3%).

In another large series reported by Gupta et al. from India, tropical appendicitis due to parasitic infestation was identified in 2.3% of pathology specimens following appendicectomies. The etiologies included enterobiasis (1.4%), amebiasis (0.5%), ascariasis (0.5%), ascariasis with trichuriasis (0.05%), and taeniasis (0.05%) (Gupta et al. 1989). Amebic trophozoites were observed on histopathological examination in 2.3% of appendectomy specimens reported from Mexico City by Guzman-Valdivia (2006).

Anisakiasis, sparganosis, gnathostomiasis, and pentastomiasis may also cause acute abdomen, manifesting as small bowel perforation or obstruction. The diagnosis of enteric anisakiasis should be considered in a patient presenting with acute abdomen after the ingestion of raw fish, such as sushi or sashimi delights (Masui et al. 2006; Yoon et al. 2004; Chikamori et al. 2004; Repiso Ortega et al. 2003; Sasaki et al. 2003; Ortega-Deballon et al. 2005; Cho et al. 1987; Dakubo et al. 2006). Angiostrongyliasis is another cause of intestinal ischemia and perforation, usually affecting the terminal ileum, cecum, and ascending colon (Loria-Cortes and Lobo-Sanahuja 1980).

The diagnosis of parasite-induced acute abdomen or parasitic eosinophilic gastroenteritis should be suspected, especially in patients presenting to emergency rooms after ingestion of seafood and in the presence of a high eosinophil count. Imaging, namely ultrasound and CT scanning, plays an important role in establishing a diagnosis of enterocolitis and eliminating other acute abdominal conditions, thus avoiding unnecessary surgery. A more specific and definitive diagnosis is usually obtained by serological tests and endoscopic biopsies. A conservative medical therapy can be instituted, while surgical exploration should be reserved for those presenting with intestinal necrosis associated with bowel perforation, or for patients with parasite-induced intestinal obstruction (Ido et al. 1998; Repiso Ortega et al. 2003; Ortega-Deballon et al. 2005; Essomba 2006).

4.13 GIP in the Immunocompromised Host

Persons with immunodeficient states, i.e., AIDS, cancer, and transplanted and splenectomized patients, have reduced immunity to parasites and are more predisposed to developing parasitic infections than the normal popu-

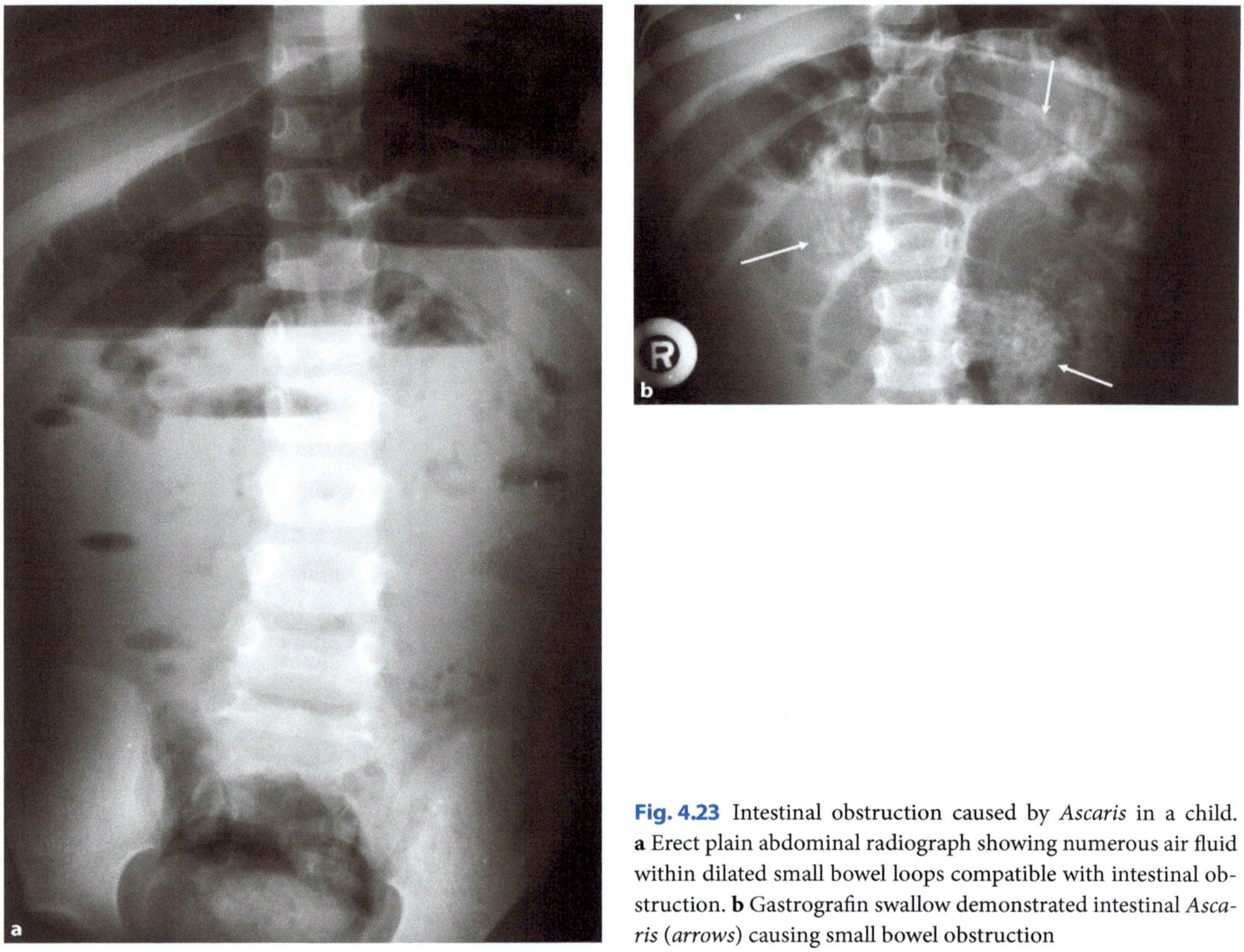

Fig. 4.23 Intestinal obstruction caused by *Ascaris* in a child. **a** Erect plain abdominal radiograph showing numerous air fluid within dilated small bowel loops compatible with intestinal obstruction. **b** Gastrografin swallow demonstrated intestinal *Ascaris* (*arrows*) causing small bowel obstruction

lation. In a retrospective review of all Ugandan cancer patients, 28% had GIP of medical importance (Robinson and Katongole-Mbidde 2006), while in the normal population, the incidence of intestinal parasites in presumably healthy subjects varies between 12.4% and 19.3% (Saab et al. 2004; Sayyari et al. 2005).

Strongyloides stercoralis is the only helminth to affect the immunocompromised patient significantly. Great proliferation of the worm from the intestine may send the filiform larva all over the body (Heyworth 1996).

Cryptosporidiasis can cause outbreaks of diarrhea and rarely cholangiopathy in HIV patients. Isosporiasis is also a common cause of diarrhea in these patients.

Hymenolepis nana may also produce a hyperinfection syndrome in the immunocompromised (Abd El Bagi et al. 2004). Another rare tropical disease that has been detected in European HIV patients is visceral leishmaniasis. The disease is now considered one of the indicators of HIV infection (Wilson and Streil 1996).

Imaging and serology, combined with endoscopic biopsies, provide a diagnosis in these patients with opportunistic hyperinfections.

4.14 Idiopathic Eosinophilic Gastroenteritis

Eosinophilic gastroenteritis is a rare disease. The pathogenesis and etiology are not very well understood, but association with seasonal allergies, food sensitivity, eczema, asthma, atopy, and elevated serum IgE levels suggests that a hypersensitivity response plays a major role in pathogenesis.

Clinically, the gastrointestinal symptoms are nonspecific, with eosinophilic gastroenteritis mimicking surgical conditions such as appendicitis and malignancies. Peripheral blood eosinophilia is present, and there is an absence of parasitic infestation.

Radiographically, eosinophilic gastroenteritis does not have a pathognomonic appearance. Radiographic changes are variable, nonspecific, and/or absent in at least 40% of patients. Ultrasound and CT scans may show thickened intestinal walls, and occasionally localized lymphadenopathy. Tc-99m HMPAO (hexamethylpropyleneamineoxime) scintigraphy helps in the detection of active inflammation in eosinophilic gastroenteritis, and in assessing response to treatment.

The differential diagnosis is other gastrointestinal diseases associated with peripheral eosinophilia such as intestinal parasites (ascariasis, taeniasis, schistosomiasis, trichuriasis, capillariasis, and strongyloidiasis), all causing eosinophilia, and can be excluded with careful examination of the stool for ova of parasites; Crohn's disease and ulcerative colitis; and idiopathic hypereosinophilic syndrome.

The definitive diagnosis of eosinophilic gastroenteritis is confirmed by endoscopic biopsies that reveal more than 20 eosinophils per high-power field on microscopic examination. Upper gastrointestinal endoscopy with biopsy of the stomach and small intestine is diagnostic in up to 80% of patients. Corticosteroid therapy is the mainstay of treatment of eosinophilic gastroenteritis (Baig et al. 2006; Chen et al. 2003b).

4.15 Conclusion

Entamoeba histolytica, G. lamblia, and *A. lumbricoides* are the commonest GIP. Malaria claims more lives than any other parasite. Prevalence of parasites is proportional to the state of hygiene, overcrowding, and literacy (Box 4.7). Transcontinental travel of tourists, military forces, refugees, and adopted children has lead to the spread of GIP. A high index of clinical suspicion is necessary to select patients for confirmatory tests. It is cheaper to treat high-risk groups like refugees and adopted children from developing countries than to perform laboratory tests. The sexual revolution has led to the proliferation of parasites. Some GIP are precancerous; some GIP are associated with malignancies, e.g., gastric carcinoma with *S. japonicum*, cholangiocarcinoma with clonorchiasis or opisthorchiasis and esophageal carcinoma with Chagas' megaesophagus. Global warming poses the threat of GIP proliferation.

Box 4.7 The millennial challenge of GIP?

- Proper hygiene
- Proper husbandry
- Proper sanitation
- Avoid overcrowding
- Human vaccine
- Live-stock vaccine
- Stop re-emerging parasites
- Mass therapy of high risks
- Stop global warming

References

Abd El Bagi ME, Al Karawi MA, Sammak B, et al. (1998) Water-enhanced "non-paralytic" transcutaneous ultrasound of the normal gastric wall layers (WETCUS). Hepatogastroenterology 45:2051–2054

Abd El Bagi ME, Sammak MB, Mohamed AE, Al Karawi MA, Al Shahed, Al Thagafi MA (2004)Gastrointestinal parasite infestation. Eur Radiol 14:E116–E131

Abu-Rumman AM (2001) Appendicitis and *entrobius vermicularis*. Sudan Med J 39:22–24

Ahmad L, El-Dib N, El-Boraey Y, Ibrahim M (1999) Capillaria phillippinensis: an emerging parasite causing severe diarrhea in Egypt. J Egypt Soc Parasitol 29:483–493

Al Karawi MA, Mohamed ARE, Yassawy I, et al. (1987) Non-surgical endoscopic transpapillary treatment of ruptured *Echinococcus* liver cyst obstructing the biliary tree. Endoscopy 19:81–83

Alkhalife IS, Hassan RR, Abdel-Hameed AA, Al-Khayal LA (2006) Diphyllobothriasis in Saudi Arabia. Saudi Med J 27(12):1901–1904

Amman RW, Eckert J (1996) *Echinococcus*. Gastroenterol Clin N Am 25:655–689

Anis MH, Shafeek H, Mansour NS, Moody A (1998) Intestinal capillariasis as a cause of chronic diarrhea in Egypt. J Egypt Soc Parasitol 28:143–147

Armignacco O, et al. (1989) *Strongyloides stercoralis* hyperinfection in acquired immunodeficiency syndrome. Am J Med 36:258

Austin DN, Mikhail MG, Chiodini PL, Murray-Lyon IM (1999) Intestinal capillariasis acquired in Egypt. Eur J Gastroenterol Hepatol 11:935–936

Baig MA, Qadir A, Rasheed J (2006) A review of eosinophilic gastroenteritis. J Natl Med Assoc 28(10):1616–1619

Barnett E (2004) Infectious disease screening for refugees resettled in the United States. Clin Infect Dis 39:833–841

Beggs I (1983) The radiological appearance of hydatid disease. Clin Radiol 34:555

Berger SA, Schwartz T, Michaeli D (1989) Infectious diseases among Ethiopian immigrants in Israel. Arch Intern Med 149(1):117–119

Botero JH, Castano A, Montoya MN, Ocampo NE, Hurtado MI, Lopera MM (2003) A preliminary study of the prevalence of intestinal parasites in immunocompromised patients with or without gastrointestinal manifestations. Rev Inst Med Trop Sao Paulo 45(4):197–200

Chao CC, Ray ML. Gastrointestinal: hookworm diagnosed by capsule endoscopy. J Gastroenterol Hepatol 21:1754

Chen L, Barnett E, Wilson M (2003a) Preventing infectious diseases during and after international adoption. Ann Intern Med 139:371–378

Chen M-J, Chu C-H, Lin S-C, Shih S-C, Wong T-E (2003b) Eosinophilic gastroenteritis: clinical experience with 15 patients. World J Gastroenterol 9(12):2813–2816

Chikamori F, Kuniyoshi N, Takase Y (2004) Intussusception due to intestinal anisakiasis: a case report. Abdom Imaging 29:39–41

Cho KJ, Lee HS, Chi JG (1987) Intramural sparganosis manifested as intestinal obstruction. J Kor Med Sci 2:137–139

Choi B, Han J, Hong S, et al. (2004) Clonorchiasis and cholangiocarcinoma: etiologic relationship and imaging diagnosis. Clin Microbiol Rev 17(3):540–552

Collins CD, Blanshard C, Cramp M, Gazzard B, Gleeson JA (1992) Case report: pneumatosis intestinalis occurring in association with cryptosporidiosis and HIV infection. Clin Radiol 46:410–411

Dairymple RB (1982) Hyperechoic liver abscess: unusual ultrasonic appearances. Clin Radiol 33:541

Dakubo JC, Etwire VK, Kumoji R, Naaeder SB (2006) Human pentastomiasis: a case report. West Afr J Med 25(2):166–168

Dunn IJ, Palmer PES (1998) Sparganosis. Semin Rontgenol 33(1):86–88

El-Dib NA, Doss WH. Intestinal capillariasis in Egypt: epidemiological background. J Egypt Soc Parasitol 32:145–154

El Sheikh Mohamed AR, Al Karawi MA, Yassawy MI (1991) Modern techniques in the diagnosis and treatment of gastrointestinal and biliary tree parasites. Hepatogastroenterology 38:180–188

Elliot DE (1996) *Schistosomiasis*, pathophysiology, diagnosis and treatment. Gastroenterol Clin N Am 25:599–625

Essomba A, Chichon Mefire A, Fokou M, Ohassouo P, Masso Misse P, Esiene A, Abolo LM, Malonga EE (2006) Acute abdomen of parasitic origin: retrospective analysis of 135 cases. Ann Chir 131:194–197

Fabijanic D, Guino L, Invani N, et al. (2001) Ultrasonographic appearance of colon taeniasis. J Ultrasound 20:275–277

Facer C, Tanner M (1997) Clinical trials of malaria vaccine. In: Baker J, Muller R, Rollingson D (eds) Advances in parasitology, vol 39. Academic, London, p 2

Farthing MJ (1996) Giardiasis. Gastroenterol Clin N Am 25:493–514

Gilles H (1995) Trichuriasis. In: Cook G (ed) Masons tropical diseases, 20th edn. Saunders, London, pp 1372–1374

Gittleman AL (2001) Guess what came to dinner? 2nd edn. Avery, Garden City Park, NY

Goldsmid J, Kibel MA, Mills AE (1992) *Entrobius vermicularis*. In: Campbell AGN, MC Intoch N (eds) Forfar and Arneil's textbook of paediatrics, 4th edn. Churchill Livingstone, London, pp 1544–1546

Gonzales de Canales Simon P, del Olmo Martinez L, Cortejaso Hernandez A, Arranz Santos T (2000) Colonic balantidiasis. Gastroenterol Hepatol 23(3):129–131

Gupta SC, Gupta AK, Keswani NK, Single PA, Tripathi AK, Krishna V (1989) Pathology of tropical appendicitis. J Clin Pathol 42:1169–1172

Guzman-Valdivia G (2006) Acute amebic encephalitis. World J Surg 30(6):1038–1042

Haddad M, Sammak B, Al-Karawi (2000) Percutaneous treatment of heterogenous predominantly solid echopattern echinoccocal cysts of the liver. Cardiovasc Intervent Radiol 23(2):121–125

Hakim SZ, Genta RM (1986) Fatal disseminated strongyloidiasis in a Vietnam War veteran. Arch Pathol Lab Med 110:809–812

Hartong WA, Gourley WK, Arvanitakis C (1979) Giardiasis: clinical spectrum and functional-structural abnormalities of the small intestinal mucosa. Gastroenterology 77:61–69

Heyworth MF (1996) Parasitic diseases in immunocompromised hosts: cryptosporidiosis, isosporiasis, and strongyloidiasis. Gastroenterol Clin N Am 25:691–707

Homeida M, Abdel-Gadir A, Cheever AQ, et al. (1988) Diagnosis of pathologically confirmed Symmer's periportal fibrosis by ultrasonography: a prospective blinded study. Am J Trop Med Hyg 38:86–91

Ido K, Yuasa H, Ide M, Kimura Km Toshimitsu K, Suzuki T (1998) Sonographic diagnosis of small intestinal anisakiasis. J Clin Ultrasound 26(3):125–130

Juniper K (1962) Acute amoebic colitis. Am J Med 33:377–386

Karawi MA, Salam I, Mohamed ARE (1989) Endoscopic diagnosis and extraction of biliary ascariasis: a case report. Ann Saudi Med 9:80–81

Katz DE, Taylor DN (2001) Parasitic infections of the gastrointestinal tract. Gastroenterol Clin N Am 30:797–815

Khoury A (1905) Le Halzoun. Arch Parasitol 9:78–94

Khuroo MS (1996) Ascariasis. Gastroenterol Clin N Am 25:553–576

Khuroo MS, Zargar SA, Mahajan R (1991) *Echinococcus granulosus* cysts in the liver: management with percutaneous drainage. Radiology 180:141–145

Kimura K, Stoopen M, Reeder M, Moncada R (1997) Amoebiasis: modern diagnostic imaging with pathological and clinical correlation. Semin Roentgenol 32:250–275

Laughon BE, Druckman DA, Vernon A, et al. (1988) Prevalence of enteric pathogens in homosexual men with and without acquired immunodeficiency syndrome. Gastroenterology 94:984–993

Leutscher Peter DC, Bagley SW (2003) Health-related challenges in United States Peace Corps volunteers serving for two years in Madagascar. J Travel Med 10(5):263

Lewall D (1998) Hydatid disease: biology, pathology, imaging and classification. Clin Radiol 53:863–874

Lewis FR, Holcroft JR, Boey J, et al. (1975) Appendicitis: a critical review, diagnosis and treatment in 1000 cases. Arch Surg 110:677

Li E, Stanley SL (1996) Amoebiasis. Gastroenterol Clin N Am 25:471–492

Liu LX, Harinasuta KT (1996) Liver and intestinal flukes. Gastroenterol Clin N Am 25(3):627–636

Loria-Cortes R, Lobo-Sanahuja JF (1980) Clinical abdominal angiostrongylosis. A study of 116 children with intestinal eosinophilic granuloma caused by Angiostrongylosis costaricensis. Am J Trop Med Hyg 29:538–544

Macedo T, MacCarty RL (2000) Eosinophilic ileocolitis secondary to *Enterobius vermicularis*: case report. Abdom Imaging 25:530–532

Macpherson CN (2005). Human behaviour and the epidemiology of parasitic zoonoses. Int J Parasitol 35(11–12):1319–1331

Magill AJ, Grogl M, Gasser R, et al. (1993) Visceral infection caused by Leishmania tropica in veterans of Operation Desert Storm. N Engl J Med 328:1383–1386

Mahmood T, Mansoor N, Quraishy S, Ilyas M, Hussain S (2001) Ultrasonographic appearance of *Ascaris lumbricoides* in the small bowel. J Ultrasound Med 20:269–274

Mansour NS, Anis MH, Mikhail EM (1990) Human intestinal capillariasis in Egypt. Trans R Soc Trop Med Hyg 84(1):114

Markell EK, Voge MA, John DT (1992) Medical parasitology, 7th edn. Saunders, Philadelphia

Marsden P (1995) American trypanosomiasis. In: Cook G (ed) Manson's tropical diseases. Saunders, London, p 1205

Martinez S, Restrepo S, Carrillo J, et al. (2005) Thoracic manifestations of tropical parasitic infections: a pictorial review. Radiographics 25:135–155

Masui N, Fujima N, Hasegawa T, Kigawa S, et al. (2006) Small bowel strangulation caused by parasitic peritoneal strand. Pathol Int 56:345–349

Mattoso LF, Reeder MM (1998) Radiological diagnosis of Chagas' disease (American trypanosomiasis). Semin Roentgenol 33:26–46

Memorias do Institutto Oswaldo Cruz, Rio de Janeiro (2001) 96:151–156

Mohamed ARE, Al Karawi MA, Yasawy MI (1990) Intestinal and hepatosplenic schistosomiasis: case series and review of the literature. J Am Med Assoc 20:241–247

Morgan AD, Brockhurst MA, Lopez-Pascua L, et al. (2007) Differential impact of simultaneous migration on coevolving hosts and parasites. BMC Evol Biol 7:1

Morsy TA, El-Sharkawy IM, Lashin AH (1999) Human nasopharyngeal linguatuliasis (Pentasomida) caused by *Linguatula serrata*. J Egypt Soc Parasitol 29(3):787–790

Nettleman MD (1996) Preparing the international traveler. Gastroenterol Clin N Am 25:451–469

Ortega-Deballon P, Carabias-Hernández A, Martín-Blázquez A, Garaulet P, Benoit L, Kretz B, Limones-Esteban M, Favre JP (2005) [Anisakiasis: an infestation to be known by surgeons]. Ann Chir 130(6–7):407–410

Palmer PES (1998) Schistosomiasis. Semin Roentgenol 33:6–25

Panet M, Viola A, Confort-Gouny S, et al. (2005) Imaging experimental cerebral malaria in vivo: significant role of ischemic brain edema. J Neurosci 25(32):7352–7358

Paolantonio P, Rengo M, Iafrate F, Martino G, Laghi A (2006) Diagnosis of Taenia saginata by MR enterography. AJR Am J Roentgenol 187(2):W238

Pedrosa I, Saiz A, Arrazola J et al. (2000) Hydatid disease: radiologic and pathologic features and complications. Radiographics 20:795–817

Phillips SC, Mildvan D, William DC, et al. (1981) Sexual transmission of enteric protozoa and helminths in a venereal disease clinic population. N Engl J Med 305:603–606

Polat P, Kantarci M, Alper F, et al. (2003) Hydatid disease from head to toe. Radiographics 23:475–494

Polenakovik H, Polenakovik S (2006) www.emedicine.com/med/topic2189.htm

Poulin R (2006) Global warming and temperature mediated increases in cercarial emergence in trematode parasites. Parasitology 132(Pt1):143–151

Poulin R, Mouritsen K (2006) Climate change, parasitism and the structure of intertidal echosystems. J Helminthol 80(2):183–191

Pulpeiro J, Armesto V, Varela J, et al. (1991) Fascioliasis: findings in 15 patients Br J Radiol 64:798–801

Reeder MM (1997) Radiological diagnosis of giardiasis. Semin Roentgenol 32:291–300

Reeder MM (1998) The radiological and US evaluation of ascariasis of the gastrointestinal, biliary and respiratory tracts. Semin Gastroenterol 33:57–58

Reeder MM, Palmer PES (1994) Parasitic disease. In: Freeny P, Stevenson GW (eds) Margulis and Burhenne's alimentary tract radiology, 5th edn. Mosby, St. Louis, pp 913–951

Repiso Ortega A, Alcantara Torres M, Gonzales de Frutos C, et al. (2003) Gastrointestinal anisakiasis. Study of a series of 25 patients. Gastroenterol Hepatol 26(6):341–346

Rha S, Ha H, Kim J, et al. (1999) CT features of intraperitoneal manifestations of parasitic infestation. AJR Am J Roentgenol 172:1289–1292

Robinson AJ, Katongole-Mbidde E (2006) Gastrointestinal parasites in Ugandan cancer patients: a retrospective departmental review. Trop Doct 365:188

Saab BR, Musharrafieh U, Nassar NT, Khogali M, Araj GF (2004) Intestinal parasites among presumably healthy individuals in Lebanon. Saudi Med J 25(1):34–37

Sammak B, Yousef B, Mohamed AR, et al. (1999) Radiological manifestations of liver and gastrointestinal parasitic infections. Hepatogastroenterology 46:1016–1022

Sangkhathat S, Patrapinyokul S, Wudhisuthimethawee P, Chedphaopan J, Mitamun W (2003) Massive gastrointestinal bleeding in infants with ascariasis. J Pediatr Surg 38(11):1696–1698

Saraswat VA, Agarwal SS, Baijal S, et al. (1992) Percutaneous catheter drainage of amoebic liver abscess. Clin Radiol 45:187–189

Sargeaunt PG, Oates JK, MacLennan I, et al. (1983) Entamoeba histolytica in male homosexuals. Br J Vener Dis 59:193–195

Sasaki T, Fukumori D, Matsumoto H, Ohmori H, Yamamoto F (2003) Small bowel obstruction caused by anisakiasis of the small bowel: report of a case. Surg Today 33:123–125

Sauvage PJ, Rabii A, Coz JM, de Carsalade GY, Thery Y, Wolf PY (2006) What is your diagnosis? J Radiol 87:1899–1901

Sayyari AA, Imanzadeh F, Bagheri Yazdi SA, Karami H, Yaghoobi M (2005) Prevalence of intestinal parasitic infections in the Islamic Republic of Iran. East Mediterr Health J 11(3):377–383

Schulze S, Chokshi R, Edavettal M, et al. (2005) Acute abdomen secondary to Ascaris lumbricoides. Am Surg 71(6):505–507

Symmer WC (1904) Note on a new form of liver cirrhosis due to the presence of ova of Bilharzia haematobium. J Pathol Bacteriol 9:237–239

Thomas A (1986) Radiological manifestations of parasitic diseases. Br J Hosp Med 35(3):303–311

Tokmak N, Koc Z, Ulusan S, Koltas SK, Bal N (2006) Computed tomographic findings of trichuriasis. World J Gastroenterol 12(26):4210–4212

Von Sinner WN (1997) Advanced medical imaging and treatment of human cystic echinococcosis. Semin Roentgenol 32:276–290

WHO (1991) Report of a World Health Organization Expert Committee on control of Chagas' disease. World Health Organization, Geneva

WHO (1995) Control of tropical diseases (CTD). World Health Organization, Geneva

WHO (1996) Ultrasound in schistosomiasis. UNDP/World Bank/WHO. Second International Workshop 22–26 October 1996. Niamey, Niger

Walsh JA (1986) Problems in recognition and diagnosis of amoebiasis: estimation of global magnitude or morbidity and mortality. Rev Infect Dis 8:288

Wilson ME, Streil JA (1996) Visceral leishmaniasis. Gastroenterol Clin N Am 25:535–551

World Bank (1993) World development report. Investing in health. Oxford University Press, Oxford

World Health Organization (1981) Intestinal protozoa and helminthic infections, technical report series 666. World Health Organization, Geneva

Yasawy MI (2004) Katayama syndrome. Saudi Med J 25(2):234–236

Yoon S-W, Yu J-S, Park M-S, Shim JY, Kim HJ, Kim KW (2004) CT findings of surgically verified acute invasive small bowel anisakiasis resulting in small bowel obstruction. Yonsei Med J 45(4):739–742

Youssef FG, Mikhail EM, Mansour NS (1989) Intestinal capillariasis in Egypt: a case report. Am J Trop Med Hyg 40:195–196

Zaman V (1984) Protozoa. In: Zaman V (ed) Atlas of medical parasitology, 2nd edn. ADIS Health Science, p 1

Zaman V, Keong LH (1990) Handbook of medical parasitology, 2nd edn. Ang, Singapore, p 1

Chapter

Imaging of Parasitic Diseases of the Hepatobiliary Tract, Pancreas, and Spleen

5

Maurice C. Haddad, Ghassan N. Al Awar

Contents

5.1 Introduction

The objective of this chapter is to increase the awareness and knowledge of tropical and especially nontropical radiologists and physicians with regard to the imaging findings of parasitic diseases that can affect the hepatobiliary system, spleen, and pancreas.

Viscerotropic parasites can reach the liver or biliary tree by several pathways (Fig. 5.1): via the arterial bloodstream (visceral leishmaniasis, malaria, babesiosis, trypanosomiasis), via the mesenteric venous plexus (amebiasis, toxoplasmosis, cryptosporidiosis, toxocariasis, strongyloidiasis, capillariasis, echinococcosis, schistosomiasis, visceral linguatulosis), by retrograde migration from the duodenum into the biliary tree (giardiasis, ascariasis, taeniasis, strongyloidiasis, clonorchiasis, opisthorchiasis, dicrocoeliasis), and penetration through the intestinal or gastric wall into the peritoneal cavity and liver capsule (fascioliasis, paragonimiasis, angiostrongyliasis, pentastomiasis, gnathostomiasis).

5.2 Protozoa

5.2.1 Amebic Liver Abscess

The parasite *Entamoeba histolytica* is prevalent worldwide. The clinical and cross-sectional imaging findings of amebic liver abscesses (ALA) are nonspecific and may be misleading. Patients with ALA may or may not have fever or gastrointestinal symptoms. On ultrasonography ALA may initially at the early presuppurative stage simulate a solid hepatic mass (Fig. 5.2a) because of its echogenic necrotic content (Ralls et al. 1982; Dairymple 1982), or more commonly at the suppurative stage shows a cystic lesion containing low-level echoes or layering debris (Fig 5.3a) simulating a type CE 1a hepatic echinococcal cyst with layering hydatid sand in its dependent portion or a hemorrhagic or infected cyst with internal low-level echoes. On CT scans (Figs. 5.2b, 5.4b), ALA has imaging features indistinguishable from a pyogenic abscess. The diagnosis is usually established by positive amebic serology and fine needle aspiration, which shows an odorless reddish brown or chocolate-colored "anchovy paste"

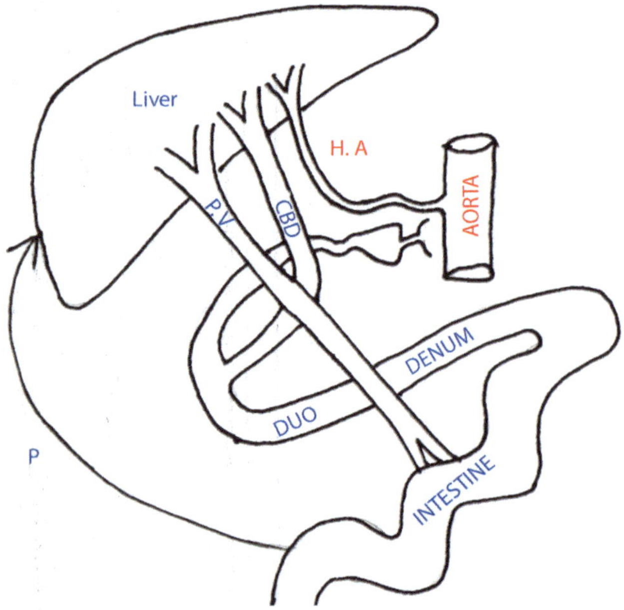

Fig. 5.1 Schematic diagram of pathways for viscerotropic parasites. *HA* hepatic artery, *CBD* common bile duct, *PV* portal venous system, *P* intestinal perforation and peritoneal migration

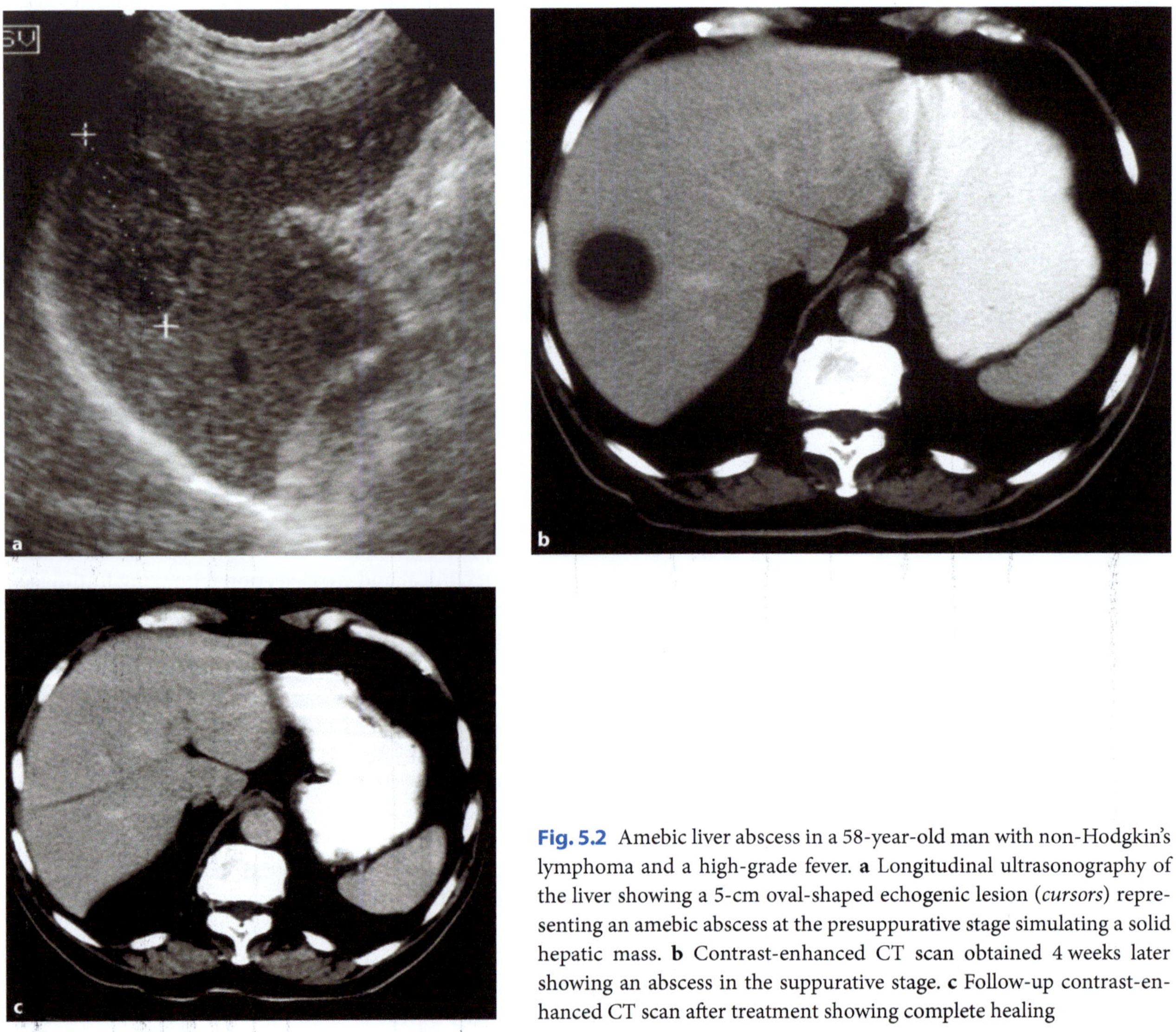

Fig. 5.2 Amebic liver abscess in a 58-year-old man with non-Hodgkin's lymphoma and a high-grade fever. **a** Longitudinal ultrasonography of the liver showing a 5-cm oval-shaped echogenic lesion (*cursors*) representing an amebic abscess at the presuppurative stage simulating a solid hepatic mass. **b** Contrast-enhanced CT scan obtained 4 weeks later showing an abscess in the suppurative stage. **c** Follow-up contrast-enhanced CT scan after treatment showing complete healing

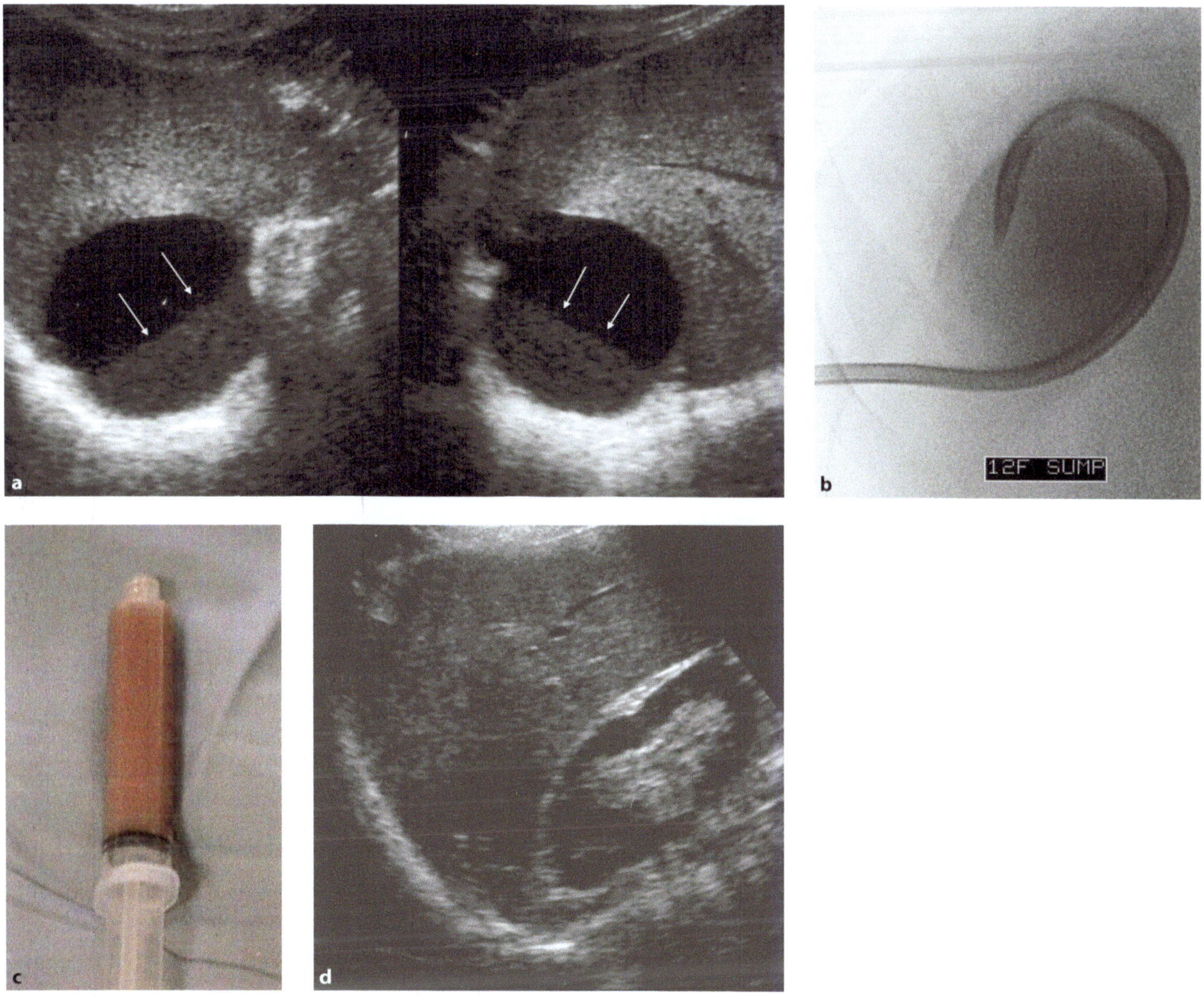

Fig. 5.3 Amebic liver abscess in a 60-year-old man with right upper quadrant pain but no fever. **a** Ultrasonography of the liver obtained in two different positions showing movable layering debris (*arrows*) within a large amebic abscess. **b** Percutaneous catheter drainage was performed. **c** Reddish-brown fluid was aspirated. Culture was negative. **d** Follow-up ultrasonography showing complete healing

pus (Figs. 5.3c, 5.4c) (Krige and Beckingham 2001). The Gram stain is negative and the culture is sterile yielding no bacterial growth. Microscopy of the aspirate may not identify the parasite because it may be present in the wall of the abscess (Krige and Beckingham 2001). Percutaneous catheter drainage combined with medical therapy is the treatment of choice for ALA larger than 5 cm in size (Fig. 5.3b). "*Restituo ad integrum*," i.e., complete healing without cicatrization following treatment (Figs. 5.2c, 5.3d, 5.4d), is a peculiar feature of ALA.

5.2.2 Visceral Leishmaniasis

Several *Leishmania* species exist in endemic regions; however, a special form of infantile visceral leishmaniasis may be encountered in the Mediterranean basin and Middle East as isolated cases due to *Leishmania infantum* (Wilson and Streit 1996; Knio et al. 2000; Nuwayri-Salti et al. 2000), which affects the reticulo-endothelium system of several organs including liver and spleen. The clinical and laboratory manifestations of visceral leishmaniasis

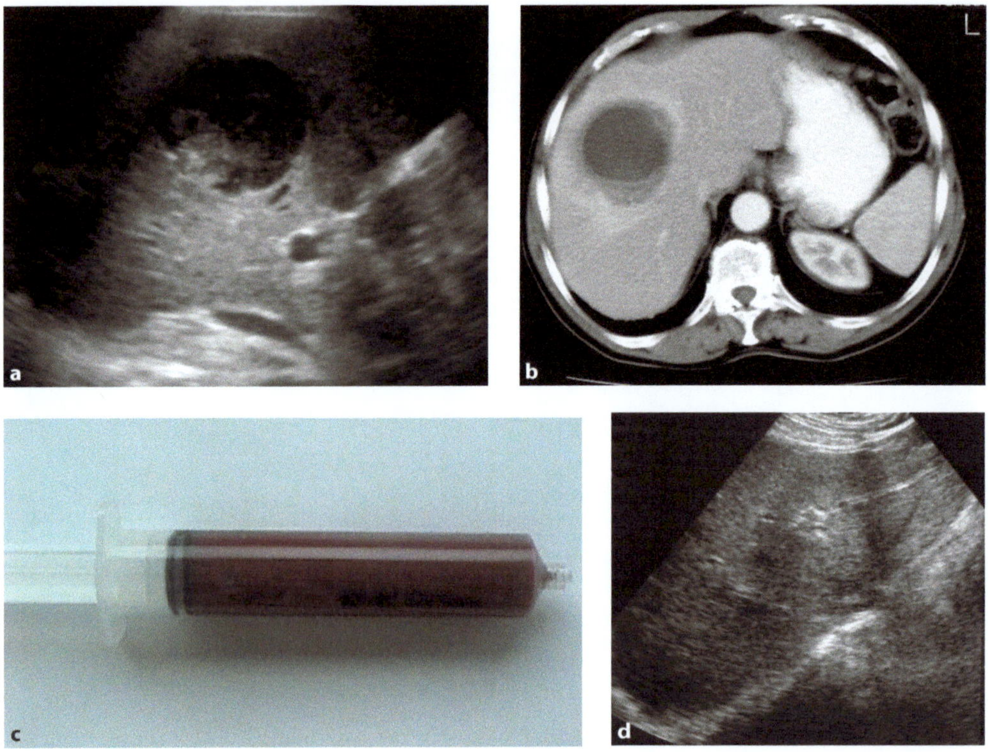

Fig. 5.4 Amebic liver abscess. **a** Ultrasound image of liver showing a round lesion with internal echoes and posterior acoustic enhancement compatible with a fluid-filled lesion. **b** Contrast-enhanced CT scan of liver demonstrating an abscess with minimal peripheral rim enhancement. **c** Chocolate-colored pus compatible with amebic liver abscess. **d** Follow-up ultrasonography of liver showing complete healing, i.e., "*restituo ad integrum*" after treatment

consist of fever, hepatosplenomegaly, lymphadenopathy, neutropenia and thrombocytopenia, and abnormal liver function tests. These findings are nonspecific and a large spectrum of diseases enter into the clinical differential diagnoses including leukemia, lymphoma, histoplasmosis, tuberculosis, salmonellosis, chronic granulomatous disease, malaria, viral infection and mononucleosis.

The imaging findings are also nonspecific, consisting of hepatosplenomegaly with prominent low density periportal tracking on contrast-enhanced CT scan indicating periportal inflammation or edema, ascites and thickened gallbladder wall, and the presence of enlarged lymph nodes (Fig. 5.5a–c). Bacterial or fungal superinfections (Fig. 5.5d,e) occur in 60% of patients because of neutropenia and severe immunodepression (Wilson and Streit 1996). Rarely, visceral leishmaniasis may show nodularity in the liver and spleen appearing on ultrasonography as solid nodules surrounded by peripheral hypoechoic halos, and on CT and MR as hypovascular lesions (Fig. 5.6) (Canalias et al. 1997; Bukte et al. 2004). Metabolic total body imaging using F-18 FDG PET/CT, showed discrete diffuse increased radioactive uptake in the skeleton and a patchy granular aspect of the increased uptake in the liver and spleen, highly suggestive of marked hypermetabolism and diffuse reticuloendothelial activation (Lupi et al. 2006).

The diagnosis can be established by enzyme-linked immunosorbent assay (ELISA) serology or skin testing with the *Leishmania* antigen, and confirmed by identification of intracellular amastigote (Farah et al. 1975) in splenic fine needle aspirate performed under imaging guidance (Fig. 5.6d), which is a highly sensitive but risky test because splenic puncture in a patient with thrombocytopenia may lead to a hemorrhagic complication. Therefore, a bone marrow or lymph node biopsy is a preferable alternative for obtaining tissue specimens.

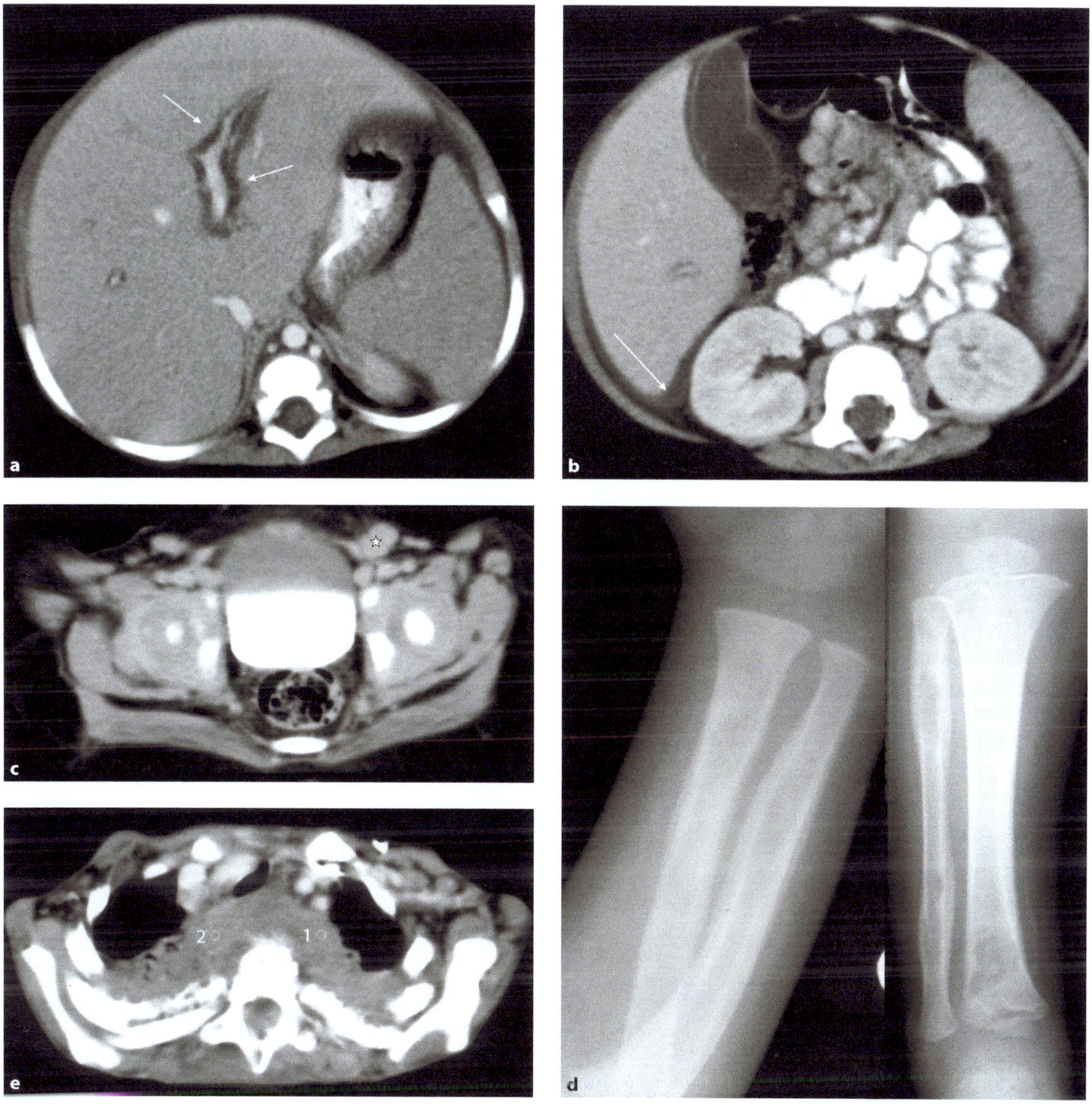

Fig. 5.5 Two-year-old boy with visceral leishmaniasis. **a–c** Contrast-enhanced CT scan images showing hepatosplenomegaly with periportal tracking (*white arrows*) due to inflammation, ascites (*white arrow*) in Morrison's pouch, and enlarged left inguinal lymph node (*star*). These changes completely healed following medical treatment. **d** Plain radiographs of the right leg and forearm showing lytic lesions of the long bones with periosteal reactions due to *Salmonella* osteomyelitis hyperinfection. **e** Contrast-enhanced CT scan of the chest showing fungal hyperinfection of the posterior chest wall by *Aspergillus*

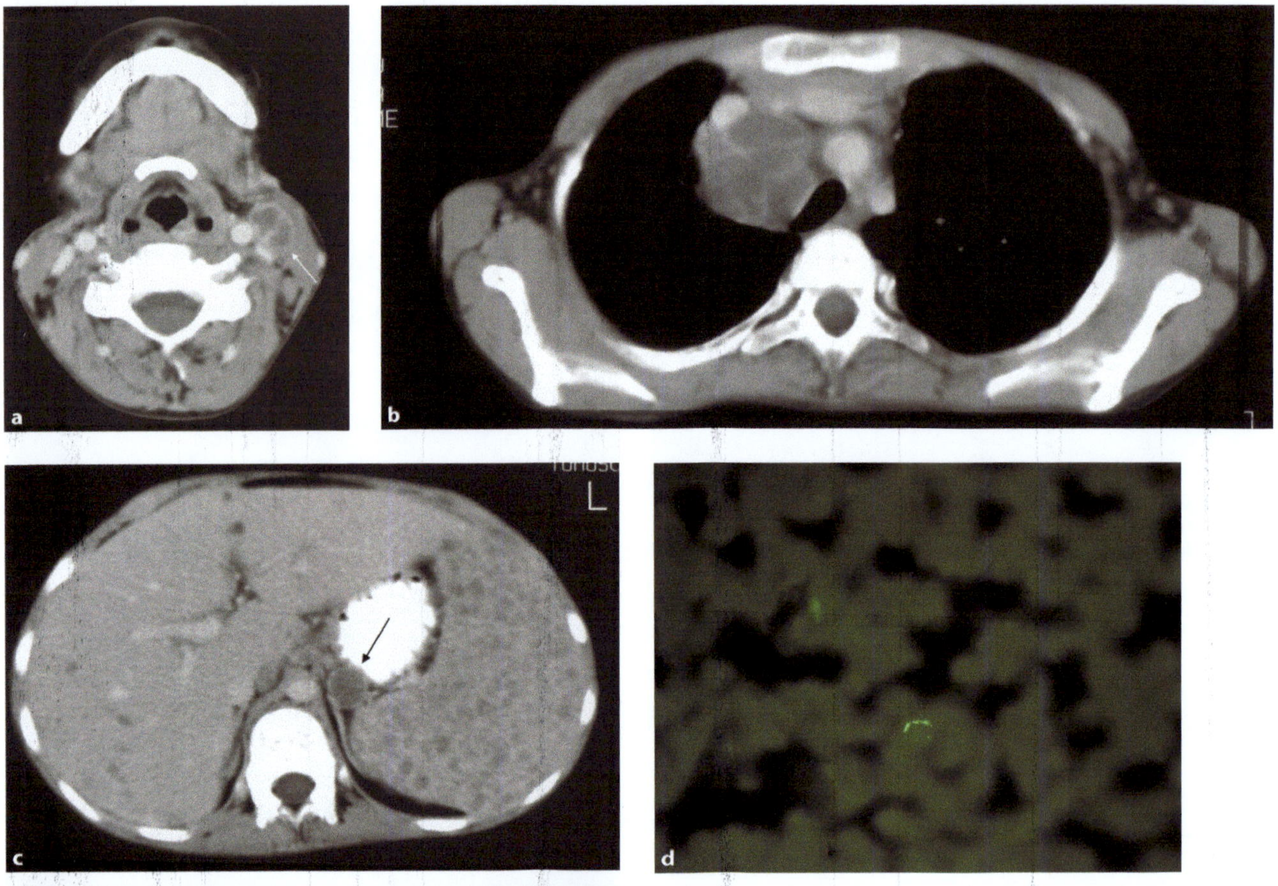

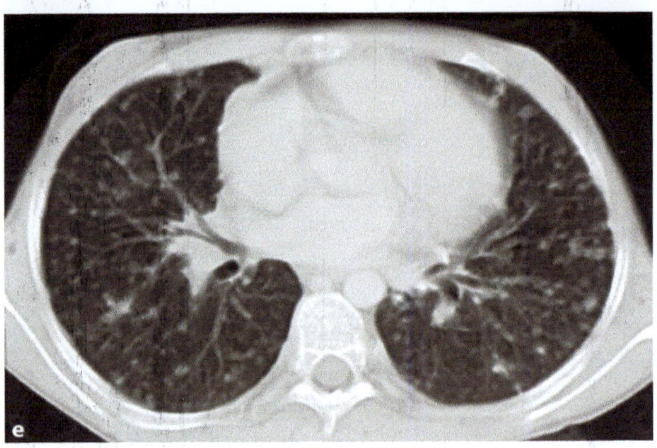

Fig. 5.6 Twelve-year-old girl with visceral leishmaniasis. **a,b** Contrast-enhanced CT scans of the neck and chest showing enlarged cervical (*arrow*) and mediastinal lymph nodes. **c** Contrast-enhanced CT scan of the abdomen showing hepatosplenomegaly with numerous hepatic and splenic small nodules, and enlarged perigastric lymph node (*arrow*). **d** Microphotograph of a splenic fine needle aspirate showing intracellular *Leishmania* organisms using immunofluorescence with rabbit anti-*Leishmania* antibodies (Courtesy of Professor Nuha Nuwayri-Salti, Human Morphology Department, American University of Beirut, Beirut, Lebanon). **e** CT scan of the chest showing hyperinfection of the lungs with miliary tuberculosis in the same patient

5.2.3 Acquired Disseminated Toxoplasmosis

Toxoplasmosis is a disease with worldwide prevalence. Acquired toxoplasmosis in the immunocompetent person is usually asymptomatic and self-limiting. However, in the immunosuppressed patient acquired disseminated toxoplasmosis may develop with involvement of multiple organs including liver, lungs, brain, bones, heart, and others. The clinical picture is nonspecific, consisting of fever and hepatosplenomegaly, it simulates other diseases such as mononucleosis, lymphoma, leukemia, malaria, salmonella, virus infection (cytomegalovirus, Epstein–Barr virus), histoplasmosis, and tuberculosis. The liver function tests are abnormal.

On the imaging of acquired disseminated toxoplasmosis (Fig. 5.7), the liver and spleen are enlarged. The liver shows prominent portal tracts due to inflammation. In the brain, characteristic but nonspecific ring-enhancing lesions may be identified in 50% of patients. A ring-enhancing lesion with eccentric nodule "asymmetric target sign" was described as a virtually pathognomonic sign seen in approximately 30% of patients with acute cerebral

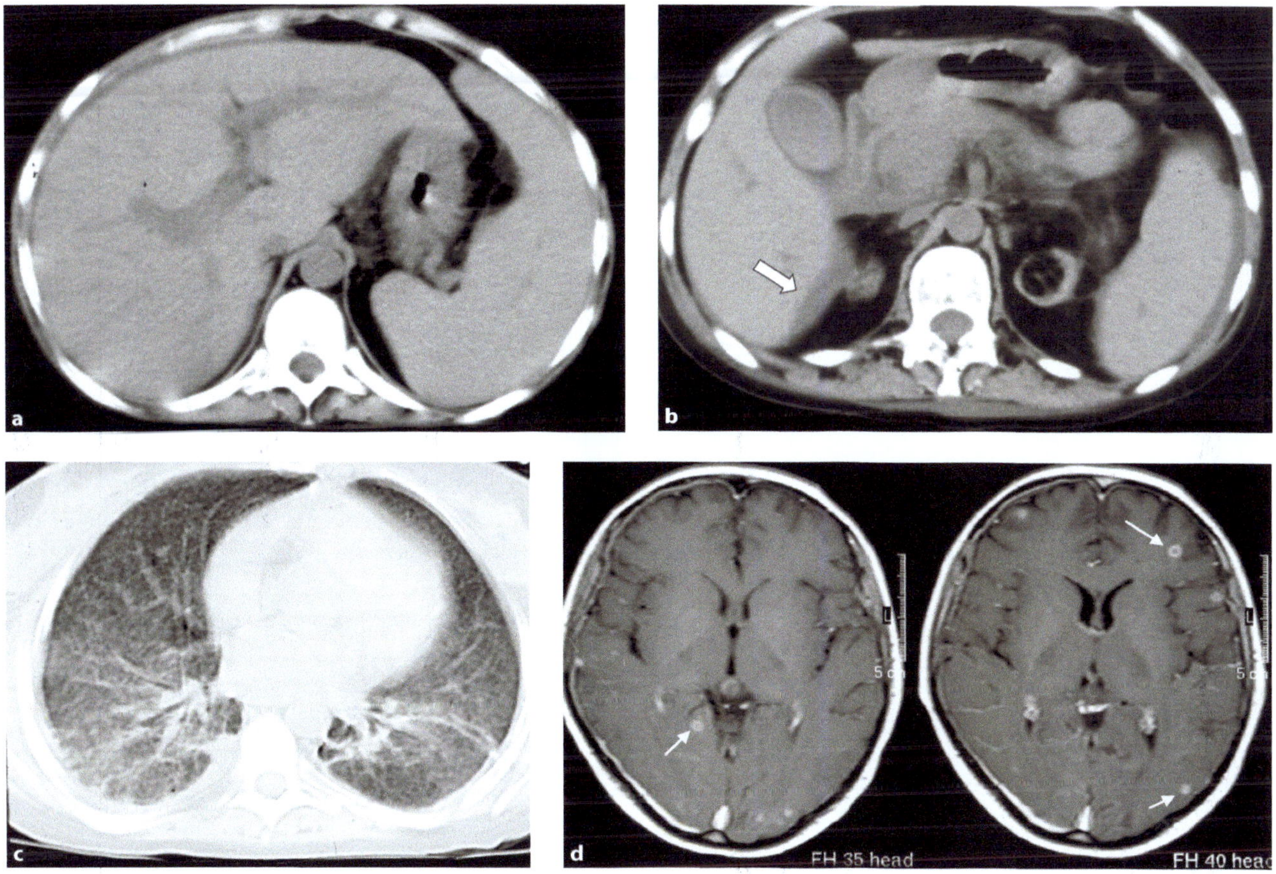

Fig. 5.7 Acquired disseminated toxoplasmosis in a 27-year-old man with renal transplant and fever. **a,b** Non-enhanced CT scan images showing hepatosplenomegaly with prominent portal tracts, ascites (*arrow*), and small end-stage kidneys. **c** Non-enhanced CT scan image of the lungs showing bilateral pulmonary infiltrates with bilateral small pleural effusions. **d** Gadolinium-enhanced T1-weighted MR images of the brain showing numerous small ring-enhancing lesions (*arrows*) compatible with microabscesses

toxoplasmosis (Dunn and Palmer 1998b; Ramsey and Geremia 1988). In the lungs, bilateral infiltrates simulating *Pneumocystis carinii* infection may be seen. The diagnosis can be confirmed by serology tests and identification of intracellular parasite from tissue biopsy specimens. Lacking a tissue biopsy for a definitive diagnosis of toxoplasmosis, a presumptive diagnosis of toxoplasmosis can be made, empirical treatment for toxoplasmosis can be started, and response to therapy assessed in 2 weeks' time.

5.2.4 Malaria

Malaria is widespread throughout the tropics. In humans, the four most frequent species are: *Plasmodium falciparum*, *P. vivax*, *P. ovale*, and *P. malariae*. The clinical findings are nonspecific, consisting of fever, hepatosplenomegaly, enlarged lymphadenopathy, and anemia. In approximately one-third of cases with malaria there may be an enlarged tender liver with jaundice and elevated liver enzymes due to malarial hepatitis (Kochar et al. 2003). The clinical differential diagnoses include leishmaniasis, histoplasmosis, tuberculosis, salmonellosis, viral infection (cytomegalovirus, Epstein-Barr virus), mononucleosis, toxocariasis, leukemia, and lymphoma. The imaging findings consist of hepatosplenomegaly with or without increased periportal echoes, gallbladder wall thickening, and ascites (Fig. 5.8) (Kachawaha et al. 2003). Rarely, a nodular liver may be observed on ultrasonography (Fig. 5.9). Poor contrast enhancement of the spleen (Fig. 5.10) (Bae and Jeon 2006) and splenic infarction (Bonnard et al. 2005) were also reported on CT scans. CT scanning demonstrates differences between a malarial spleen and a bilharzial spleen (Fig. 5.10). The diagnosis should be thought of in a patient who has traveled or lived in endemic tropical regions presenting with fever and anemia, and confirmed by identification of the parasite within red blood cells on a blood smear (Fig. 5.11).

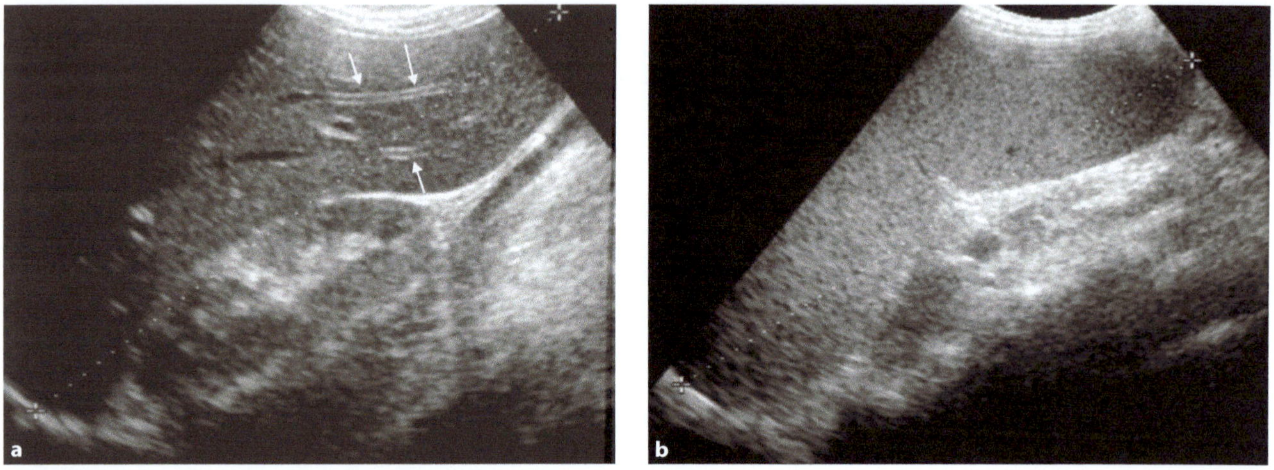

Fig. 5.8 Thirty-two-year-old woman living in Africa, presenting with fever and anemia due to malaria. **a,b** Longitudinal ultrasound images demonstrating hepatosplenomegaly with slight prominence of the portal tracts (*arrows*)

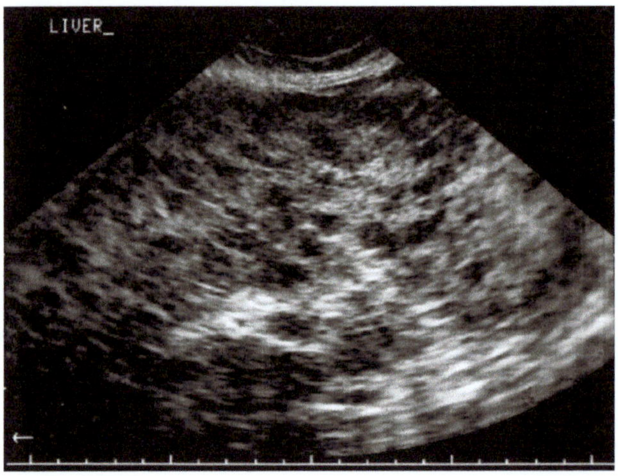

Fig. 5.9 Ultrasonography of the liver showing innumerable small hepatic nodules in a patient with malarial hepatitis (Courtesy of Dr. Nabil Ammouri, Tel Chiha Hospital, Zahleh, Lebanon)

5.2.5 Babesiosis

Babesiosis is an intraerythrocytic protozoan infection, characterized by malaria-like symptoms, i.e., fever and hemolytic anemia. It is a disease with worldwide prevalence, with isolated cases of human infections caused by *Babesia microti* in Northern America, *Babesia divergens*, and *Babesia bovis* in Europe. It occurs in splenectomized and immunosuppressed patients, but it has been also described in immunocompetent individuals with a normal spleen.

The laboratory diagnosis is established by identification of the intraerythrocytic parasite on thick and thin blood smears with Giemsa staining, the *Babesia* closely resembling the malarial parasite but contains no pigment. Specific serological tests are also available.

Imaging has little to contribute to the diagnosis; occasionally there may be hepatomegaly, which can be confirmed by ultrasound or CT scan (Dunn and Palmer 1998a).

5.2.6 Hepatobiliary Giardiasis

Giardiasis is prevalent worldwide. *Giardia lamblia* usually inhabits the small bowel, namely the jejunum; rarely, it may invade retrogradely the biliary tree and gallbladder causing abnormal liver function tests, jaundice, and

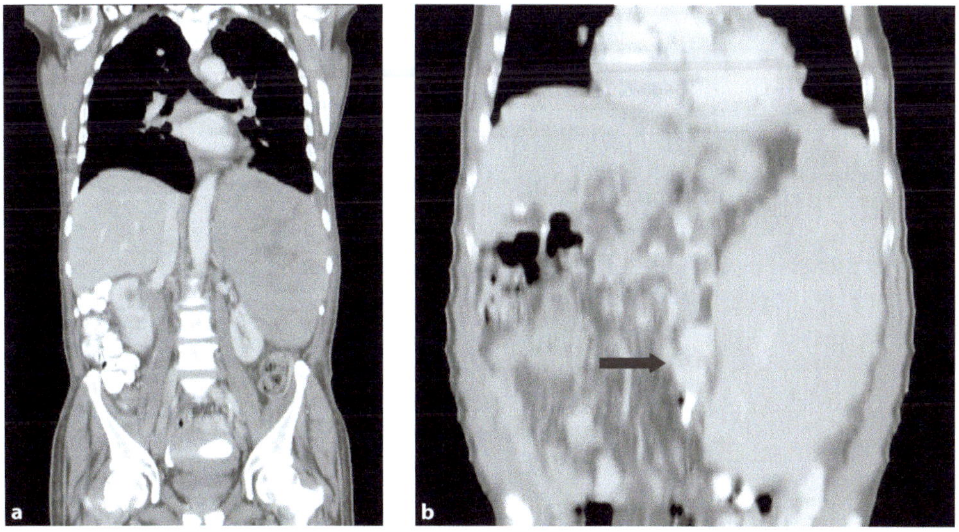

Fig. 5.10 Differentiation between malarial and bilharzial spleen. **a** Coronal reconstruction image of a contrast-enhanced CT scan showing splenomegaly due to malaria with characteristic poor arterial inhomogeneous enhancement of the spleen. The liver is of normal size. No varices are present. **b** Coronal reconstruction image of a contrast-enhanced CT scan showing splenomegaly with homogeneous enhancement with a small contracted liver due to periportal fibrosis, and numerous giant varices (*arrow*) and collaterals due to portal hypertension in a patient with schistosomiasis

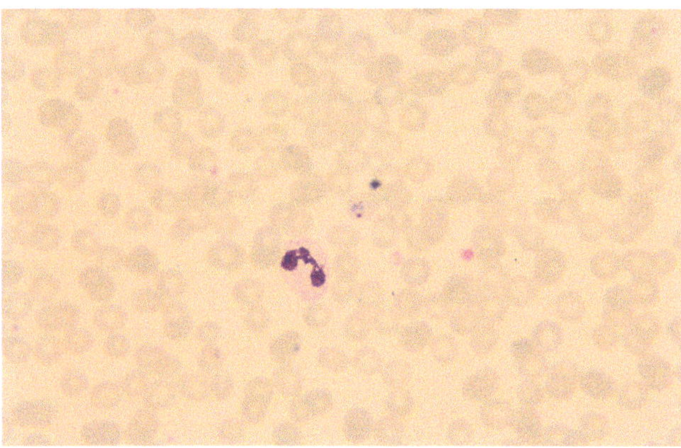

Fig. 5.11 Microphotograph of a malarial blood smear showing intraerythrocytic amastigotes

chronic cholecystitis with thickening of the gallbladder wall seen on ultrasound examination and dilatation with luminal irregularities of the bile ducts demonstrated by endoscopic retrograde cholangiopancreatography (ERCP). The diagnosis of biliary giardiasis is confirmed by demonstration of trophozoites and cysts in the bile aspirates (Aronson et al. 2001; Dominguez et al. 1998). In a study by Sotto and Gra (1985) in 25 patients with intestinal giardiasis confirmed by duodenal intubation aspirates, 60% of patients had histologic changes consisting of granulomatous inflammatory lesions and chronic hepatitis on liver biopsy specimens. Hepatic lesions regressed with antiparasitic treatment.

5.2.7 Biliary Cryptosporidiosis

Cryptosporidium parvum is a parasitic protozoan that occurs worldwide and affects primarily the epithelial cells of the gastrointestinal tract, including the small and large bowel, causing diarrhea. In immunocompetent patients it causes only mild illness, but in immunosuppressed patients, namely AIDS and transplant patients, it can produce a severe, debilitating diarrhea with or without multiorgan involvement including the respiratory and biliary tracts. *Cryptosporidia* involve the biliary tract in 10% of AIDS patients. At least half of cases with AIDS-related diarrhea or cholangiopathy are due to *Cryptosporidium*, with the other infections caused by *Cytomegalovirus*, the

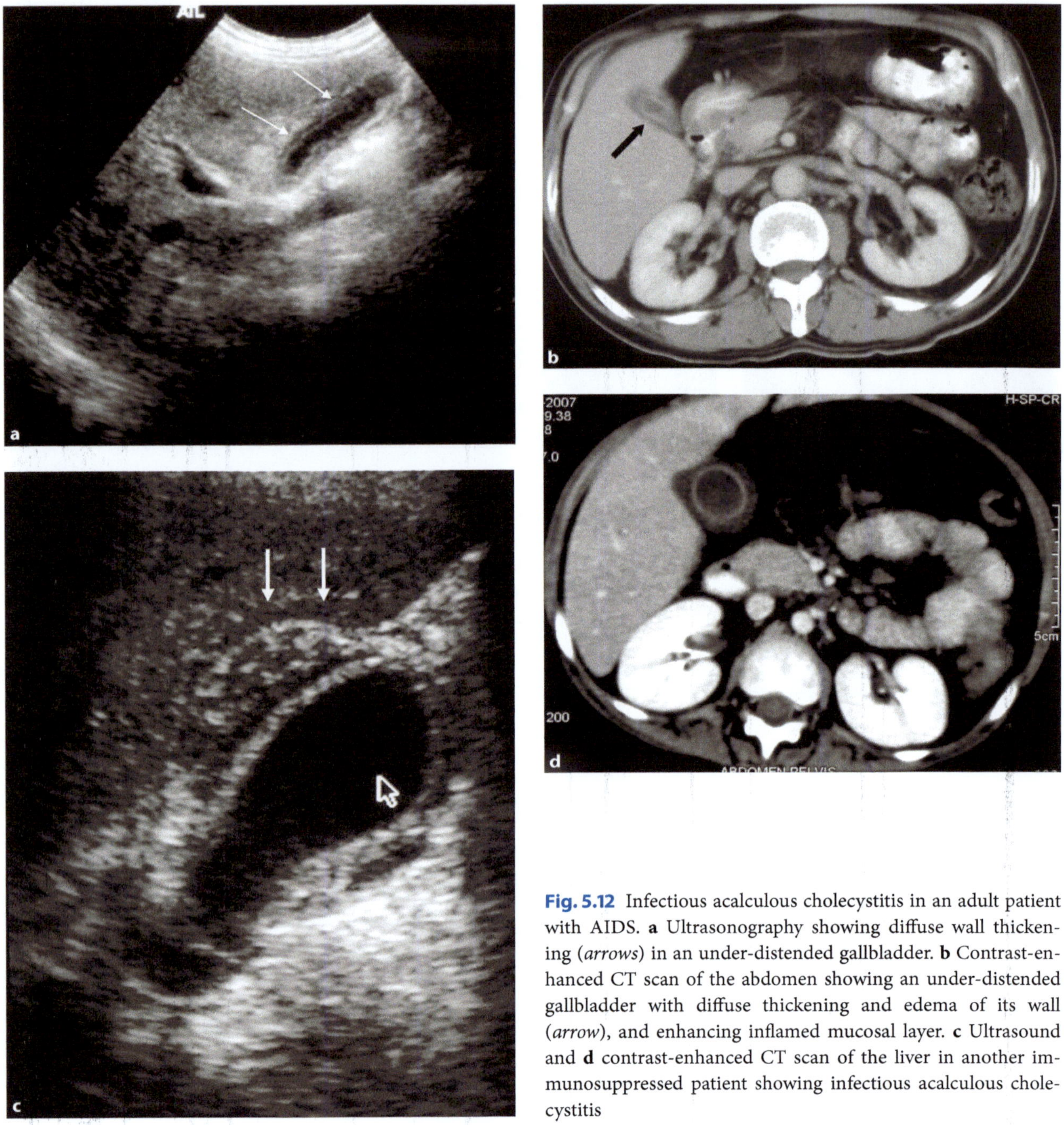

Fig. 5.12 Infectious acalculous cholecystitis in an adult patient with AIDS. **a** Ultrasonography showing diffuse wall thickening (*arrows*) in an under-distended gallbladder. **b** Contrast-enhanced CT scan of the abdomen showing an under-distended gallbladder with diffuse thickening and edema of its wall (*arrow*), and enhancing inflamed mucosal layer. **c** Ultrasound and **d** contrast-enhanced CT scan of the liver in another immunosuppressed patient showing infectious acalculous cholecystitis

Mycobacterium avium complex, and other organisms responsible for the remaining cases.

Clinically, patients present with right upper quadrant pain, fever, nausea and vomiting, and a cholestatic jaundice with abnormal liver function tests. On imaging, the appearance of AIDS-related cholangitis is similar to acalculous cholecystitis, i.e., gallbladder wall thickening and pericholecystic fluid on ultrasound and CT scans (Fig. 5.12), sclerosing cholangitis, i.e., attenuation and pruning of the intrahepatic bile ducts with some beading and dilatation of the common bile duct on cholangiograms, or papillary stenosis. The diagnosis of cryptosporidiosis can be confirmed by isolation of the organism from stool, bile, and biopsy specimens (Teixidor et al. 1991).

5.2.8 American Trypanosomiasis (Chagas' Disease)

Chagas' disease is confined to the American continent spreading from the south of the USA to Argentina. It is a protozoan infection caused by *Trypanosoma cruzi*. In the acute phase of the disease, hepatosplenomegaly and

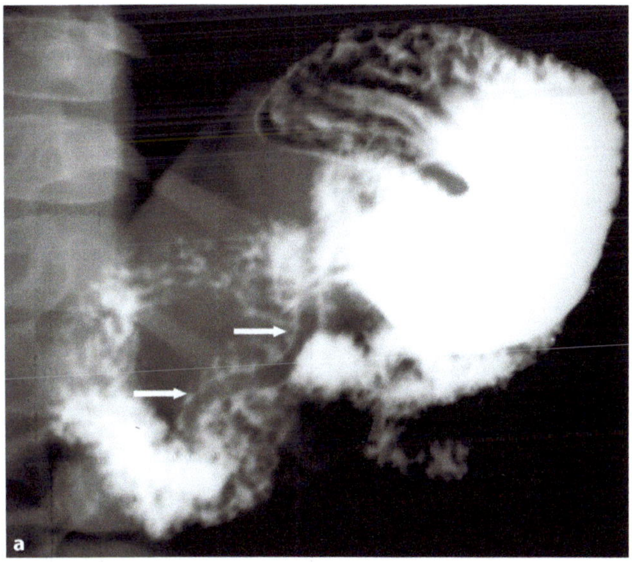

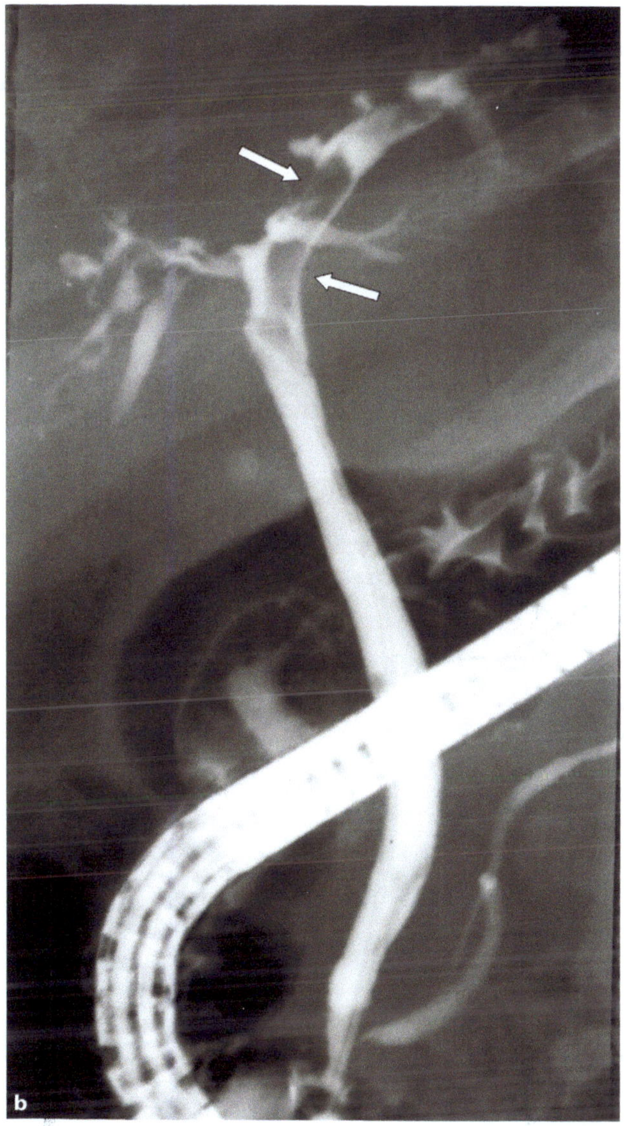

Fig. 5.13 *Ascaris* (*arrows*) by **a** barium meal and **b** endoscopic retrograde cholangiopancreatography (ERCP) (Courtesy of Dr. Halim Saad, Hôpital Sacré-Coeur, Hazmieh, Lebanon)

enlarged abdominal lymph nodes with fever are seldom observed. In the chronic phase of the disease so-called "mega" phase because of the presence of visceromegaly, i.e., dilatation and enlargement of hollow viscera, namely, megaesophagus and dilated cardiomyopathy. Ultrasound is useful in detecting a rare mega-gallbladder and in the identification of biliary stones present in up to 7% of Chagasic patients (Gharbi et al. 1998).

5.3 Helminths – Roundworms (Nematodes)

5.3.1 Hepatobiliary and Pancreatic Ascariasis

Ascaris lumbricoides is a major cause of intestinal parasitism worldwide. The parasite usually inhabits the small bowel, but occasionally it can migrate retrogradely into the biliary tree and pancreatic duct, causing complications such as biliary obstruction and jaundice with or without cholangitis and *Ascaris* induced pancreatitis. In endemic regions, for example in Syria, pancreatic-biliary ascariasis was identified in 18% of ERCP examinations (Sandouk et al. 1997b).

The imaging appearances of the *Ascaris* worm are very characteristic on barium studies and ERCP (Fig. 5.13), appearing as round and elongated filling defects. Ultrasound (Fig. 5.14) and magnetic resonance cholangiopancreatography (MRCP) are noninvasive imaging techniques capable of diagnosing *Ascaris* worms in the gallbladder and common bile duct (Khuroo et al. 1992; Ng et al. 1999; Hwang et al. 2001; Danaci et al. 1999). *Ascaris*-induced hepatic intraparenchymal abscesses were also described on imaging studies (Javid et al. 1999; Akata et al. 1999). ERCP plays a diagnostic and thera-

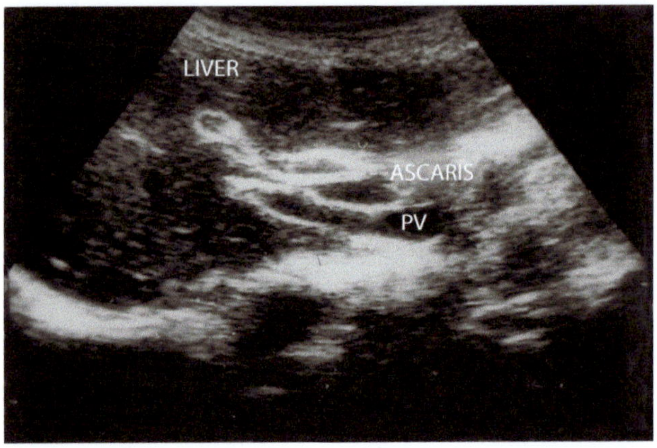

Fig. 5.14 Ultrasonography showing an *Ascaris* within the common bile duct (Courtesy of Dr. Fayez Sandouk, Department of Gastroenterology, University of Damascus and Al-Mouassat University Hospital, Damascus, Syria)

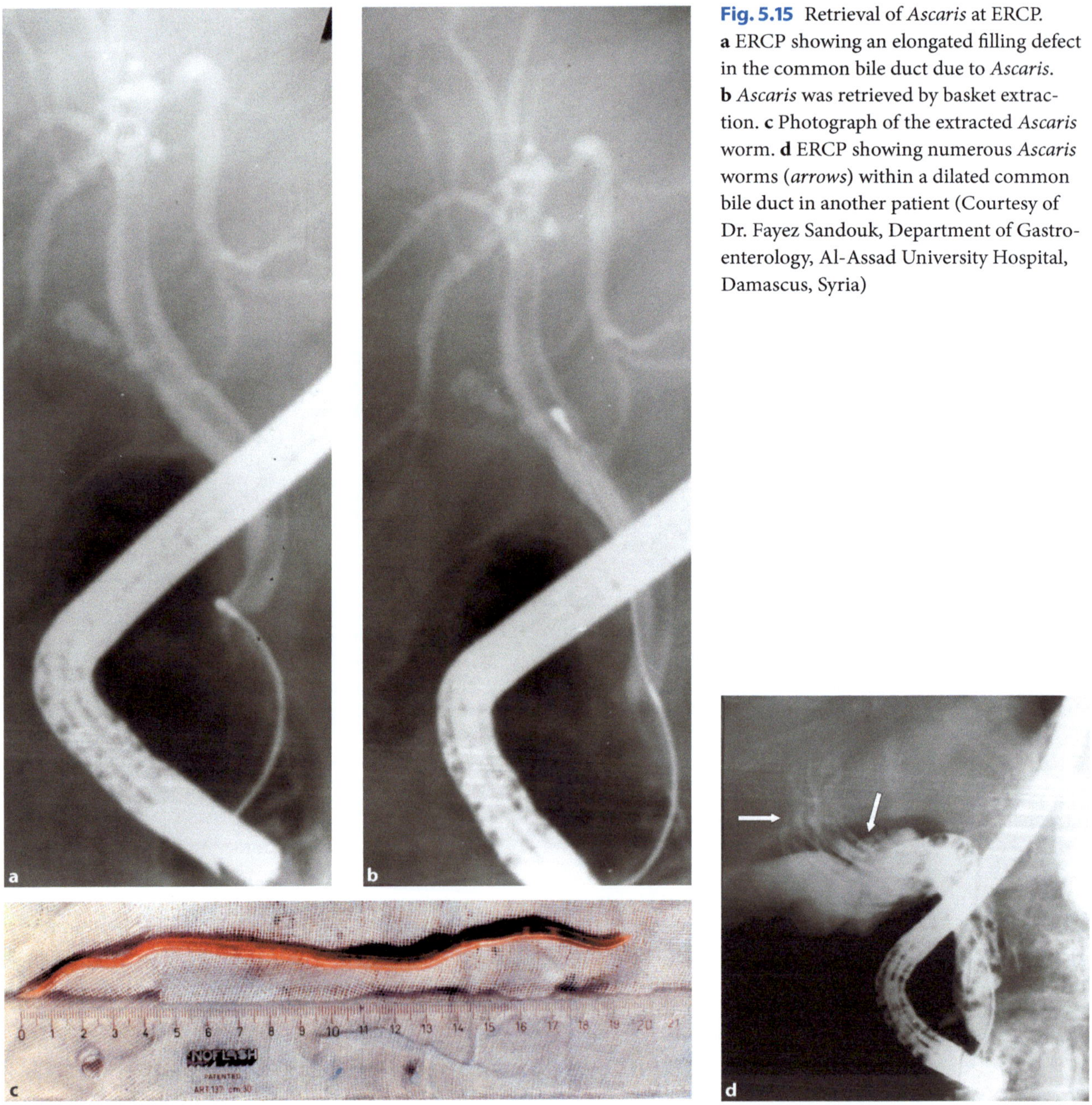

Fig. 5.15 Retrieval of *Ascaris* at ERCP. **a** ERCP showing an elongated filling defect in the common bile duct due to *Ascaris*. **b** *Ascaris* was retrieved by basket extraction. **c** Photograph of the extracted *Ascaris* worm. **d** ERCP showing numerous *Ascaris* worms (*arrows*) within a dilated common bile duct in another patient (Courtesy of Dr. Fayez Sandouk, Department of Gastroenterology, Al-Assad University Hospital, Damascus, Syria)

peutic role (Fig. 5.15) for relief of biliary and pancreatic ductal obstruction by endoscopic removal of the parasite (Al-Karawi et al. 1989, 1999; Sandouk et al. 1997a). Percutaneous transhepatic management of biliary ascariasis can be attempted as an alternative to surgery when endoscopic extraction fails (Ozcan et al. 2003).

Ascaris suum, once considered a subtype of *A. lumbricoides*, is now thought to be a separate species morphologically and immunoserologically from *A. lumbricoides*. It can migrate to the liver and other organs through the portal venous system, causing visceral larval migrans (VLM). In the liver, it induces small nodular inflammatory eosinophilic pseudotumors or infiltration, appearing hypoechoic on ultrasonography and hypodense on contrast-enhanced CT scans, simulating hepatic metastases or lymphoma. These imaging findings are nonspecific and the diagnosis is usually confirmed by positive specific immunoserologic test, elevated peripheral blood eosinophil count or elevated immunoglobulin (IgE) level. In biopsy specimens of the liver lesions, larvae are not generally detected. The liver lesions completely disappear after medical treatment (Kakihara et al. 2004; Hayashi et al. 1999).

5.3.2 Toxocariasis (Visceral Larva Migrans)

Related ascarids, *Toxocara canis* and *T. cati*, the roundworms of the dog and cat respectively, cause visceral larval migrans (VLM) in humans, i.e., Loeffler's syndrome. VLM is a disease that occurs worldwide, and is characterized clinically by fever, hepatosplenomegaly, lymphadenopathy, with or without central nervous system or other organ manifestations. The laboratory findings consist of hypereosinophilia, abnormal liver function tests, and hyperglobulinemia (Ishibashi et al. 1992). On imaging, hepatomegaly with low-density areas representing inflammatory eosinophil granulomas may be seen on contrast-enhanced CT scans (Fig. 5.16), and appear

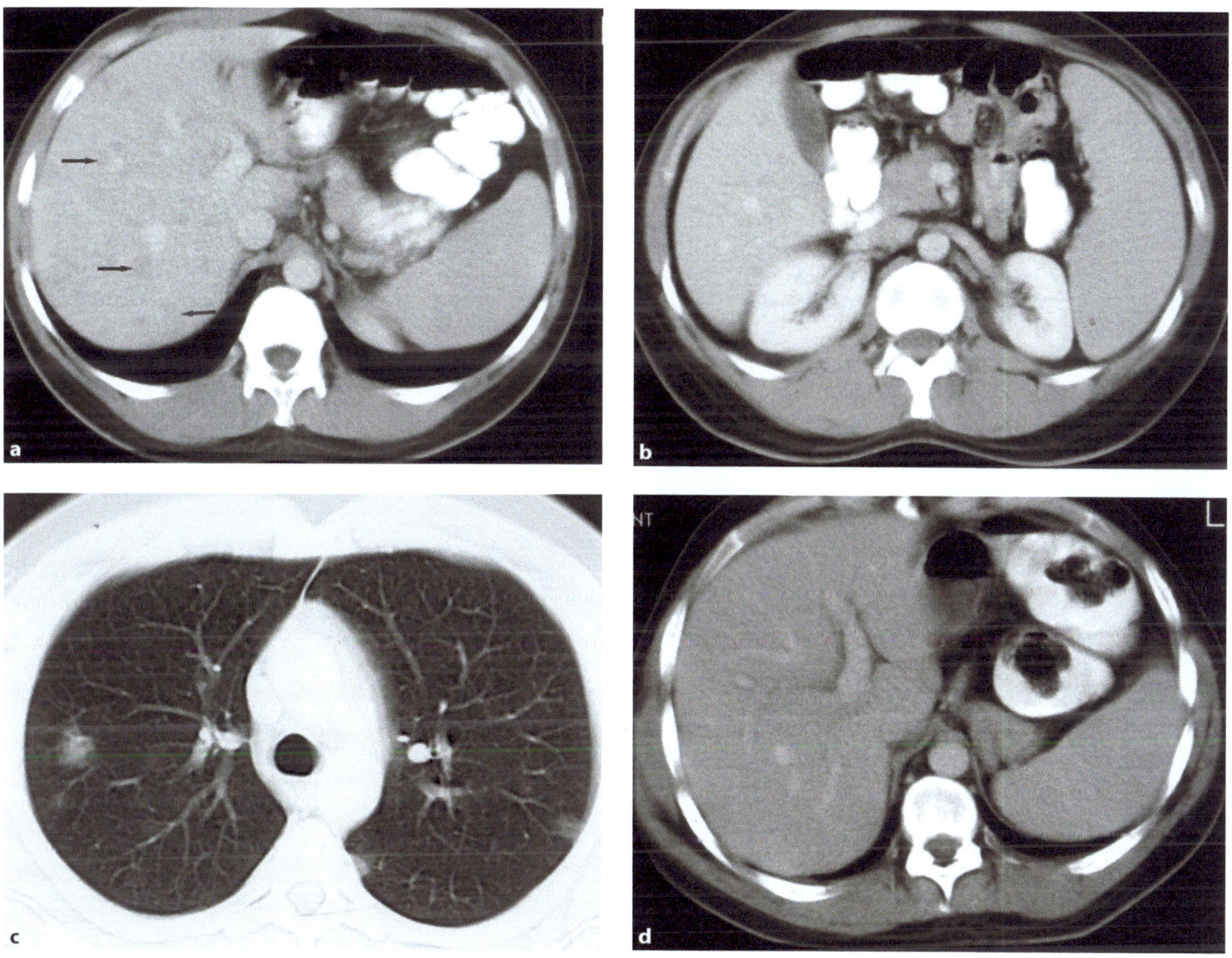

Fig. 5.16 Thirty-year-old man with Loeffler's syndrome and eosinophilia caused by toxocariasis, confirmed by positive blood serology. **a**,**b** Contrast-enhanced CT scan of the abdomen showing splenomegaly and numerous ill-defined low density lesions (*arrows*) in the liver. **c** Multiple patches of peripheral pulmonary infiltrates were also noted. **d** The liver and pulmonary lesions completely healed following treatment

as small hypoechoic nodular lesions on ultrasonography (Ishibashi et al. 1992; Azuma et al. 2002; Kabaalioglu et al. 2005; Leone et al. 2006; Chang et al. 2006). The diagnosis can be confirmed by positive specific ELISA serology tests and liver tissue biopsy demonstrating focal eosinophil necrosis; however, the larvae themselves are very difficult to find, they can be visualized in approximately 20% of cases.

5.3.3 Hepatobiliary Strongyloidiasis

Strongyloidiasis is an intestinal parasitic disease that is prevalent worldwide and affects the submucosa and lamina propria of the duodenum and upper jejunum, and rarely the large bowel. Occasionally, extraintestinal hyperinfection with *Strongyloides stercoralis* occurs in immunocompromised patients, the parasite enters the mesenteric venules producing hepatitis with focal inflammatory lesions (Rawat and Simons 1993). Occasionally, intestinal strongyloidiasis may be associated with obstructive jaundice caused by ampullary stenosis at the involved segment of the duodenum (Astagneau et al. 1994).

On imaging, the focal inflammatory hepatic lesions have a nonspecific appearance mimicking metastatic deposits. They appear hypoechoic on ultrasonography and hypodense on contrast-enhanced CT scan.

The diagnosis is established by duodenal or jejunal aspirate and biopsy for the identification of alive rhabditiform larvae. The hematologic profile shows eosinophilia. Fine needle aspiration biopsy of hepatic lesions is unrevealing, but it can be performed to exclude malignancy or metastatic disease by showing no evidence of malignant cells. Liver biopsy usually fails to demonstrate the parasite.

5.3.4 Gnathostomiasis

Gnathostoma spinigerum is a roundworm endemic in the Far East. Humans acquire the disease by eating infected raw or undercooked fish, meat, chicken or pork. Clinically, two stages of the disease are recognized. First, a visceral larva migrans (VLM) stage due to migration of the parasite through the stomach wall into the peritoneal cavity and then through the liver and other deep organs to the skeletal muscles and subcutaneous tissues, forming the second cutaneous larva migrans stage of the disease where it provokes a creeping eruption with intermittent or migratory subcutaneous swellings with inflammation and edema. During the first VLM stage, it can induce marked peripheral eosinophilia, right upper quadrant pain, and tender hepatomegaly with abnormal liver function tests. Often during this stage there is peritoneal irritation, which can be mistaken clinically for acute abdominal conditions such as cholecystitis, appendicitis, and peptic ulcer perforation. In addition, it can provoke eosinophilic inflammatory masses of the deep organs including the colon and ovary, simulating malignancies.

The specific serological ELISA test for the detection of antibodies against *Gnathostoma* is not universally available; it is only available in endemic countries.

The radiological findings are as nonspecific as the clinical manifestations often misinterpreted for acute abdominal conditions and malignancies.

The definitive diagnosis of gnathostomiasis is established by isolation or retrieval of the parasite by resection and not by biopsy of skin swellings. As isolation of the parasite for definitive diagnosis is often impossible, the diagnosis of gnathostomiasis is often a presumptive diagnosis based on a characteristic clinical triad of intermittent or migratory skin and subcutaneous tissues swellings, peripheral eosinophilia, history of travel to endemic regions, and eating infected food, with the serological tests if available used as supportive evidence (Rusnack and Lucey 1993; Dow et al. 1998).

5.3.5 Angiostrongyliasis

Angiostrongyliasis costaricensis causes a disease first observed in Costa Rican children, characterized by eosinophilic gastroenteritis involving the terminal ileum, cecum, appendix, and ascending colon. The involvement of other organs such as lymph nodes, liver, and testicles may be observed. Larvae penetrate the cecal and appendiceal walls and invade the peritoneal cavity, then reach the liver by penetration of Glisson's capsule, inducing an inflammatory eosinophilic reaction, with necrosis of liver tissue. The diagnosis is usually established at liver biopsy (Vasquez et al. 1994).

5.3.6 Hepatic Capillariasis

Human hepatic capillariasis is a rare disease caused by the nematode *Capillaria hepatica*. It predominantly affects children aged 1–4 years, due to the frequent soil-to-hand-to-mouth contact in this age group. The disease is characterized by the clinical triad of fever, hepatomegaly, and hypereosinophilia. The diagnosis is made by needle biopsy of the liver, demonstrating the presence of typical intracellular eggs. Pathologically, there is a granulomatous inflammation leading to interstitial fibrosis (Choe et al. 1993; Pannenbecker et al. 1990; Berger et al. 1990).

5.4 Helminths – Tapeworms (Cestodes)

5.4.1 Hepatic Echinococcosis

Unilocular or cystic echinococcosis (CE) is caused by *Echinococcus granulosus*, while alveolar echinococcosis (AE) is due to *Echinococcus multilocularis* and polycystic echinococcosis is due to *Echinococcus vogeli*. Hepatic echinococcosis is endemic in rural parts of the world. Echinococcosis can affect any organ of the human body from head to toe (Polat et al. 2003). Mass screening in hyperendemic regions using hand-held portable ultrasound scanners and specific serological tests have been applied to detect the early stage of the disease in the asymptomatic population. An international classification of cystic echinococcosis has been recently proposed by the WHO Informal Working Group on echinococcosis in 2003 (WHO Informal Working Group on Echinococcosis 2003), which is a modified form of the first described and widely used Gharbi's classification (Gharbi et al. 1981), based on ultrasonographic patterns that correlate with the natural evolution and viability of the cyst. Cyst viability much depends on the presence of fluid content within the cyst. Cysts were also categorized into small (<5 cm), medium-sized (5–10 cm), and large (>10 cm) which can produce a mass effect on adjacent structures.

On imaging, a unilocular cystic lesion (type CL) with no visible cyst wall is a nonspecific finding that may represent a simple nonparasitic cyst, or other fluid-filled hepatic lesions including a parasitic cyst.

Type CE1 (Fig. 5.17) corresponds to a type I Gharbi's classification, which describes a unilocular cyst with a visible cyst wall and may contain hydatid sand (snow flake sign). Type CE2 (Fig. 5.18) corresponds to a type III Gharbi's classification, consisting of a multivesicular or multiseptated hydatid cyst with internal daughter cysts. Type CE3 corresponds to type II Gharbi's classification, i.e., a cyst with a floating or detached laminated membrane (Fig. 5.19), and to type IV Gharbi's classification, i.e., a cyst with heterogeneous echo-patterns and containing few peripheral daughter cysts (Fig. 5.20). Type CE4 corresponds to a type IV Gharbi's classification consisting of a degenerated solidified cyst that has no fluid component but having a pseudotumoral or tumor-like appearance (Fig. 5.21). Type CE5 corresponds to type V Ghar-

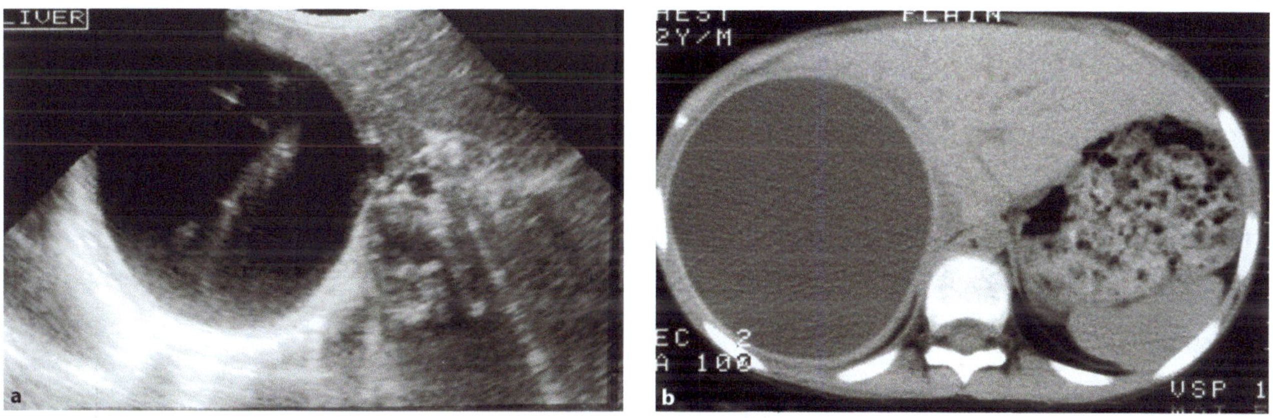

Fig. 5.17 Type CE1 unilocular hepatic hydatid cyst by **a** ultrasound and **b** CT scan

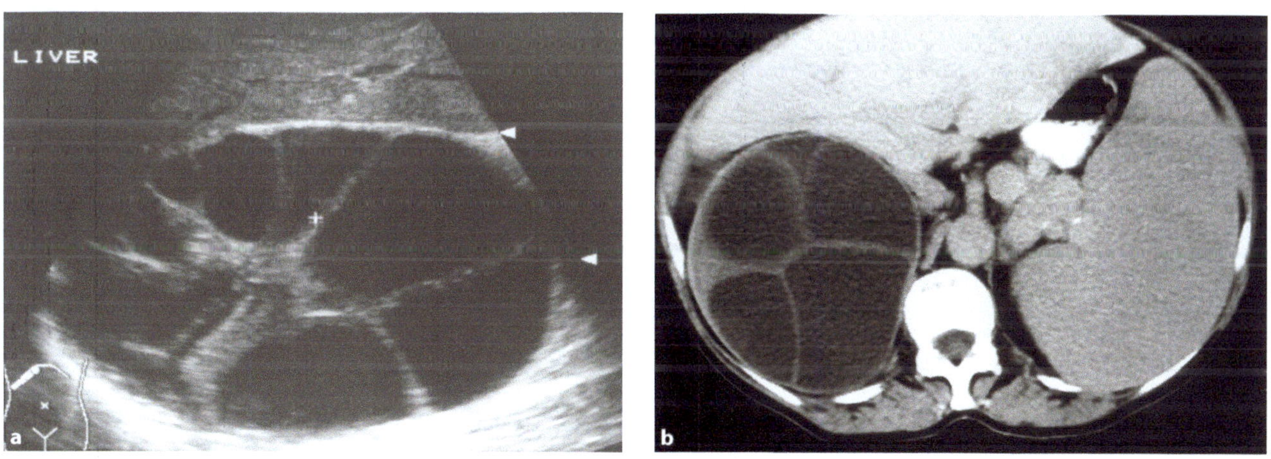

Fig. 5.18 Type CE2 multivesicular hydatid cyst by **a** ultrasound and **b** CT scan

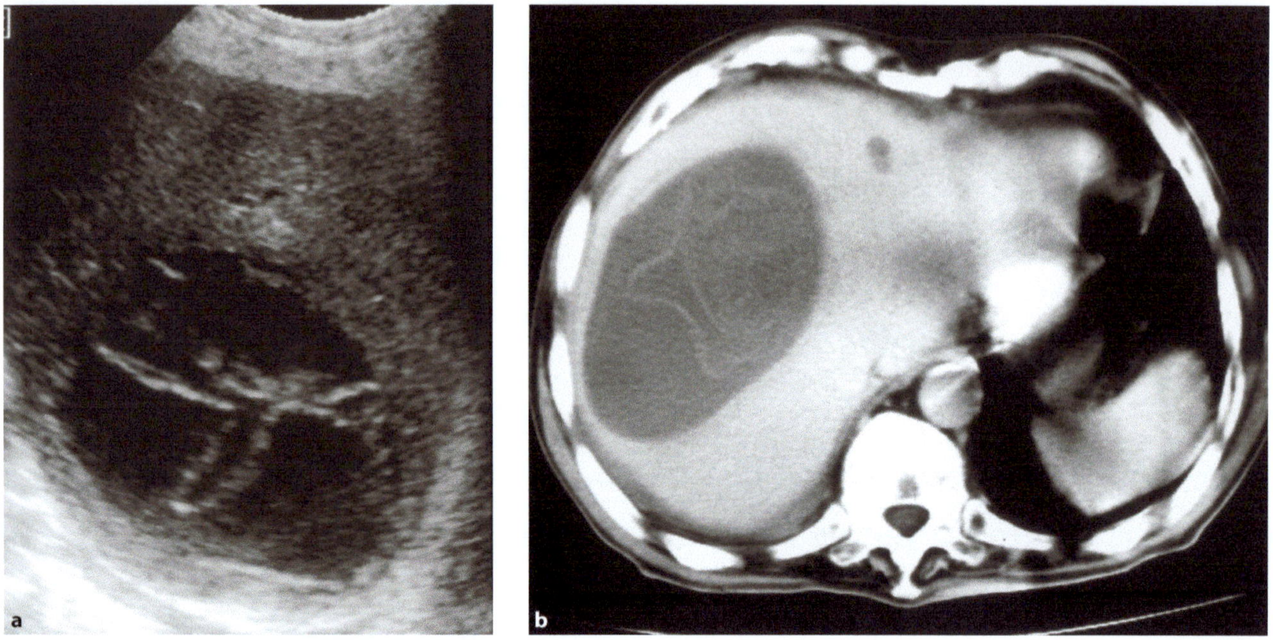

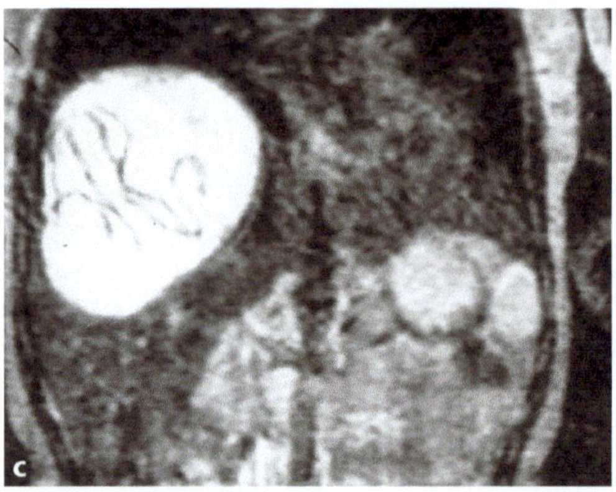

Fig. 5.19 Type CE3 with floating detached membrane by **a** ultrasound, **b** CT scan, and **c** MRI

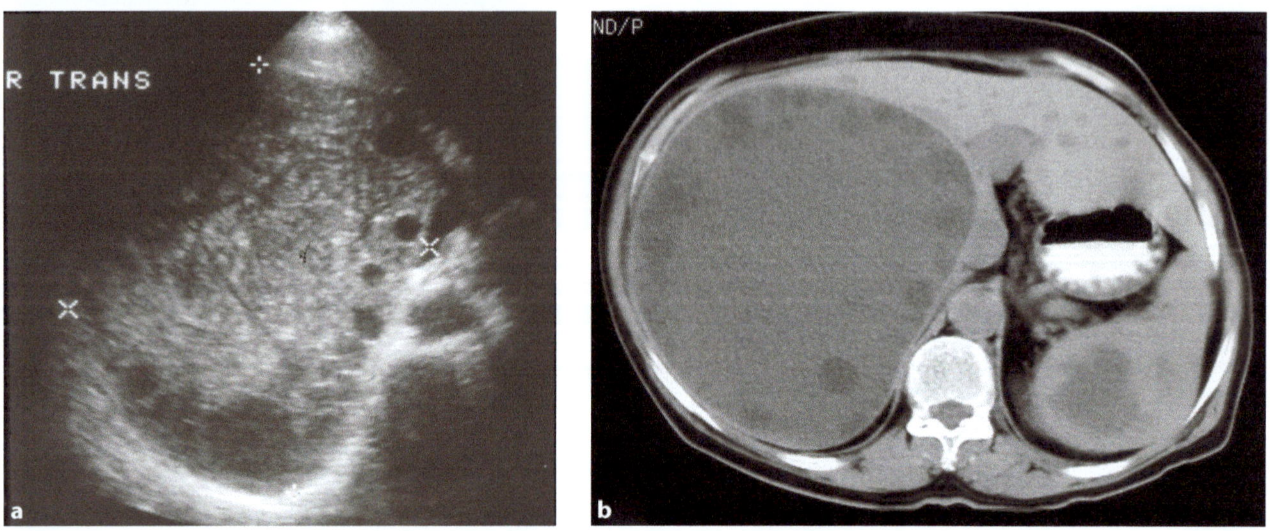

Fig. 5.20 Type CE3 with heterogeneous echo-pattern and few peripheral daughter cysts by **a** ultrasound and **b** CT scan. Note also the presence of a splenic hydatid cyst in **b**

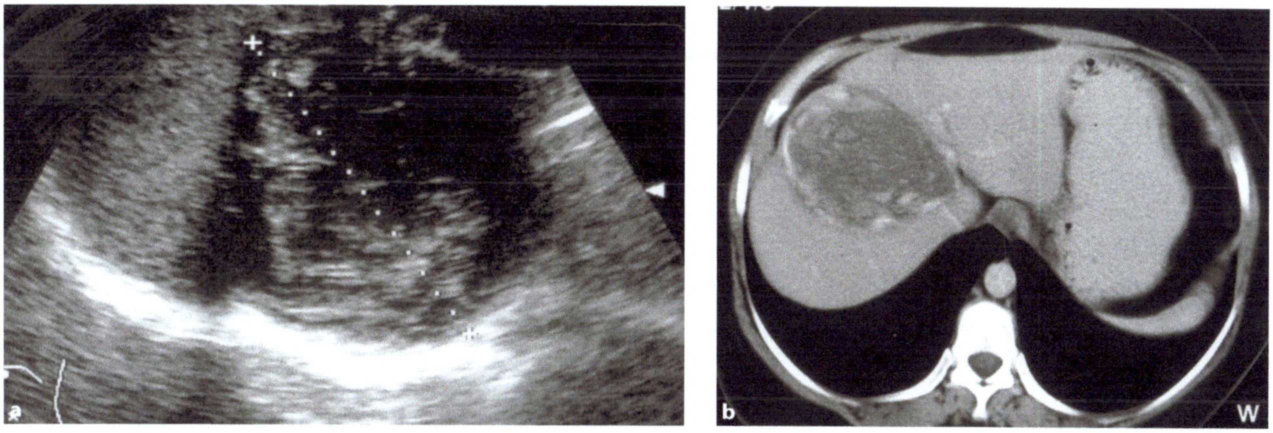

Fig. 5.21 Type CE4 with a degenerated solidified cyst that has no fluid component and a pseudotumoral appearance on **a** ultrasound and **b** CT scan, and peripheral calcification on CT scan

bi's classification, consisting of a cyst with thick reflecting walls (Fig. 5.22). The five types of cystic echinococcosis classified by the WHO Informal Working Group (2003) were also grouped into three groups: Group 1 (CE1 and CE2) consisting of active and fertile cysts; Group 2 (CE3) consisting of transitional cysts that have started to degenerate, but may still contain viable protoscoleces; and Group 3 (CE4 and CE5) consisting of inactive and infertile cysts.

Some of the imaging features are pathognomonic, allowing a diagnosis of CE in the majority of cases. However, in a very small number of patients with atypical imaging features of the cysts and negative combined serology tests (indirect hemagglutination and ELISA), a fine needle aspiration biopsy of the cyst may be required for a definitive diagnosis.

The management of cystic echinococcosis depends largely on guidelines established by the World Health Organization (WHO) in 1996 (WHO Informal Working Group on Echinococcosis 1996) and in 2001 (WHO-IGWE 2001; Filice et al. 2000), and on local expertise. The main goals of the most appropriate treatment is to ablate the cyst while preserving normal liver tissue using a minimally invasive therapy that gives the best results with the lowest rates of morbidity and mortality. Long-term medical therapy with benzimidazolic drugs used alone (Fig. 5.23) has a low cure rate, estimated at 30% (WHO Informal Working Group on Echinococcosis 1996). This is why chemotherapy is preferably used as an adjuvant therapy to surgery, which remains the optimal treatment of choice for hydatidosis that has the potential to remove the cyst and lead to a complete cure. There is a tendency toward the application of laparoscopic surgery for uncomplicated superficial cysts larger than 5 cm in size more often than open surgery, simply because of its lower morbidity and mortality rates and the advantage of a shorter hospital stay compared with open surgery. The PAIR (puncture, aspiration, injection, reaspiration) technique with concomitant medical therapy is a viable and safe alternative to surgery that is applicable to inoperable patients with cyst types CE1–CE3 that have a predominantly fluid component and viable scoleces (Fig. 5.24). Percutaneous catheter drainage may also be successfully applied in all cyst types CE1–CE3 (Fig. 5.25), including type CE3 corresponding to Gharbi's type IV cyst with a predominantly solid heterogeneous echo-pattern (Haddad et al. 2000).

The incidence of intrabiliary rupture of hepatic echinococcal cyst is estimated at 8.2% (Haddad et al. 2001). It occurs with the hypermature cyst types CE2 and CE3. Patients present with obstructive jaundice, which may sometimes be subclinical with or without cholangitis or focal pancreatitis, which can simulate a pancreatic head malignancy. The diagnosis of intrabiliary rupture is based on characteristic ultrasonographic (Fig. 5.26) and CT imaging features and demonstration of biliocystic communication on cystography, MRCP, technetium hepatobiliary scintigraphy, or ERCP, which is the diagnostic and therapeutic method (Fig. 5.27) of optimal choice.

Alveolar echinococcosis (AE) is not endemic in the Middle East, but is prevalent in Northern Europe and America. It typically appears as a multiloculated cystic lesion (Fig. 5.28) or occasionally as an infiltrative tumor-like lesion simulating primary or secondary hepatic malignancy or abscesses. Characteristic clusters of calcifications are seen in approximately 50% of cases (Didier et al. 1985). The diagnosis is established by identification of typical imaging features and positive serologic tests. However, an image-guided biopsy may be required for atypical lesions with negative serology.

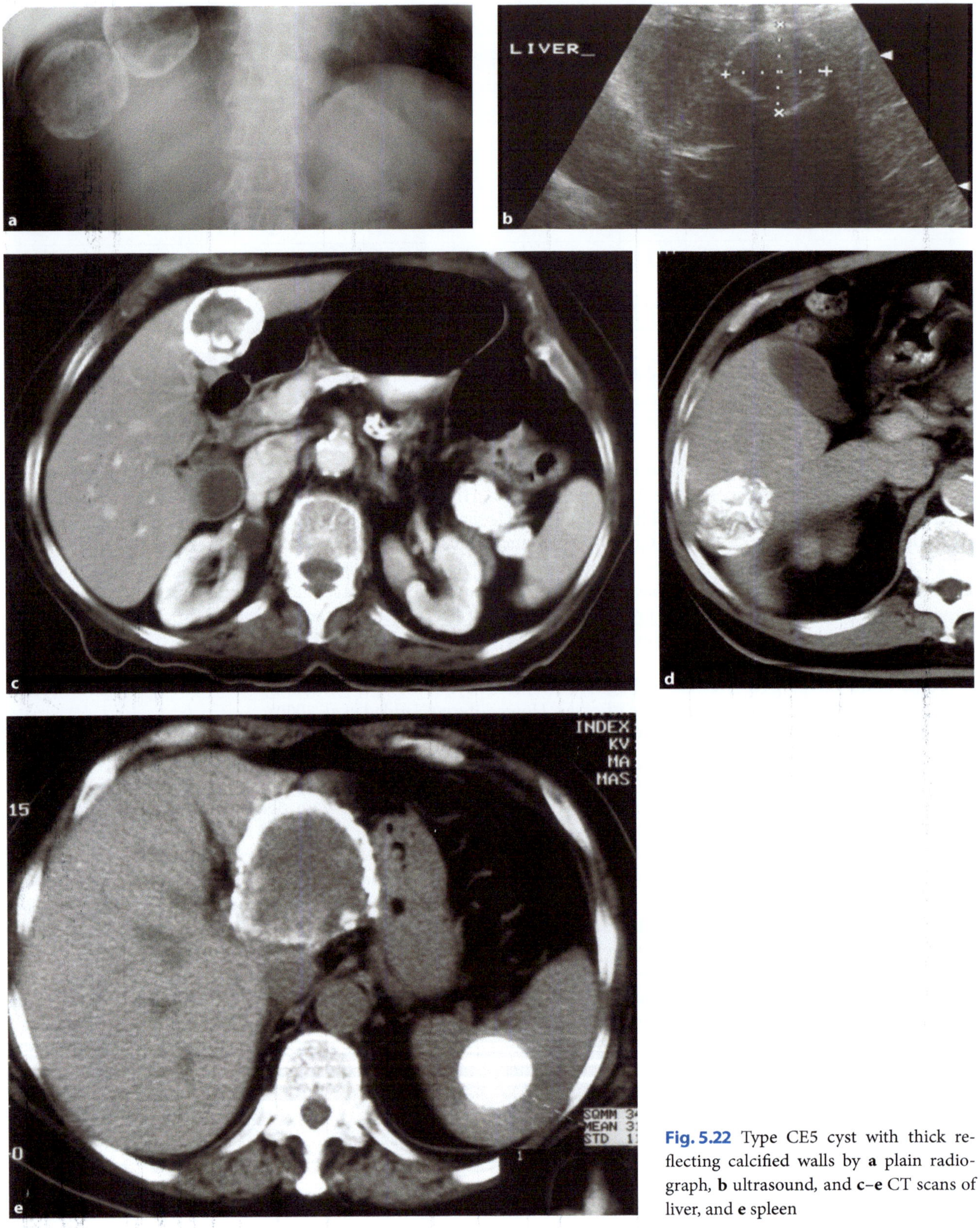

Fig. 5.22 Type CE5 cyst with thick reflecting calcified walls by **a** plain radiograph, **b** ultrasound, and **c–e** CT scans of liver, and **e** spleen

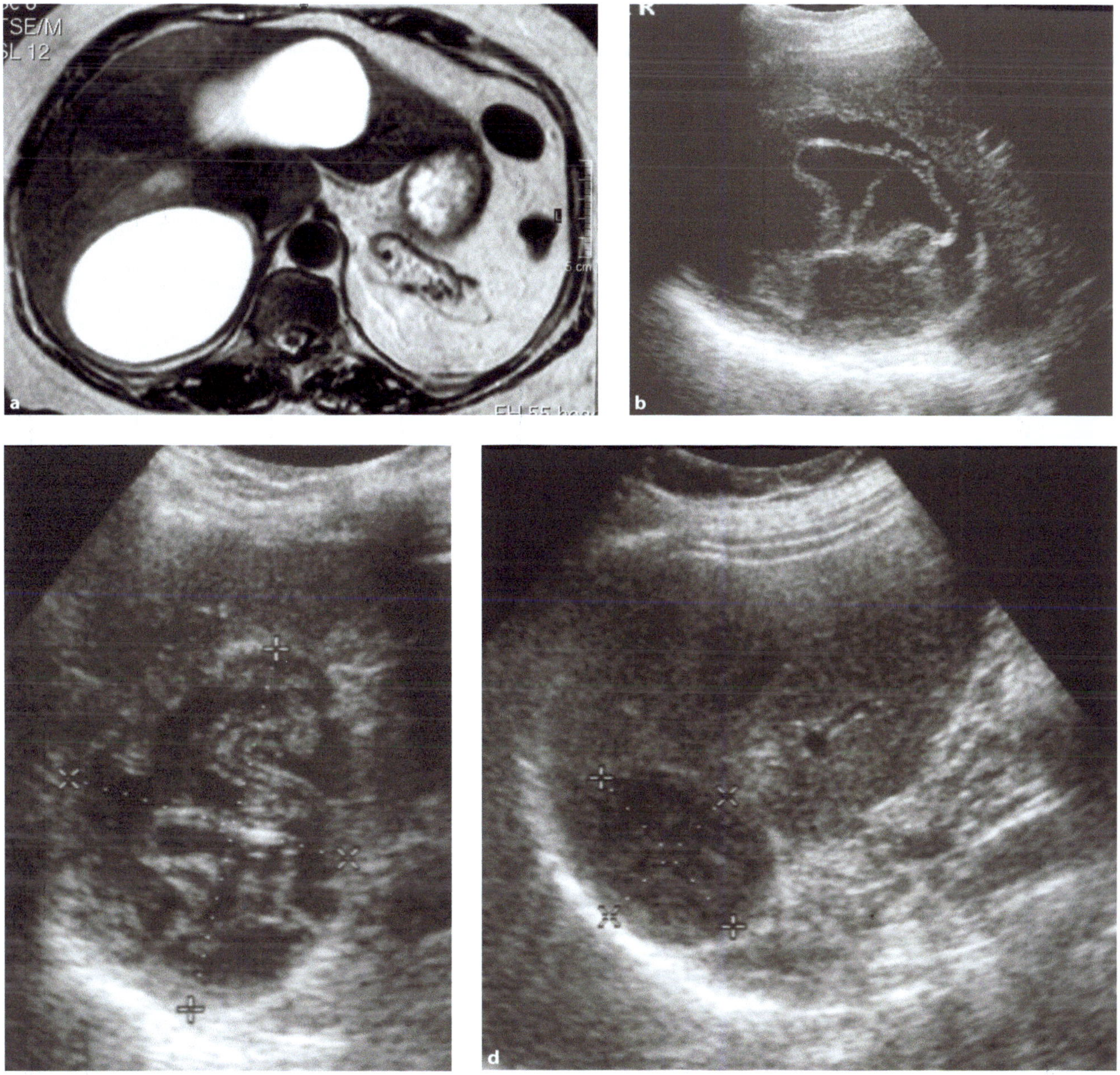

Fig. 5.23 Successful result with medical treatment using benzimidazolic drugs. **a** Initial T2-weighted MR image obtained at presentation, showed a large unilocular hepatic hydatid cyst. **b** Follow-up ultrasound image obtained after 9-month medical therapy, showing intracystic detachment of the membrane or endocyst. **c** Another follow-up ultrasound image obtained at 15 months, showed partial solidification of the cyst. **d** Last follow-up ultrasonography obtained after a 2-year interval showed complete solidification and reduction in the size of the cyst

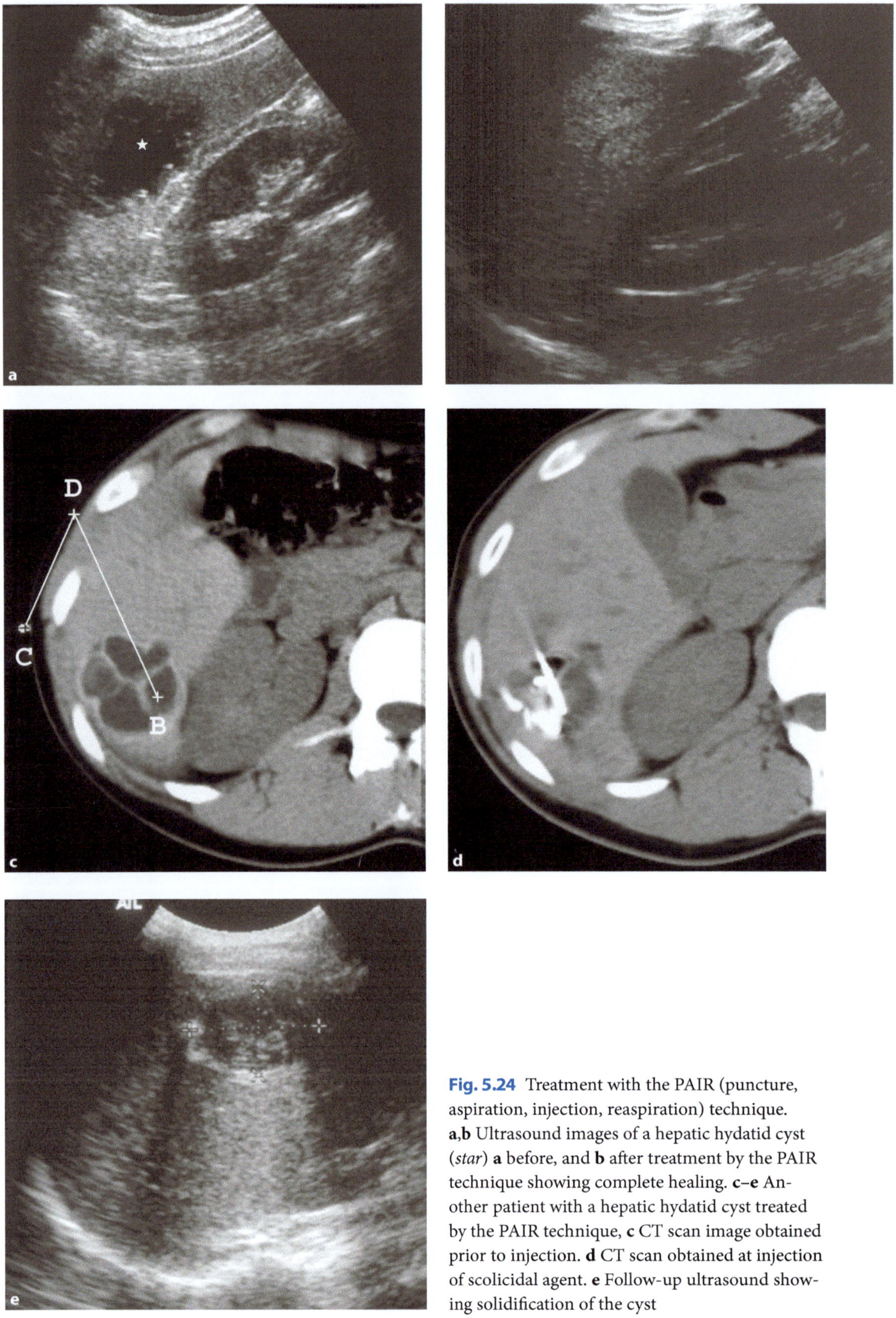

Fig. 5.24 Treatment with the PAIR (puncture, aspiration, injection, reaspiration) technique. **a,b** Ultrasound images of a hepatic hydatid cyst (*star*) **a** before, and **b** after treatment by the PAIR technique showing complete healing. **c–e** Another patient with a hepatic hydatid cyst treated by the PAIR technique, **c** CT scan image obtained prior to injection. **d** CT scan obtained at injection of scolicidal agent. **e** Follow-up ultrasound showing solidification of the cyst

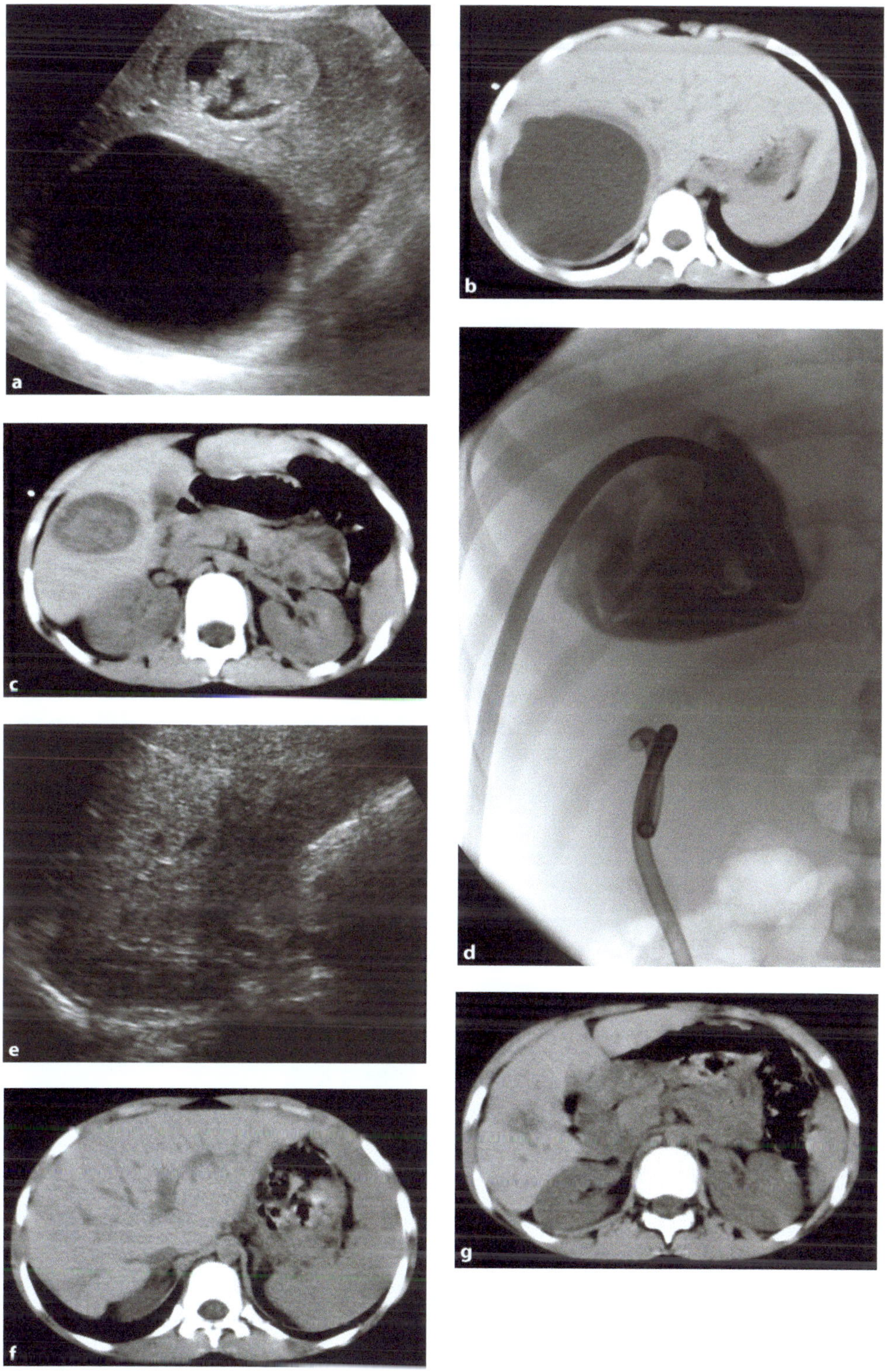

Fig. 5.25 Ten-year-old girl with hepatic echinococcal cysts treated successfully by percutaneous catheter drainage and ablation combined with medical anti-helminthic therapy. She had previous open surgery for liver hydatid disease. **a** Ultrasound and **b,c** CT scan images of the liver demonstrating an 8-cm anechoic type CL (cystic lesion) unilocular cyst, and a smaller cyst of type CE3 containing detached floating membranes compatible with echinococcal cysts. **d** Percutaneous drainage and ablation of the cysts were performed by means of two large bore 12F sump catheters. **e** Follow-up ultrasound and **f,g** CT scan images of the liver showing complete healing

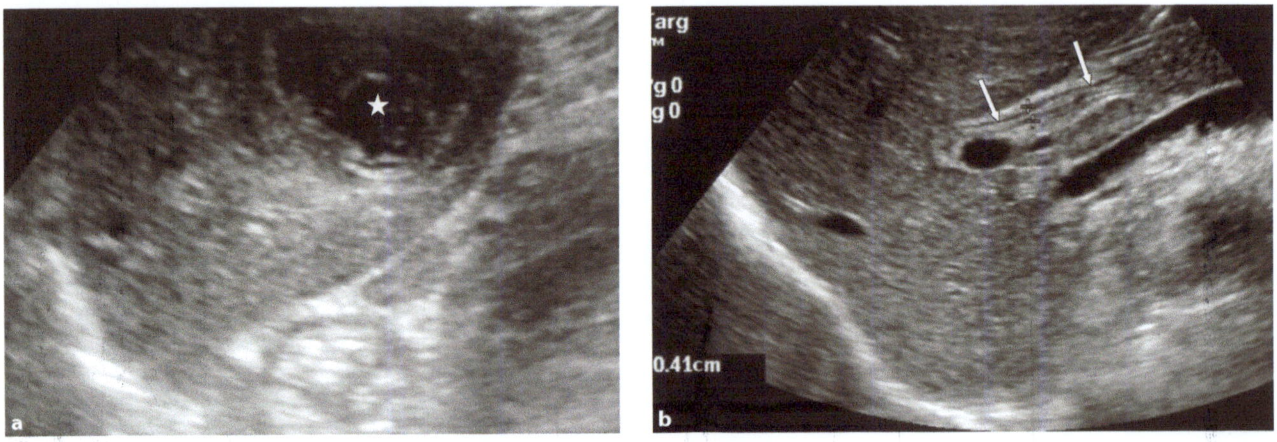

Fig. 5.26 Hepatic echinococcal cyst complicated by intrabiliary rupture. **a** Ultrasound image of the liver demonstrating a hydatid cyst (*star*). **b** Ultrasound image of the common bile duct (CBD) showed intraluminal echogenic structures (*arrows*) within a nondilated CBD (*cursors*) representing membranes

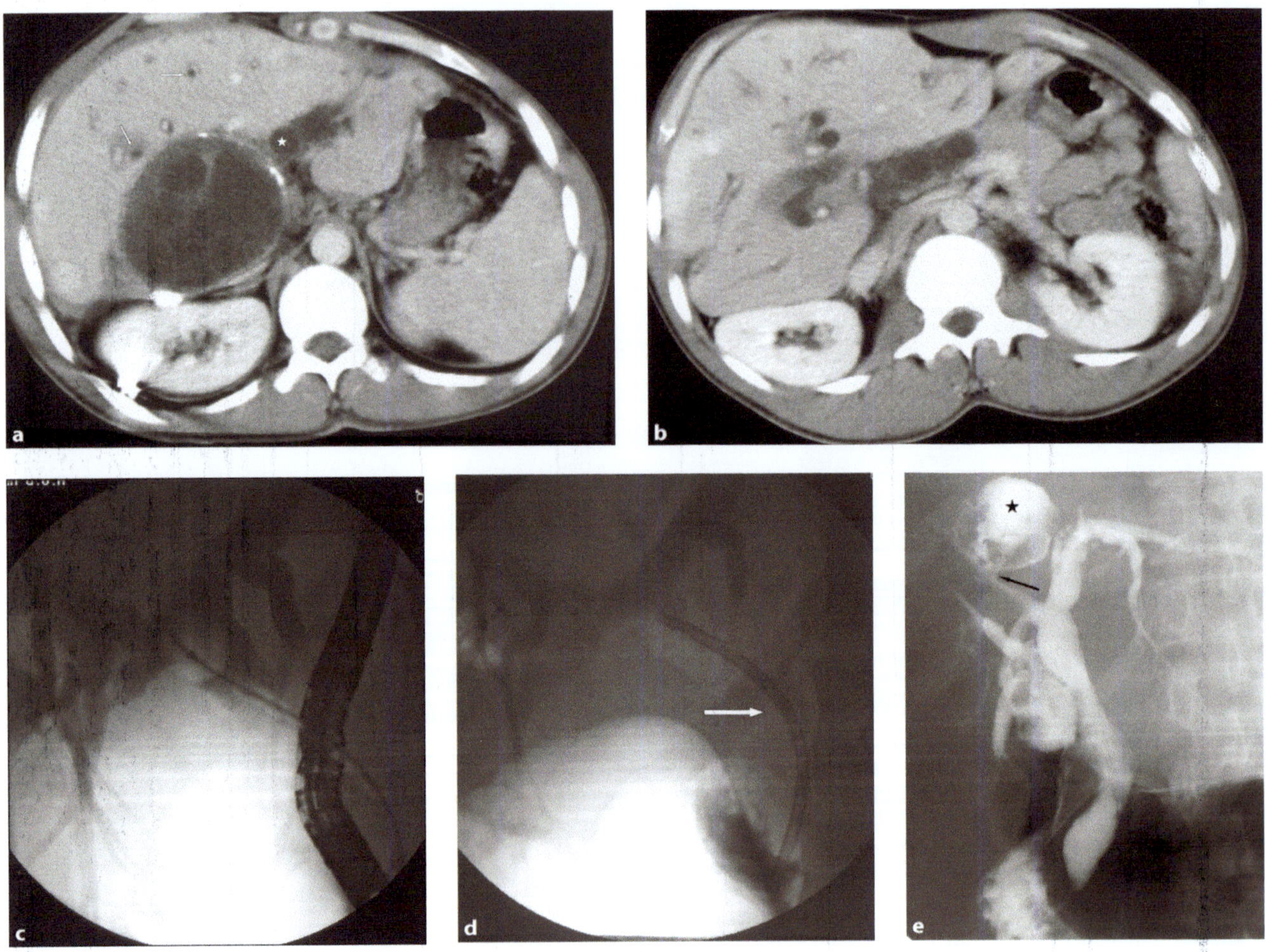

Fig. 5.27 Endoscopic retrograde cholangiopancreatography as a diagnostic and therapeutic tool for biliary obstruction caused by intrabiliary rupture of hepatic echinococcal cyst. **a,b** Contrast-enhanced CT scans of the liver demonstrating a hepatic echinococcal cyst, intra- (*arrows*) and extrahepatic (*star*) biliary ductal dilatation due to biliary obstruction caused by intrabiliary rupture of the cyst. **c,d** ERCP with a plastic stent or biliary endoprosthesis (*arrow*) deployment following a balloon sweep of the membranes or small daughter cysts from the CBD to relieve biliary obstruction. **e** ERCP in another patient demonstrating biliocystic communication (*arrow*)

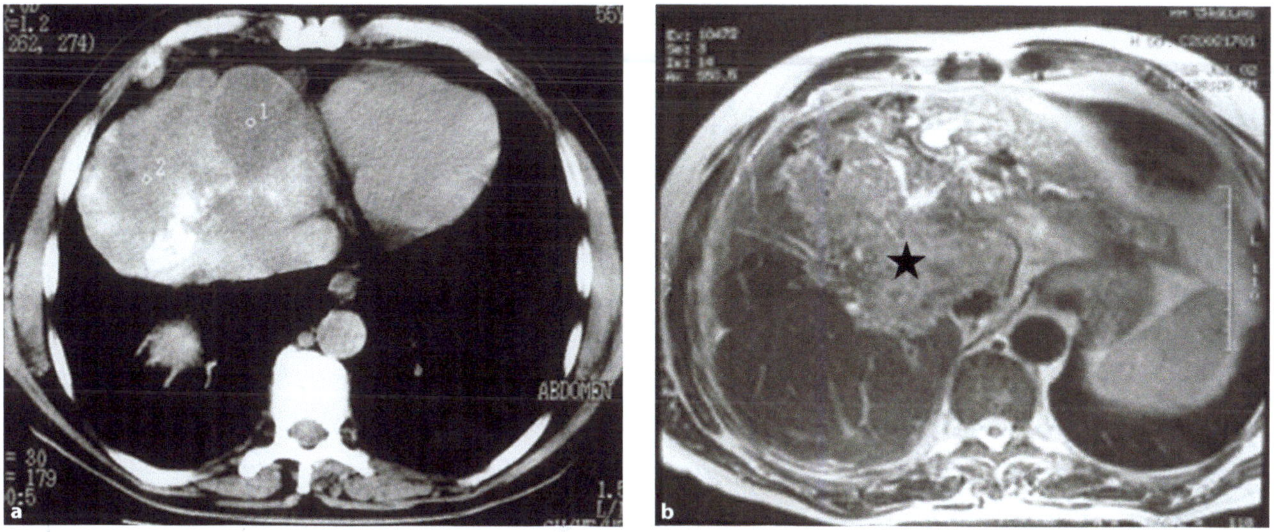

Fig. 5.28 **a** Contrast-enhanced CT scan and **b** T2-weighted MR images showing alveolar echinococcosis (*star*) of the liver (Courtesy of Dr. Menezes da Silva, Portugal)

5.4.2 Taeniasis

Occasionally, acalculous cholecystitis may be induced by *Taenia saginata*, which is a tapeworm that inhabits the jejunum (Daou et al. 1998). The worm migrates retrogradely from the small bowel through the ampulla of Vater into the biliary tree, causing biliary or pancreatic complications.

5.5 Helminths – Flukes (Trematodes)

5.5.1 Hepatobiliary Schistosomiasis

In tropical and subtropical areas *Schistosoma mansoni*, with its predilection for the inferior mesenteric artery territory, i.e., the descending colon and sigmoid, prevalent in the Middle East, and *Schistosoma japonicum*, with its predilection for the superior mesenteric artery territory, i.e., the duodenum and jejunum, prevalent in the Far East, affect the liver and biliary tree.

Two clinical and pathological stages may be identified that correlate with the radiological findings. First, an acute reversible and compensated stage in which a granulomatous inflammatory reaction around *Schistosoma* eggs develops in the liver or gallbladder. Radiologically, a schistosomal hepatic granuloma (Fig. 5.29) appears as a focal hypoechoic solid lesion on ultrasonography, and a hypervascular nodule on contrast-enhanced CT scans. The imaging features of schistosomal hepatic granuloma are nonspecific and mimic many other more common diseases, in particular primary or secondary malignancies. Schistosomal granulomatous cholecystitis occurs in approximately 4% of patients with hepatosplenic schistosomiasis (El Sheikh Mohamed et al. 1994). The inflamed gallbladder is not over-distended and shows marked diffuse thickening of its wall on ultrasonography and CT scans, with marked enhancement of the mucosa on contrast-enhanced CT scans compatible with an infectious acalculous cholecystitis (Sharara et al. 2001). Another pattern of acute parasitic injury may be observed consisting of early periportal granulomatous inflammation with thickened portal venous tracts. In the chronic irreversible or decompensated stage of the disease, periportal fibrosis, known as "Symmer's periportal fibrosis" (Figs. 5.30, 5.31) occurs, leading to presinusoidal portal hypertension and splenomegaly. Previously, Abdel-Wahab et al. (1992, 1993) developed a grading system and scoring parameter values for periportal fibrosis and portal hypertension respectively by ultrasonography in adults with hepatosplenic schistosomiasis that correlate well with endoscopic esophageal grade and bleeding. An ultrasound score of greater than 5 correlates with the presence of esophageal varices grade 2 or greater on endoscopy with a sensitivity of 91.3% and a specificity of 94.7%. In 1991, a first WHO consensus meeting was held in Cairo (Egypt), followed by a second meeting in Niamey (Niger) in 1996, and a third meeting in Belo Horizonte (Brazil) in 1997, which have led to the establishment of practical guidelines and protocols to the standardized use of ultrasonography for the assessment of pathological changes induced by schistosomiasis-related morbidity (WHO 1991; Cairo Working Group 1992; Niamey Working Group 2000; Richter et al. 2001). In large-scale surveys conducted according to WHO coding guidelines for ultrasound in schistosomiasis, the use of alternative height-indexing of portal vein diameter (PVD), image patterns in liver parenchyma plus PVD findings predicted that 15% of Egyptians and 2.5% of Kenyans were at risk of variceal bleeding (King et al. 2003). Contrast-enhanced

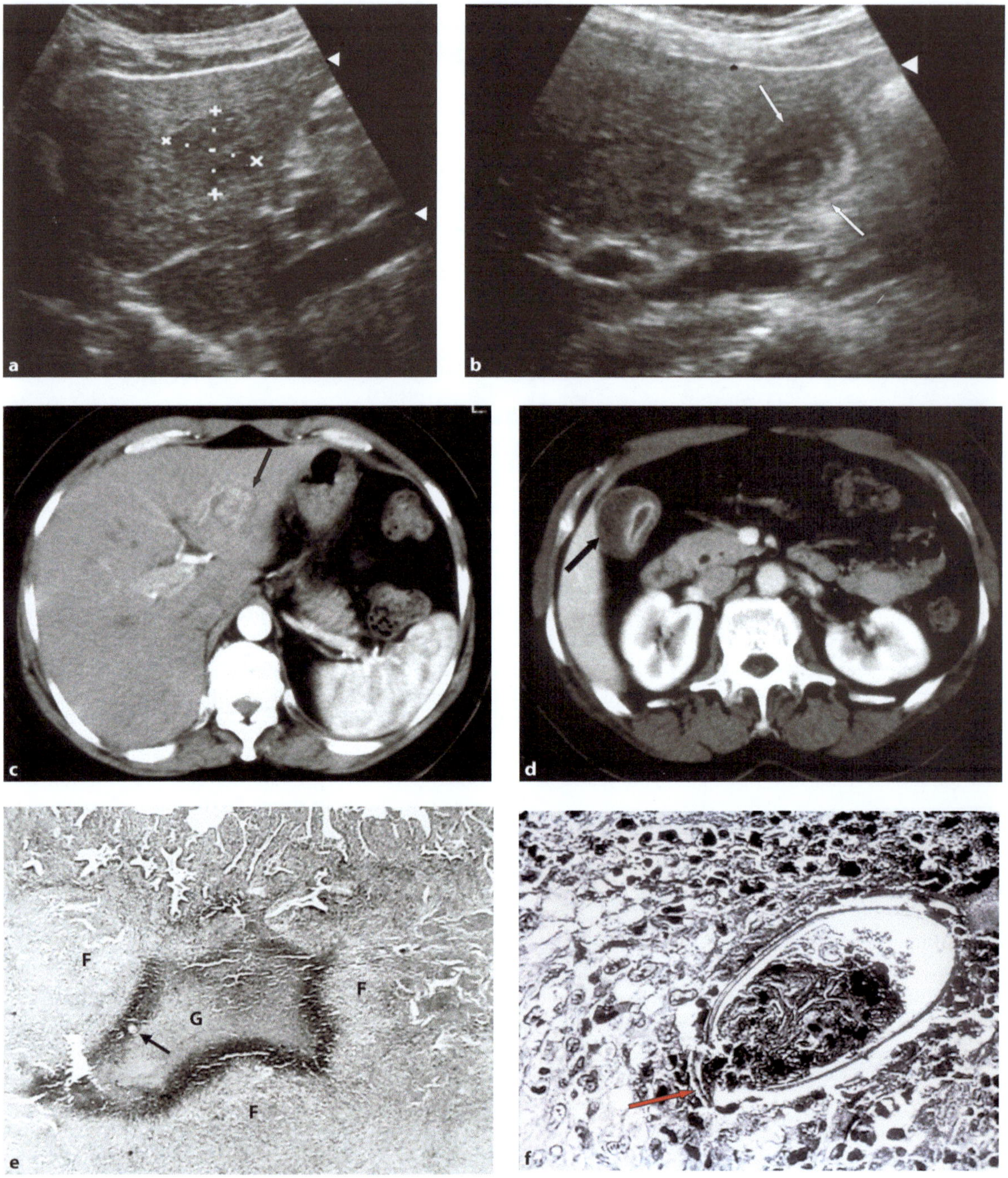

Fig. 5.29 Forty-eight-year-old Lebanese woman with hepatic schistosomal granuloma and schistosomal cholecystitis. **a,b** Ultrasound images of the liver and gallbladder showing a small hypoechoic lesion (*cursors*) in the left hepatic lobe, and under-distended gallbladder (*arrows*) with diffuse thickening of its wall. **c,d** Arterial phase of a contrast-enhanced CT scan demonstrating a hypervascular nodule (*arrow*) in **c** the liver, and **d** diffuse thickening of the gallbladder wall (*arrow*) with enhancement of the mucosa. **e** Microphotograph of the microscopic histologic examination of the gallbladder specimen following cholecystectomy, showing a necrotizing granuloma (*G*) and surrounding fibrosis (*F*) in the gallbladder wall. A parasite egg is indicated by the *arrow*. (H&E stain; original magnification, ×20). **f** High magnification of a *Schistosoma* ovum with its lateral spine (*red arrow*; H&E stain; original magnification ×400). **g,h** *see next page*

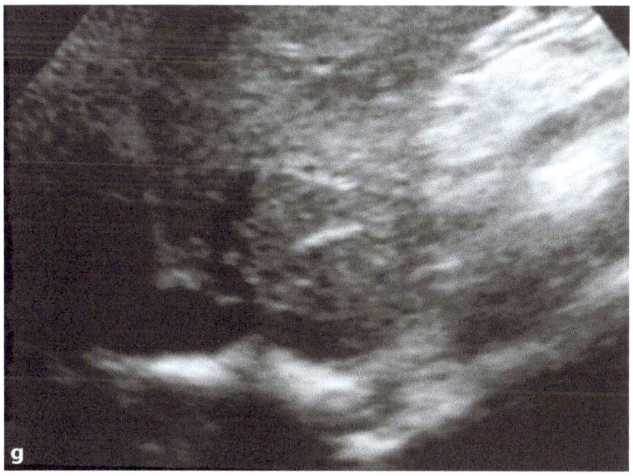

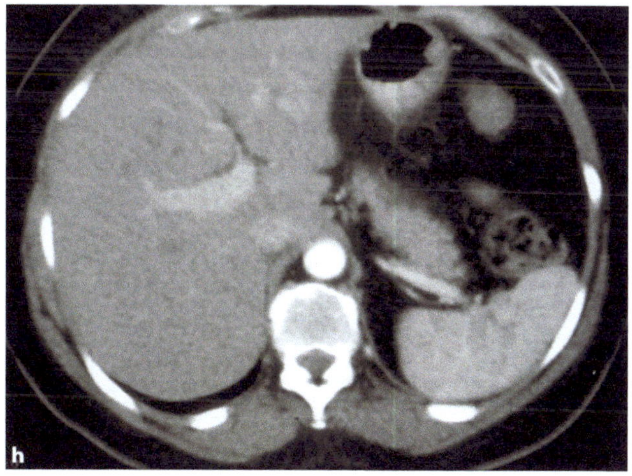

Fig. 5.29 (*continued*) Forty-eight-year-old Lebanese woman with hepatic schistosomal granuloma and schistosomal cholecystitis. **g,h** Follow-up ultrasound and CT scan images of the liver obtained after adjuvant medical treatment for schistosomiasis, showing a significant reduction in the size of the left hepatic nodule (Courtesy of Dr. Ala Sharara, Department of Internal Medicine, American University of Beirut Medical Center, Beirut, Lebanon; reproduced with kind permission from Lippincott Williams & Wilkins)

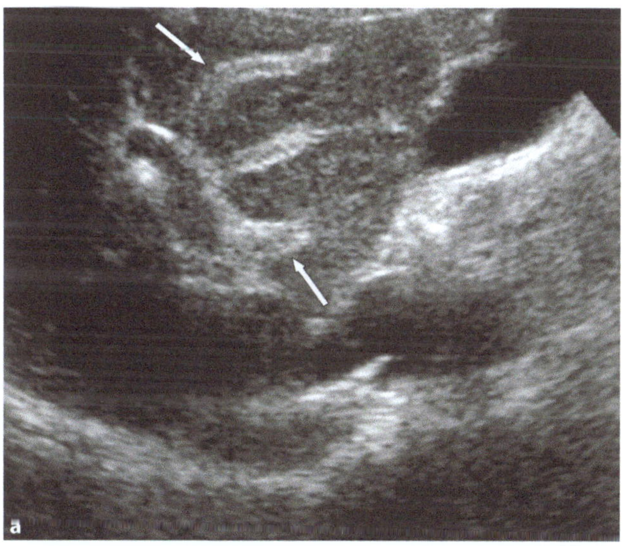

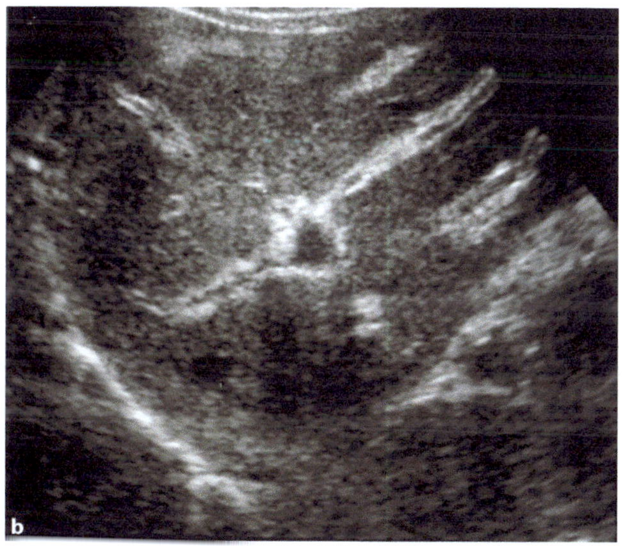

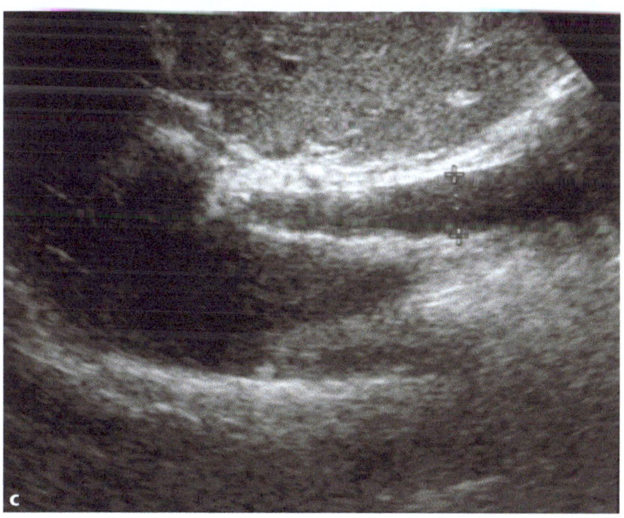

Fig. 5.30 Forty-two-year-old Egyptian man with schistosomal periportal fibrosis. **a–c** Ultrasonography of the liver demonstrating increased periportal echoes (*arrows*) compatible with periportal fibrosis, and **c** dilated portal vein (*cursors*) due to portal hypertension

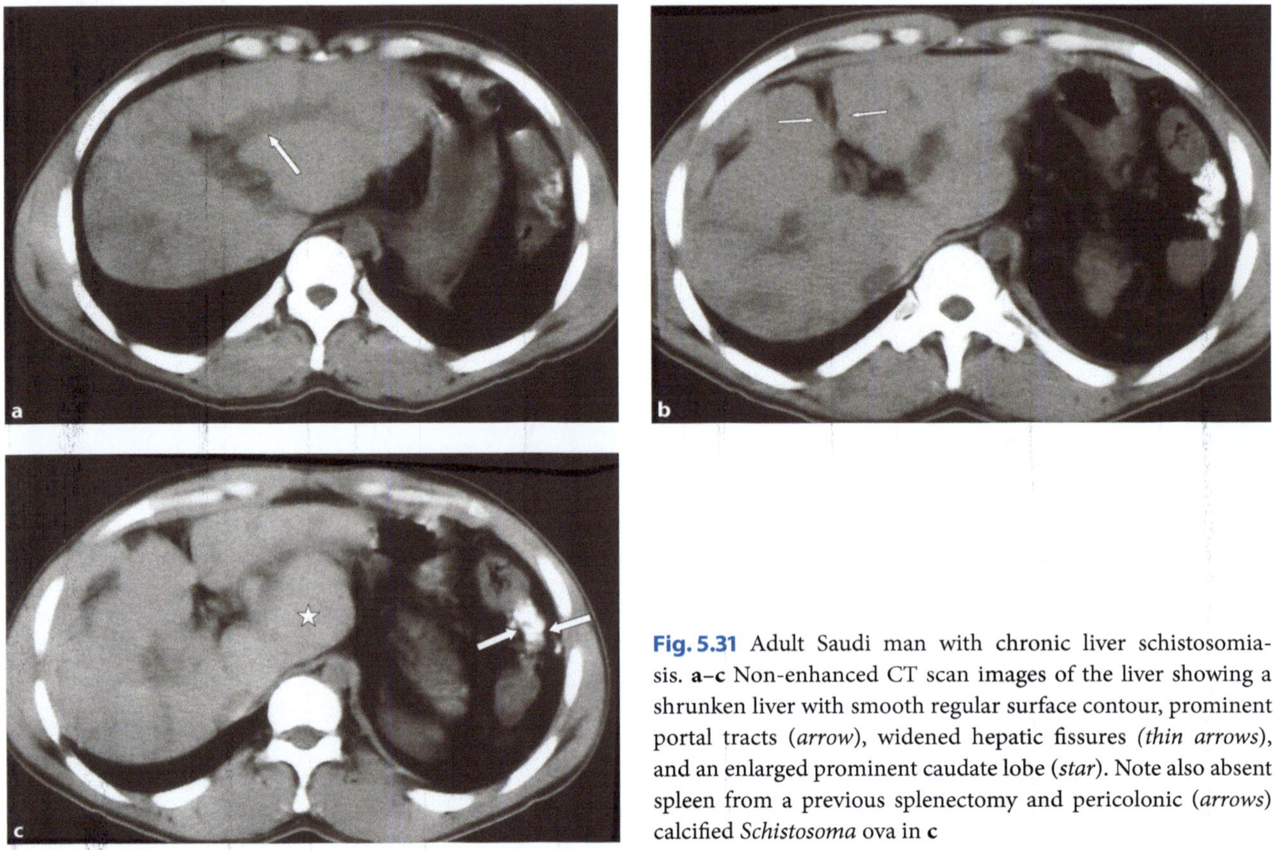

Fig. 5.31 Adult Saudi man with chronic liver schistosomiasis. **a–c** Non-enhanced CT scan images of the liver showing a shrunken liver with smooth regular surface contour, prominent portal tracts (*arrow*), widened hepatic fissures (*thin arrows*), and an enlarged prominent caudate lobe (*star*). Note also absent spleen from a previous splenectomy and pericolonic (*arrows*) calcified *Schistosoma* ova in **c**

CT or MR scans are useful techniques for imaging the early active periportal inflammatory stage. On CT and MR scans early in the disease process the periportal inflammation enhances on contrast-enhanced CT scans and shows increased signal on T2-weighted MR images. As the periportal fibrotic reaction progresses, enhancement on CT decreases, as would the T2 signal on MRI; thus, T2-weighted spin echo sequences may be helpful in assessing the activity of periportal inflammation (Sammak et al. 1999; Willemsen et al. 1995; Lambertucci et al. 2004). With *S. japonicum* hepatic septal fibrosis is characterized by the irregular surface outline of "turtle-back" liver with or without capsular calcifications (Araki 1985), whilst with *S. mansoni* the liver surface remains smooth and regular without calcifications of the liver capsule.

The diagnosis of schistosomiasis is based on the identification of *Schistosoma* eggs or ova in stool and urine examinations, and on positive specific serology tests. If these tests are negative then a rectal biopsy becomes necessary. In the acute stage of the disease a liver biopsy of the schistosomal granuloma can be performed to demonstrate schistosoma eggs and to exclude malignancy, whilst in the chronic stage of liver schistosomal fibrosis, the ultrasound and CT findings are so characteristic and diagnostic that liver biopsy is usually unnecessary (Cerri et al. 1984; Abdel-Wahab et al. 1989; Cheung et al. 1996; Richter et al. 2003).

5.5.2 Liver Flukes (Clonorchiasis, Opisthorchiasis, Fascioliasis, Dicrocoeliasis) and Paragonimiasis (Lung Fluke)

Biliary clonorchiasis, caused by *Clonorchis sinensis*, and opisthorchiasis, caused by *Opisthorchis viverrini*, are raw-fish eating infestations found in certain endemic regions, particularly in the Far East. Radiologically, clonorchiasis shows characteristically intrahepatic bile duct dilatation with filling defects caused by small adult flukes, periductal changes consisting of fibrous thickening of the bile ducts or periductal fibrosis showing increased periductal echogenicity on ultrasonography, with no or minimal dilatation of the extrahepatic bile duct (Lim 1990).

Recurrent pyogenic cholangitis, which is also known as oriental cholangiohepatitis or intrahepatic pigment stone disease (Fig. 5.32), is characterized by intrahepatic formation of pigmented bilirubinate, noncalcium-containing stones with recurrent exacerbation and remission of abdominal pain frequently associated with jaundice, chills, and fever. The cause of the disease is not known, but associations with clonorchiasis, ascariasis, and nutritional deficiency have been suggested (Lim 1991). Also, clonorchiasis predisposes the host to the development of cholangiocarcinoma (Choi et al. 2004).

With opisthorchiasis characteristic cystic or saccular intrahepatic biliary ductal dilatation with or without

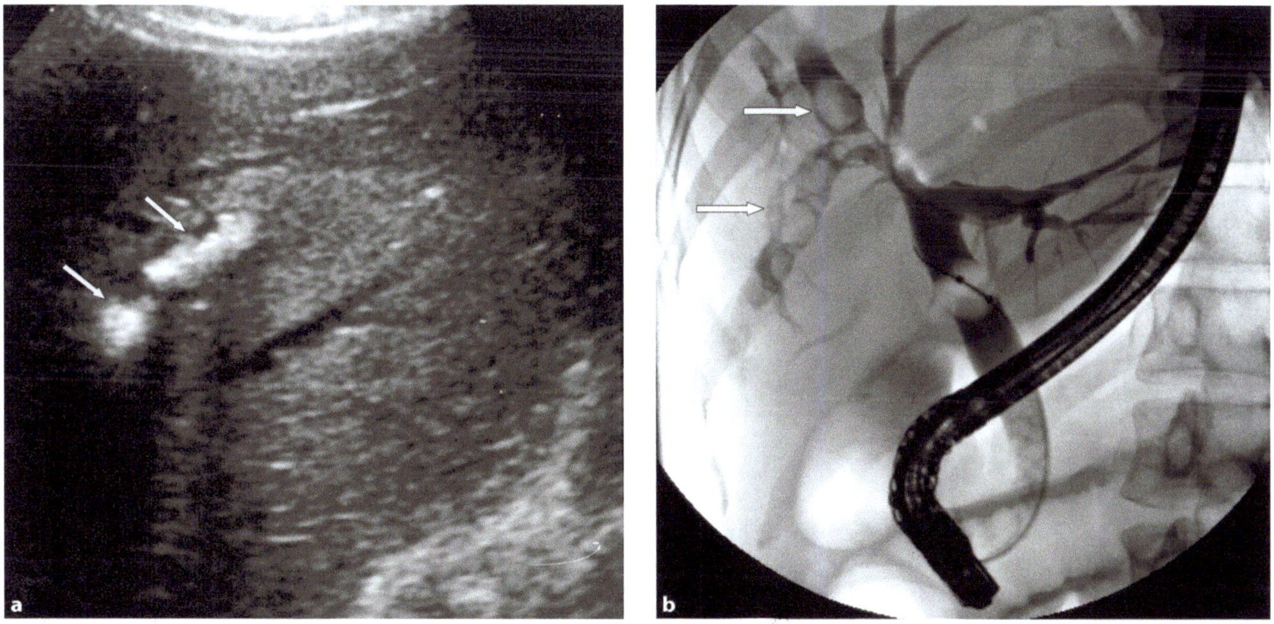

Fig. 5.32 Thirty-two-year-old woman from the Philippines with a history of recurrent attacks of abdominal pain and fever. **a** Ultrasound image of the liver showing intrahepatic echogenic foci (*arrows*) casting faint posterior acoustic shadowing. The gallbladder was unremarkable. **b** ERCP image demonstrating dilated right intrahepatic ducts with intraluminal filling defects (*arrows*) and minimally dilated common bile duct

stone formation may be identified (Harinasuta et al. 1993).

Hepatobiliary fascioliasis is a zoonosis of the liver and bile duct that has worldwide prevalence and is caused by the large adult fluke *Fasciola hepatica*. Two phases of the disease process can be identified, which correlate well with the radiological changes. An acute parenchymal phase (Fig. 5.33) of larval migration in the liver characterized by multiple, small, peripheral, often subcapsular lesions or channels corresponding to microabscesses and/or larger eosinophilic granulomas best seen on CT scans or MRI of the liver, representing migratory tracts left by the flukes. These changes regress or disappear after treatment (Fig. 5.34). In the chronic biliary phase of fascioliasis (Fig. 5.35) dilatation of the bile ducts occurs, with irregular thick walls due to hyperplasia, and the parasite is best visualized by ultrasonography and ERCP.

Humans are very rarely infested with *Dicrocoelium dentriticum* causing biliary sludge or gallstones (Mohammed 1990), or occasionally biliary obstruction (Bourgeon et al. 1974; Karadag et al. 2005).

Hepatic paragonimiasis is a rare form of ectopic infestation caused by the lung fluke *Paragonimus westermani*, which penetrates the intestinal wall into the peritoneal cavity and migrates into the peritoneal cavity to reach the liver or penetrates the diaphragm to reach the pleural cavity and lung. During this migratory phase, it induces liver parenchymal changes similar to fascioliasis (Kim et al. 2004).

The diagnosis of liver flukes should be suspected in patients presenting with the clinical triad consisting of right upper quadrant pain, fever, and eosinophilia. The infection is confirmed by positive serologic tests, identification of fluke eggs from duodenal or bile aspirates using endoscopy, and retrieval of flukes at ERCP (Birjawi et al. 2002). Alternatively, the diagnosis of biliary fascioliasis can be established by ultrasound-guided gallbladder needle aspiration with demonstration of parasite eggs in the bile sample on microscopy (Kabaalioglu et al. 1999).

5.6 Arthropods

5.6.1 Pentastomiasis

Pentastomiasis is a zoonosis caused by the arthropod parasite *Armillifer armillatus*, found in certain endemic regions, namely in Central and West Africa. Clinically, the majority of infested people are asymptomatic, occasionally patients with heavy infestation may present with acute abdomen due to peritoneal irritation by live worms, or with a granulomatous reaction in the liver leading to hepatic fibrosis. Laboratory tests may show mild eosinophilia. Typical or characteristic C-shaped, 4- to 8-mm, scattered calcifications may be seen throughout

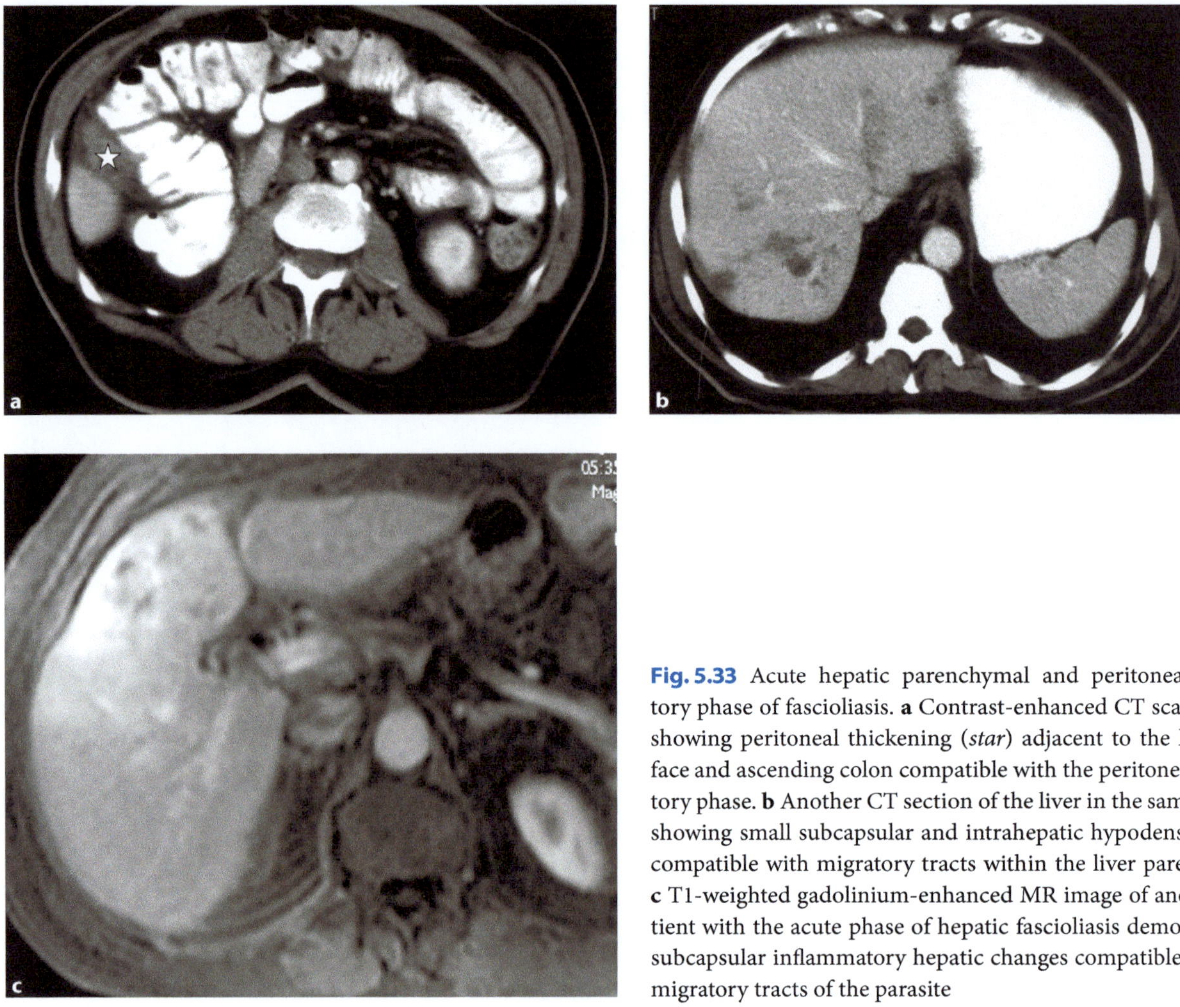

Fig. 5.33 Acute hepatic parenchymal and peritoneal migratory phase of fascioliasis. **a** Contrast-enhanced CT scan images showing peritoneal thickening (*star*) adjacent to the liver surface and ascending colon compatible with the peritoneal migratory phase. **b** Another CT section of the liver in the same patient showing small subcapsular and intrahepatic hypodense lesions compatible with migratory tracts within the liver parenchyma. **c** T1-weighted gadolinium-enhanced MR image of another patient with the acute phase of hepatic fascioliasis demonstrating subcapsular inflammatory hepatic changes compatible with the migratory tracts of the parasite

the liver (Fig. 5.36), spleen, peritoneum, and mesentery, representing calcified dead larvae (Bouchaud and Matheron 1996; Steinbach and Johnstone 1957). The diagnosis is usually confirmed at laparotomy performed for an acute abdomen, by identification of viable worms in the peritoneum or encysted worms (Obengui et al. 1999).

5.6.2 Visceral Linguatulosis

Among different species, *Linguatula serrata* infects man and is found worldwide. Humans can become infected either by ingesting the eggs or larvae of the parasite shed on consumed vegetables by nasal secretions of dogs or other canids, or by ingesting encysted nymphs in viscera, namely raw liver of infected sheep or goat.

When eggs shed by infected canids on vegetables are consumed, larvae encyst in the viscera, producing visceral linguatulosis. Encysted larvae in the viscera of humans are a dead-end and they eventually die with granuloma formation (Lapierre et al. 1976), which may be mistaken for a tumorous process or deposit. Occasionally, it can produce a liver abscess containing a nympha of the parasite encysted and calcified; the pus material is sterile on culture with no growth (Latrive et al. 1980).

5.7 Hepatic Involvement in Hypereosinophilic Syndrome

Several diseases may cause hypereosinophilia, including parasitic infestations (schistosomiasis, strongyloidiasis, gnathostomiasis, toxocariasis, trichinosis, filariasis, echinococcosis, cysticercosis, dicrocoeliasis, fascioliasis and other liver flukes, pentastomiasis), autoimmune diseases, hypersensitivity or allergic diseases, and malignancies. In some rare instances, hypereosinophilia is idiopathic, i.e., without a demonstrable cause despite extensive investigation, so-called hypereosinophilic syndrome (HES). The criteria used for diagnosis of HES include persistent eosinophilia of 1,500 eosinophils/mm^3 for longer than 6 months, evidence of organ involvement, with no demonstrable cause (Hardy and Anderson 1968; Chusid et al. 1975). The clinical disease consists of flu-like symp-

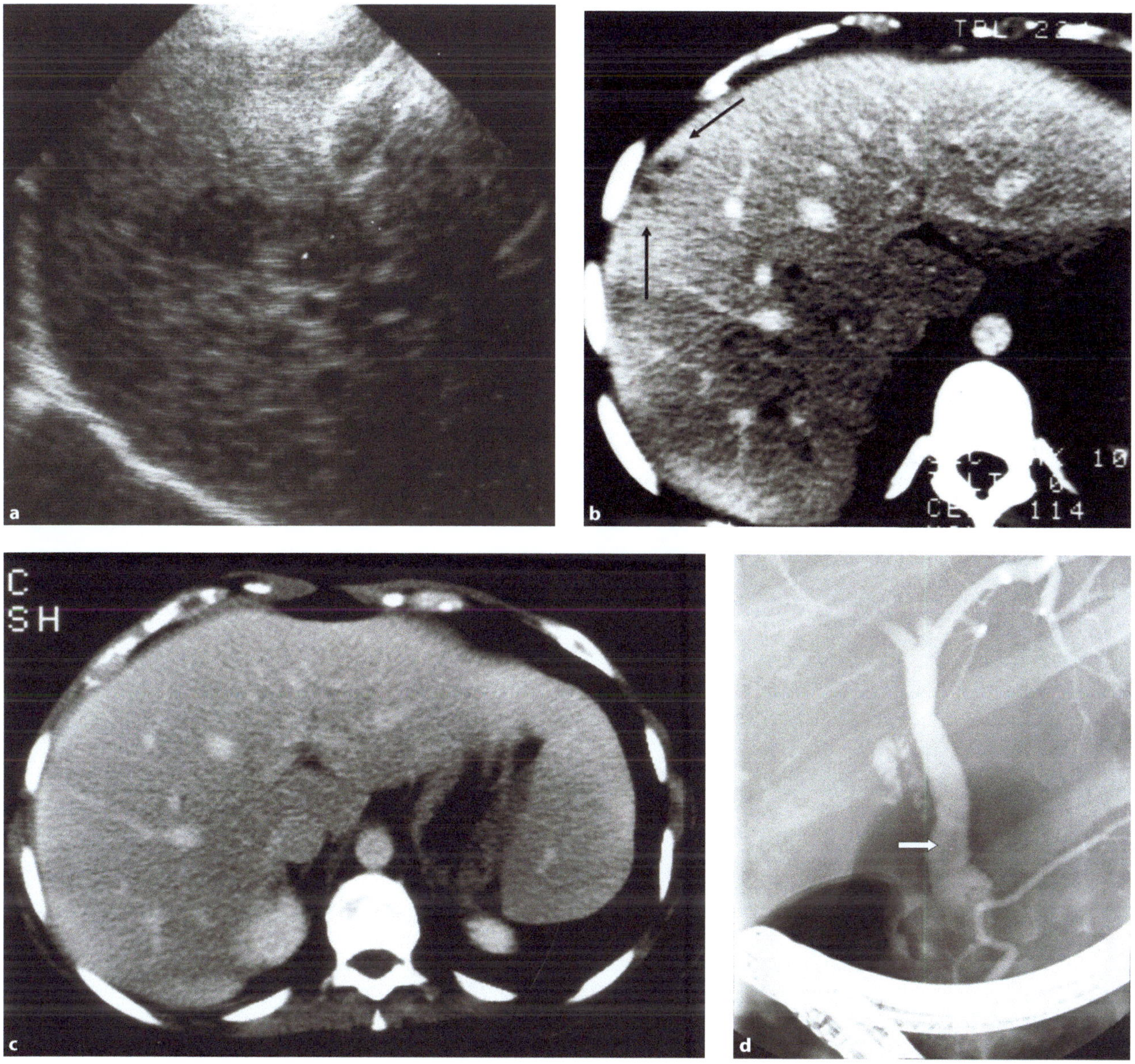

Fig. 5.34 Twenty-five-year-old woman with hepatobiliary fascioliasis. **a** Ultrasound and **b** contrast-enhanced CT scan images of the liver showing inhomogeneity of liver echotexture and small subcapsular hypodense lesions on a CT scan (*black arrows*), representing acute parenchymal larval migratory phase of fascioliasis. **c** Follow-up contrast-enhanced CT scan examination obtained 5 years later showing complete healing of the hepatic parenchymal changes. **d** ERCP image demonstrating a filling defect in the distal segment of the common bile duct (*white arrow*) representing the adult fluke, compatible with the chronic biliary phase of fascioliasis

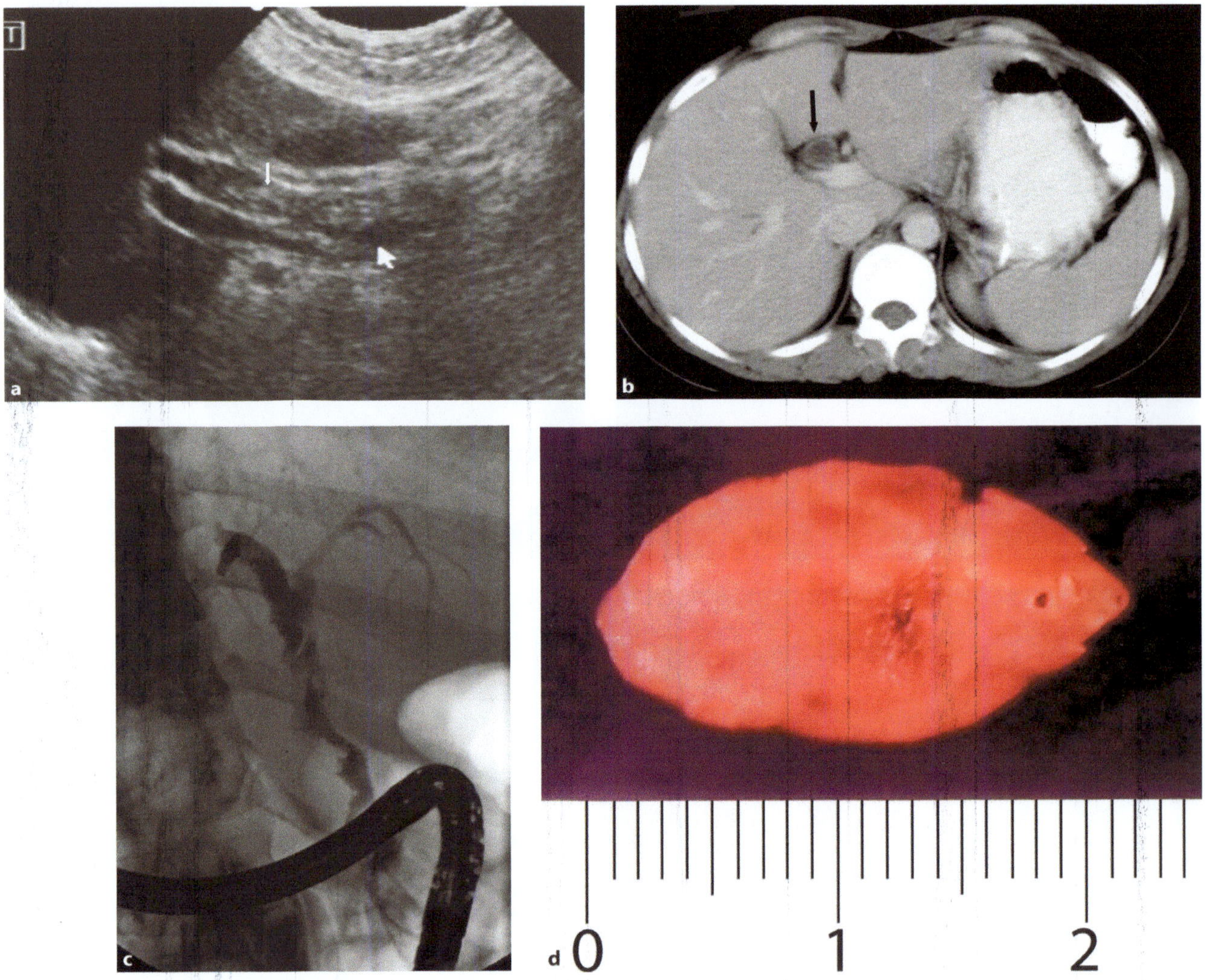

Fig. 5.35 Chronic biliary phase of fascioliasis. **a** Ultrasound and **b** CT scan images of the liver showing a normal liver parenchyma; however, there is minimal intra- and extrahepatic biliary ductal dilatation (*black arrow*) with evidence of an intraluminal echogenic structure (*white arrows*) within the CBD casting no acoustic shadowing. **c** ERCP demonstrating irregularities of CBD due to hyperplasia, and **d** a filling defect on ERCP compatible with the *Fasciola hepatica* parasite that was extracted (Courtesy of Dr. Ghina Birjawi, Department of Diagnostic Radiology, American University of Beirut Medical Center, Beirut, Lebanon; reproduced with kind permission of the Lebanese Medical Journal)

toms (fever, arthralgia, myalgia), hepatosplenomegaly, lymphadenopathy, high peripheral eosinophil count (30–70% eosinophils), and abnormal liver function tests. HES may cause eosinophil-related damage to various organs, including the liver, due to eosinophilic infiltration.

Hepatosplenomegaly with or without solid liver lesions and enlarged lymph nodes may be identified on cross-sectional imaging (Kim et al. 1993; Nam et al. 1999; Lim et al. 2000; Sun et al. 2005). The imaging findings are nonspecific, mimicking primary or metastatic malignant disease. The diagnosis is usually confirmed by bone marrow biopsy demonstrating eosinophilic hyperplasia or biopsy of the organs involved showing eosinophilic infiltration or focal eosinophil necrosis (FEN) with no evidence of malignant cells or parasites or its eggs. There is complete resolution of liver changes in 2–6 months following corticosteroids and antihistamine therapy (Fig. 5.37).

5.8 Conclusion

The liver and biliary tree are the second commonest organs involved with parasites after the gastrointestinal tract. Imaging is essential for the identification of abnormalities in the hepatobiliary tract, pancreas, and spleen. Some imaging findings are characteristic and diagnostic, while atypical findings may be misinterpreted for other pathologies. Laboratory and serology tests, combined with biopsies or retrieval of the parasite, help to confirm the diagnosis.

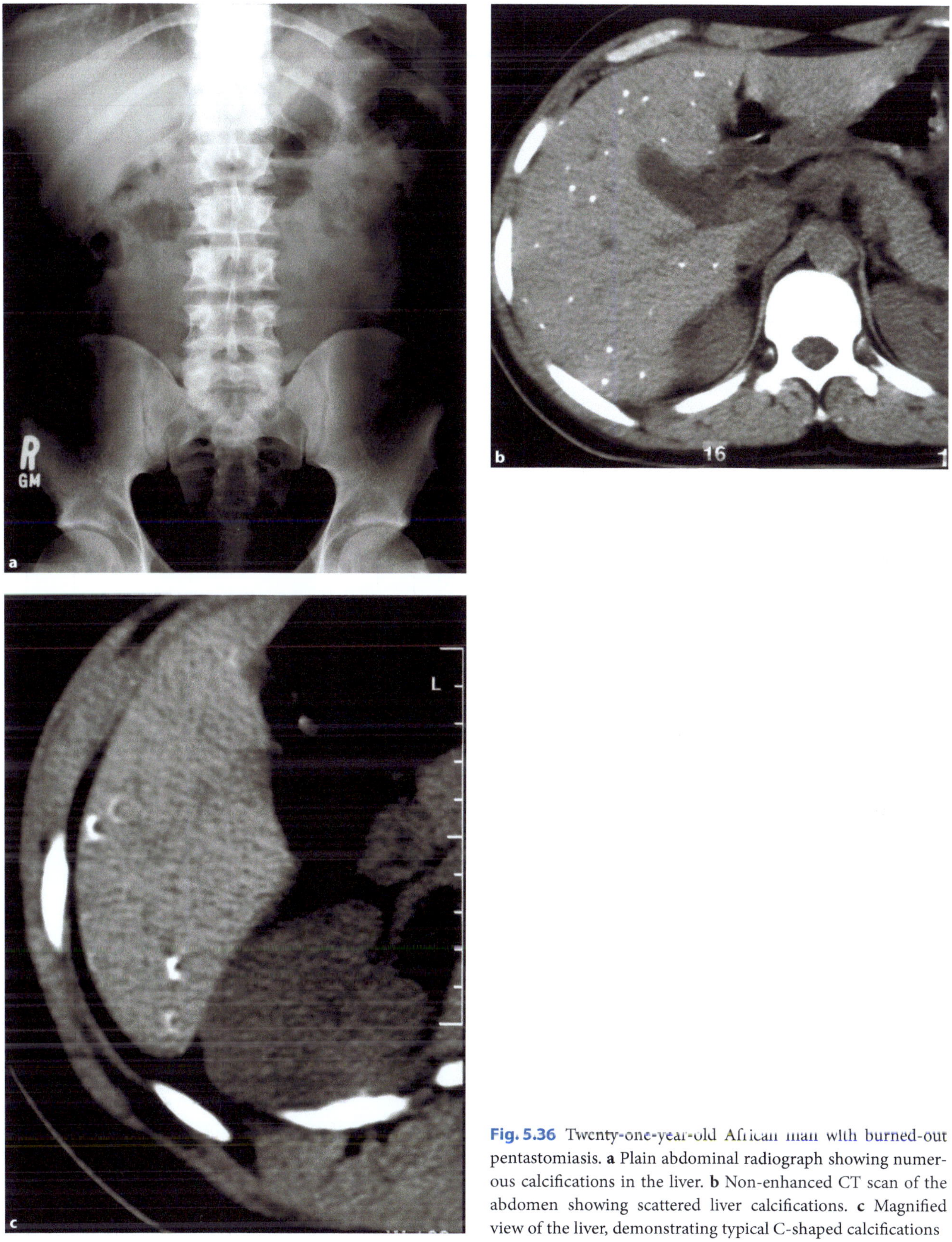

Fig. 5.36 Twenty-one-year-old African man with burned-out pentastomiasis. **a** Plain abdominal radiograph showing numerous calcifications in the liver. **b** Non-enhanced CT scan of the abdomen showing scattered liver calcifications. **c** Magnified view of the liver, demonstrating typical C-shaped calcifications

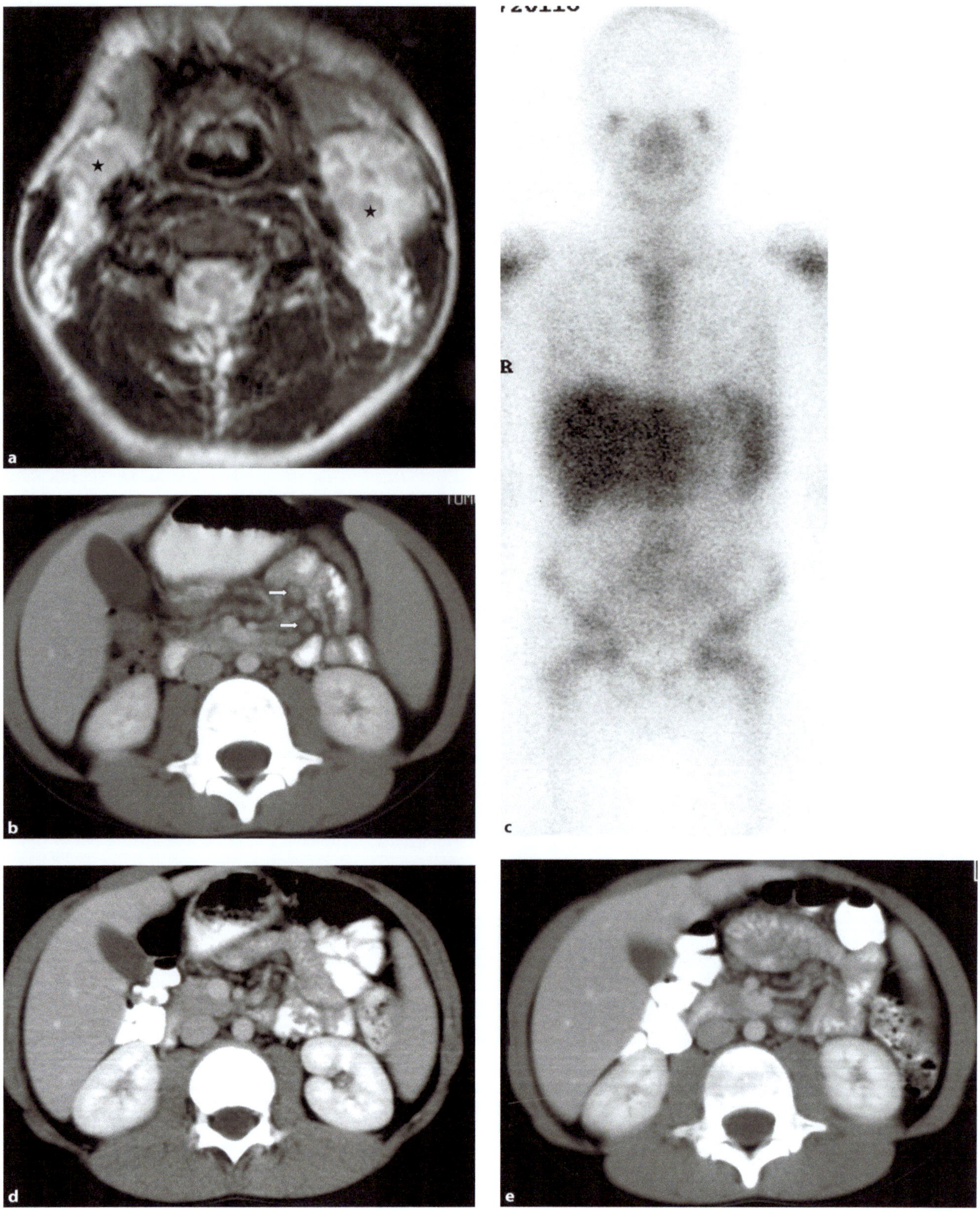

Fig. 5.37 Ten-year-old boy with fever, adenopathy, leukocytosis, and a high eosinophil count. **a** T2-weighted MR image of the neck, **b** CT scan of the abdomen, and **c** a gallium 67 citrate scan obtained at presentation. There is evidence of bilateral enlargement of the cervical lymph nodes (*stars*) on MRI, enlarged spleen and mesenteric lymph nodes (*arrows*) on the CT scan. No abnormal uptake of the radiotracer is seen on the radioisotope scan. **d,e** Follow-up CT scan images of the abdomen showing complete resolution of the splenomegaly and mesenteric lymphadenopathy following corticosteroid therapy

References

Abdel-Wahab MF, Esmat G, Milad M, Abdel-Razek S, Strickland GT (1989) Characteristic sonographic pattern of schistosomal hepatic fibrosis. Ann J Trop Med Hyg 40(1):72–76

Abdel-Wahab MF, Esmat G, Farrag A, El-Boraey YA, Strickland GT (1992) Grading of hepatic schistosomiasis by the use of ultrasonography. Am J Trop Med Hyg 46(4):403–408

Abdel-Wahab MF, Esmat G, Farrag A, El-Boraey Y, Strickland GT (1993) Ultrasonographic prediction of esophageal varices in schistosomiasis mansoni. Am J Gastroenterol 88(4):560–563

Akata D, Ozmen MN, Kaya A, Akhan O (1999) Radiological findings of intraparenchymal liver *Ascaris* (hepatobiliary ascariasis). Eur Radiol 9:93–95

Al-Karawi MA, Salam I, Mohamed AS (1989) Endoscopic diagnosis and extraction of biliary ascaris: a case report. Ann Saudi Med 9:310–311

Al-Karawi MA, Sanai FM, Yasawy MI, Mohamed AE (1999) Biliary strictures and cholangitis secondary to ascariasis: endoscopic management. Gastrointest Endosc 50:695–697

Araki T (1985) Hepatic schistosomiasis japonica identified by CT. Radiology 157:757–760

Aronson NE, Cheney C, Rholl V, Burris D, Hadro N (2001) Biliary giardiasis in a patient with human immunodeficiency virus. J Clin Gastroenterol 33(2):167–170

Astagneau ED, Hadengue A, Degott C, Vilgrain V, Erlinger S, Benhamon JP (1994) Biliary obstruction resulting from *Strongyloides stercoralis* infection. Report of a case. Gut 35:705–706

Azuma K, Yashiro N, Kinoshita T, Yoshigi J, Ihara N (2002) Hepatic involvement of visceral larva migrans due to *Toxocara Canis:* a case report – CT and MR findings. Radiat Med 20:89–92

Bae K, Jeon KN (2006) CT findings of malarial spleen. Br J Radiol 79(946):e145–e147

Berger T, Degremont A, Gebbers JO, Tonz O (1990) Hepatic capillariasis in a 1-year-old child. Eur J Pediatr 149:333–336

Birjawi GA, Sharara AI, Al-Awar GN, Tawil AN, Moukaddam H, Khouzami RA, Haddad MC (2002) Biliary fascioliasis: case report and review of the literature. J Med Liban 50(1–2):60–62

Bonnard P, Guiard-Schmid J-B, Develoux M, Rosenbaum W, Pialoux G (2005) Splenic infarction during acute malaria. Trans R Soc Trop Med Hyg 99:82–86

Bouchaud O, Matheron S (1996) Radiologic diagnosis for a Gabonese case. Bull Soc Pathol Exot 89(1):31–32

Bourgeon R, Borelli JP, Koch G, Le Fichoux Y, Brisard M (1974) Letter: biliary tract fluke: a surgical first. Nouv Presse Med 3(25):1616

Bukte Y, Nazaroglu H, Mete A, Yilmaz F (2004) Visceral leishmaniasis with multiple nodular lesions of the liver and spleen: CT and sonographic findings. Abdom Imaging 29:82–84

Cairo Working Group (1992) The use of diagnostic ultrasound in schistosomiasis-attempts at standardization of methodology. In: Hatz C, Jenkins JM, Tanner M (eds) Special issue: ultrasound in schistosomiasis. Acta Trop 51:45–63

Canalias J, Falco J, Martin J, Jurado I (1997) Macronodular hepatic granulomas due to visceral leishmaniasis in an AIDS patient: imaging findings. J Comput Assist Tomogr 21(4):677–679

Cerri CG, Alves VA, Magalhaes A (1984) Hepatosplenic schistosomiasis mansoni: ultrasound manifestations. Radiology 153(3):777–780

Chang S, Lim JH, Choi D, Park CK, Kwon NH, Cho SY, Choi DC (2006) Hepatic visceral larva migrans of *Toxocara canis*: CT and sonographic findings. AJR Am J Roentgenol 187(6): W622–W6229

Cheung H, Lai YM, Loke TK, Lee KC, Ho WC, Choi WC, Metreweli C (1996) The imaging diagnosis of hepatic schistosomiasis japonicum sequelae. Clin Radiol 51(1):51–55

Choe G, Lee HS, Seo JK, Chai JY, Lee SH, Eom KS, Chi JG (1993) Hepatic capillariasis: first case report in the Republic of Korea. Am J Trop Med Hyg 48(5):610–625

Choi BI, Han JK, Hong ST, Lee KH (2004) Clonorchiasis and cholangiocarcinoma: etiologic relationship and imaging diagnosis. Clin Microbiol Rev 17(3):540–552

Chusid MJ, Dale DC, West BC, Wolf SM (1975) The hypereosinophilic syndrome: analysis of fourteen cases with review of the literature. Medicine 54:1–27

Dairymple RB (1982) Hyperechoic liver abscesses, unusual ultrasonic appearances. Clin Rad 33:541

Danaci M, Belet U, Polat V, Incesu L (1999) MR imaging features of biliary ascariasis. AJR Am J Roentgenol 173(2):503

Daou R, Achram M, Abousalbi M, Dannaoui M (1998) Acute acalculous cholecystitis due to *Taenia saginata.* Chirurgie 123:195–197

Didier D, Weiler S, Rohmer P, Lassegue A, Deschamps JP, Vuitton D, Miguet JP, Weill F (1985) Hepatic alveolar echinococcosis: correlative US and CT study. Radiology 154(1):179–186

Dominguez S, Hillaire S, Molas G, Degott C, Valla DC, Erlinger S (1998) Hepato-biliary involvement in lambliasis. Gastroenterol Clin Biol 22(6–7):647–648

Dow C, Chiodini PL, Haines AJ, Michelson SMC (1998) Human gnathostomiasis. J Infect 17:147–149

Dunn IJ, Palmer PE (1998a) Babesiosis. Semin Roentgenol 33:89–90

Dunn IJ, Palmer PE (1998b) Toxoplasmosis. Semin Roentgenol 33:81–85

El Sheikh Mohamed AR, Al Karawi MA, Yasawy MI (1994) Organ involvement in hepatointestinal schistosomiasis. Hepatogastroenterology 41:370–376

Farah FS, Samra SA, Nuwayri-Salti N (1975) The role of the macrophage in cutaneous leishmaniasis. Immunology 29:755–764

Filice C, Brunetti E, Bruno R, Crippa FG (2000) Percutaneous drainage of echinococcal cysts (PAIR—puncture, aspiration, injection, reaspiration): results of a worldwide survey for assessment of its safety and efficacy. WHO-Informal Working Group on Echinococcosis-Pair Network. Gut 47(1):156–157

Gharbi HA, Hassine W, Brauner MW, Dupuch K (1981) Ultrasound examination of the hydatic liver. Radiology 139:459–463

Gharbi HA, Moussa-Haddad N, Hammou A, De Oliveira Cerri L, Cerri GG (1998) US in tropical diseases: what indications can we promote? JEMU 19(2/3):64–70

Haddad MC, Sammak BM, Al-Karawi M (2000) Percutaneous treatment of heterogenous predominantly solid echo-pattern echinococcal cysts of the liver. Cardiovasc Interv Radiol 23:121–125

Haddad MC, Al-Awar G, Huwaijah SH, Al-Kutoubi AO (2001) Echinococcal cysts of the liver: a retrospective analysis of clinico-radiological findings and different therapeutic modalities. J Clin Imaging 25:403–408

Hardy WR, Anderson RE (1968) The hypereosinophilic syndrome. Ann Intern Med 68:1220–1229

Harinasuta T, Pungpak S, Keystone JS (1993) Trematode infections: opisthorchiasis, clonorchiasis, fascioliasis, and paragonimiasis. Infect Dis Clin North Am 7:699–716

Hayashi K, Tahara H, Kurobi K, et al. (1999) Hepatic imaging studies on patients with visceral larva migrans due to probable *Ascaris Suum* infection. Abdom Imaging 24:465–469

Hwang CM, Kim TK, Ha HK, Kim PN, Lee MG (2001) Biliary ascariasis: MR cholangiography findings in two cases. Korean J Radiol 2:175–178

Ishibashi H, Shimamura R, Hirata Y, Kudo J, Onizuka H (1992) Hepatic granuloma in toxocaral infection: role of ultrasonography in hypereosinophilia. J Clin Ultrasound 20:204–210

Javid G, Wani NA, Gulzar GM, Khan BA, Shah AH, Shah OJ, Khan M (1999) *Ascaris*- Kabaalioglu A, Apaydin A, Sindel T, Luleci E (1999) US-guided gallbladder aspiration: a new diagnostic method for biliary fascioliasis. Eur Radiol 9:880–882

Kabaalioglu A, Ceken K, Alimoglu E, Saba R, Apaydin A (2005) Hepatic toxocariasis: US, CT and MRI findings. Ultraschall Med 26:329–332

Kachawaha S, Pokharana R, Rawat N, Garg P, Badjatiya H, Kochar DK (2003) Ultrasonography in malarial hepatitis. Indian J Gastroenterol 22(3):110

Kakihara D, Yoshimitsu K, Ishigami K, et al. (2004) Liver lesions of visceral larva migrans due to *Ascaris Suun* infection: CT findings. Abdom Imaging 29:598–602

Karadag B, Bilici A, Doventas A, Kantarci F, Selcuk D, Dincer N, Oner YA, Erdincler DS (2005) An unusual case of biliary obstruction caused by *Dicrocœlium dendriticum*. Scand J Infect Dis 37(5):385–388

Khuroo MS, Zargar SA, Yattoo GN, Dar MY, Javid G, Khan BA, Boda MI, Mahajan R (1992) Sonographic findings in gallbladder ascariasis. J Clin Ultrasound 20:587–591

Kim EA, Juhng SK, Kim HW, Kim GD, Lee YW, Cho HJ, Won JJ (2004) Imaging findings of hepatic paragonimiasis: a case report. J Korean Med Sci 19:759–762

Kim GB, Kwon JH, Kang DS (1993) Hypereosinophilic syndrome: imaging findings in patients with hepatic involvement. AJR Am J Roentgenol 161:577–580

King CH, Magak P, Abdel Salam E, Ouma JH, Kariuki HC, Blanton RE (2003) Measuring morbidity in schistosomiasis mansoni: relationship between image pattern, portal vein diameter and portal branch thickness in large-scale surveys using new WHO coding guidelines for ultrasound in schistosomiasis. Trop Med Int Health 8(2):109–117

Knio KN, Baydoun E, Tawk R, Nuwayri-Salti N (2000) Isoenzyme characterization of *Leishmania* isolates from Lebanon and Syria. Am J Trop Med Hyg 63(1–2):43–47

Kochar DK, Agarwal P, Kochar SK, Jain R, Rawat N, Pokharna RK, Kachhawa S, Srivastava T (2003) Hepatocyte dysfunction and hepatic encephalopathy in *Plasmodium falciparum* malaria. Q J Med 96:505–512

Krige JEJ, Beckingham IJ (2001) Liver abscesses and hydatid disease. BMJ 322:537–541

Lambertucci JR, dos Santos Silva LC, Andrade LM, de Queiroz LC, Pinto-Silva RA (2004) Magnetic resonance imaging and ultrasound in hepatosplenic schistosomiasis mansoni. Rev Soc Bras Med Trop 37(4)333–337

Lapierre J, Tourte-Schaefer C, Hien TV, Holler C, Bouchard J, Deslignieres S, Chapuis YL. A case of human hepatic linguatulosis. Bull Soc Pathol Exot Filiales 1976 69(5):450–456

Latrive JP, Hy TD, Sang HT, Huguier M, Le Quintrec Y (1980) Liver abscess and visceral linguatulosis with *Linguatula serrata*. A case report with radiologic-histologic studies. Sem Hop 56(11–12):567–569

Leone N, Baronio M, Todros L, David E, Brunello F, Artioli S, Rizzetto M (2006) Hepatic involvement in larva migrans of *Toxocara Canis*: report of a case with pathological and radiological findings. Dig Liver Dis 38:511–514

Lim JH (1990) Radiologic findings of clonorchiasis. AJR Am J Roentgenol 155:1001–1008

Lim JH (1991) Oriental cholangiohepatitis: pathologic, clinical, and radiologic features. AJR Am J Roentgenol 157:1–8

Lim JH, Lee WJ, Lee DH, Nam KJ (2000) Hypereosinophilic syndrome: CT findings in patients with hepatic lobar or segmental involvement. Korean J Radiol 1:28–103

Lupi A, Todeschini G, Zanco P (2006) Diffuse metabolic activation of reticuloendothelium on F-18 FDG PET imaging in a case of visceral leishmaniasis. Clin Nucl Med 31(1):34–36

Mohammed AE (1990) Human dicrocoeliasis. Report of 208 cases from Saudi Arabia. Trop Geog Med 42(2):1–7

Nam KJ, Jung WJ, Choi JC, Koo BS, Park BH, Lee KN, Han SY, Shin WW, Han SS (1999) Hepatic involvement in hypereosinophilic: sonographic findings. J Ultrasound Med 18:475–479

Ng KK, Wong HF, Kong MS, Chiu LC, Tan CF, Wan YL (1999) Biliary ascariasis: CT, MR cholangiopancreatography, and navigator endoscopic appearance – report of a case of acute biliary obstruction. Abdom Imaging 24:470–472

Niamey Working Group (2000) Ultrasound in schistosomiasis: a practical guide to the standardized use of ultrasonography for the assessment of schistosomiasis-related morbidity. WHO, Geneva www.int/tdr/publications/publications/ultrasound.htm

Nuwayri-Salti N, Baydoun E, El-Tawk R, Fakhoury Makki R, Knio K (2000) The epidemiology of leishmaniases in Lebanon. Trans R Soc Trop Med Hyg 94(2):164–166

Obengui, Moyen G, Mbika-Cardorelle A, Assambo-Kieli C (1999) Porocephalosis: still a rare diagnosis. Santé 9(6):357–360

Ozcan N, Erdogan N, Kucuk C, Ok E (2003) Biliary ascariasis: percutaneous transhepatic management. J Vasc Interv Radiol 14:391–393

Pannenbecker J, Miller TC, Muller J, Jeschke R (1990) Severe capillaria hepatica infestation in a young child. Monatsschr Kinderheilkd 138:767–771

Polat P, Kantarci M, Alper F, Suma S, Koruyucu MB, Okur A (2003) Hydatid disease from head to toe. Radiographics 23:475–494

Ralls PW, Colletti PM, Quinn MF, Halls J (1982) Sonographic findings in hepatic amebic abscess. Radiology 145(1):123–126

Ramsey R, Geremia GK (1988) CNS complications of AIDS: CT and MR findings. AJR Am J Roentgenol 151:449–454

Rawat B, Simons ME (1993) *Strongyloides stercoralis* hyperinfestation: another cause of focal hepatic lesions. Clin Imaging 17:274–275

Richter J, Domingues AL, Barata CH, Prata AA, Lambertucci JR (2001) Report of the Second Satellite Symposium on Ultrasonography in Schistosomiasis. Mem Inst Oswaldo Cruz 96 [Suppl]:151–156

Richter J, Hatz C, Haussinger D (2003) Ultrasound in tropical and parasitic diseases. Lancet 362:900–902

Rusnack JM, Lucey DR (1993) Clinical gnathostomiasis: case report and review of the English-language literature. Clin Infect Dis 16:33–50

Sammak B, Youssef B, Mohamed AR, Abdel Bagi M, Al Shahed M, Ghandour Z, Al Karawi M (1999) Radiological manifestations of liver and gastrointestinal parasitic infections. Hepatogastroenterology 46:1016–1022

Sandouk F, Anand BS, Graham DY (1997a) The whirlpool jet technique for removal of pancreatic duct ascaris. Gastrointest Endosc 46(2):180–182

Sandouk F, Haffar S, Zada M, Graham D, Anaud B (1997b) Pancreatic-biliary ascariasis: experience of 300 cases. Am J Gastroenterol 92:2264–2267

Sharara AI, Abi-Saad G, Mansour A, Haddad M, Tawil A (2001) Acute granulomatous cholecystitis due to *Schistosoma mansoni*. Eur J Gastroenterol Hepatol 13:1001–1003

Sotto A, Gra B (1985) Hepatic manifestations in giardiasis. Acta Gastroenterol Latinoam 15(2):89–94

Steinbach HL, Johnstone HG (1957) The roentgen diagnosis of armillifer infection (porocephalosis) in man. Radiology 68:234–237

Sun JS, Kim JK, Won JH, Lee KM, Cheong JY, Kim YB (2005) MR findings in eosinophilic infiltration of the liver. J Comput Assist Tomogr 29(2):191–194

Teixidor HS, Godwin TA, Ramirez EA (1991) Cryptosporidiosis of the biliary tract in AIDS. Radiology 180:51–56

Vasquez JJ, Sola JJ, Boils PL (1994) Hepatic lesions induced by *Angiostrongylus costaricensis*. Histopathology 25(5):489–491

WHO (1991) Meeting on ultrasonography in schistosomiasis: proposal for a practical guide to the standardized use of ultrasound in the assessment of pathological changes. World Health Organization, Geneva

WHO Informal Working Group on Echinococcosis (1996) Guidelines for treatment of cystic and alveolar echinococcosis in humans. Bull World Health Organ 74(3):231–242

WHO Informal Working Group on Echinococcosis (2001) PAIR: puncture, aspiration, injection, re-aspiration. Geneva WHO, 2001: www.who.int/emc-documents/zoonoses/whocdscraph 20016.html

WHO Informal Working Group on Echinococcosis (2003) International classification of ultrasound images in cystic echinococcosis for application in clinical and field epidemiological settings. Acta Trop 85:253–261

Willemsen UF, Pfluger T, Zoller WG, Kueffer G, Hahn K (1995) MRI of hepatic schistosomiasis mansoni. J Comput Assist Tomogr 19:811–813

Wilson ME, Streit JE (1996) Visceral leishmaniasis. Gastroenterol Clin North Am 25:535–551

Chapter

Imaging of Parasitic Diseases of the Genitourinary System

6

Tarek A. El-Diasty,
Ahmad Farouk El-Sherbiny

Contents

6.1 Introduction

Parasitic infections of the genitourinary system are a heterogeneous group of diseases that have some common features. Most parasitic infections are chronic, and the host's immune response reacts to the different stages of the parasite lifecycle involving different parasite antigens. Although renal disease is not one of the common presenting features, many parasitic infections are associated with glomerular lesions. While many parasites wander into the urinary tract, only three parasitic infections are relatively common, namely schistosomiasis, echinococcosis, and filariasis. Other parasites may also rarely infest the genitourinary system such as malaria, leishmaniasis, trypanosomiasis, babesiosis, toxoplasmosis, trichinosis, dioctophymiasis, microsporidiasis, sparganosis, fascioliasis, genital amebiasis, toxocariasis, strongyloidiasis, and genital flagellates.

6.2 Protozoa

6.2.1 Malaria

Malaria is one of the most prevalent infectious diseases in the world. It was the first parasitic infection clearly shown to be associated with nephrotic syndrome (Kibukamusoke et al. 1967). Moreover, areas of the world with a high incidence of nephrotic syndrome overlap with those where *Plasmodium malariae* occur (Saggie and Dwomoa 1988). Four species of *Plasmodia* are responsible for malaria. Only two of the malaria parasites, namely *P. malariae* (quartan malaria) and *P. falciparum* (tertian malaria), are clearly associated with renal disease, and this occurs in only a small percentage of patients. Renal involvement in the course of malaria is generally characterized by nephrotic syndrome (Eiam-Ong 2003; Mehta et al. 2001). A membranoproliferative type of glomerulonephritis with relatively sparse proliferation of endothelial and mesangial cells is the most common type of glomerular lesion encountered in malaria. Focal and segmental glomerulosclerosis can be seen as well.

6.2.2 Leishmaniasis

Glomerular lesions are observed with visceral leishmaniasis (kala-azar) caused by *Leishmania donovani*. Cutaneous or mucocutaneous leishmaniasis caused by other *Leishmania* species is not associated with renal disease. A prospective study has shown that 60% of patients with kala-azar or visceral leishmaniasis have mild proteinuria with benign changes in the urinary sediment, i.e., microscopic hematuria and leukocyturia (Dutra et al. 1985). The pathological picture is glomerulonephritis with focal and segmental collapse of capillary loops, or interstitial nephritis leading to oliguric renal failure (Caravaca et al. 1991; Sartori et al. 1987).

Cutaneous leishmaniasis is usually characterized by chronic localized ulceration developing at the site of inoculation by sand-fly bites. Genital cutaneous lesions are rare, but have been described in men and women in South America, among miners and farmers. The diagnosis is confirmed by demonstrating the presence of *Leishmania* amastigotes in blood smear or biopsy material (Richens 2004; Cabello et al. 2002; Castro-Coto et al. 1987; Blickstein et al. 1993).

6.2.3 Trypanosomiasis

African trypanosomiasis is a protozoal disease caused by motile hemoflagellates of the genus *Trypanosoma*. The clinical stages of trypanosomiasis range from the trypanosomal chancre that appears at the site of inoculation, to febrile attacks, diffuse intravascular coagulation, lymphadenopathy, and eventually progressive brain dysfunction leading to sleeping sickness, cachexia, and death. Glomerular disease associated with American trypanosomiasis, i.e., Chagas' disease, is limited to an occasional report (Costa et al. 1991).

6.2.4 Toxoplasmosis

Toxoplasmosis is caused by *Toxoplasma gondii*. Infection occurs by the ingestion of cysts or oocysts, or by the transplacental or hematogenous routes. Most recent reports about renal disease associated with *T. gondii* infection deal with the problem of acute renal failure due to sulfadiazine crystal deposition, i.e., crystalluria in the urinary tract after treatment of *Toxoplasma* encephalitis with the drug. Renal ultrasound shows diffuse bilateral echogenic material with acoustic shadowing in both dilated and nondilated systems compatible with renal stones, whereas X-ray examination possesses a low diagnostic sensitivity. In some patients with hydronephrosis and renal obstruction, a percutaneous nephrostomy may be required. Urinalysis typically shows "sheaves of wheat" crystalluria (Kane et al. 1996; De Sequera et al. 1996; Becker et al. 1996).

Another form of urinary involvement in AIDS patients with acute or acquired disseminated toxoplasmosis is the presence of associated acute glomerulonephritis (Ginsburg et al. 1974; Holch et al. 1993), or toxoplasmosis localized to the bladder (Besnier et al. 1995; Chemlal et al. 1996). In neonates with congenital toxoplasmosis, association with a congenital nephrotic syndrome has been described (Shahin et al. 1974; Roussel et al. 1987).

6.2.5 Babesiosis

Babesia is a tick-borne intraerythrocytic parasite. In the US and Europe, *Babesia bovis* and *divergens* are transmitted from cattle to humans. Asplenic persons living in rural areas are particularly susceptible to this disease. The onset of the disease is characterized by a high-grade fever, malaise, arthralgia and myalgia. Approximately 40% of patients develop serious complications that can be fatal such as acute respiratory failure, disseminated intravascular coagulation, congestive heart failure, hemoglobinuria and renal failure. Intraerythrocytic pleomorphic parasites are usually observed in stained thin blood smears (Hatcher et al. 2001; Brasseur and Gorenflot 1992).

6.2.6 Disseminated Microsporidiasis

Microsporidia have emerged as important opportunistic infections in AIDS patients. In disseminated microsporidiasis all organs can be affected, including the central nervous system, heart, respiratory, alimentary and urinary tracts, liver, spleen, bone marrow, and lymph nodes. The disease is fatal, and at autopsy necrotizing and sclerosing microsporidiasis is identified at tissue examination (Yachnis et al. 1996).

6.2.7 Amebiasis

Genital amebiasis is a rare sexually transmitted disease, characterized by a foul bloody discharge from ulcers that affect the vagina, cervix, uterus, and fallopian tubes in women mimicking a genital organ cancer, and the penis in men mimicking a penile carcinoma. The diagnosis is made by biopsy, smear or culture, and serological tests (Richens 2004; Antony and Lopez-Po 1999; Othman and Ismail 1993; Calore et al. 2002).

Immune complex glomerulonephritis associated with the *Entamoeba histolytica* liver abscess has been described (Margolis et al. 1971; Lecuit et al. 1997; Westendorp et al. 1990).

6.2.8 Genital Flagellates

Trichomonas hominis in men and *Trichomonas vaginalis* in women are genital infections that cause urethral and vaginal discharge secondary to urethritis. A nephrotic syndrome with hematuria was described in Italian soldiers stationed in Ethiopia between 1934 and 1939, who were infected with *Trichomonas* (Bellinghieri et al. 2002).

6.3 Helminths – Nematodes (Roundworms)

6.3.1 Filariasis, Loiasis and Onchocerciasis

Filarial infections are widespread in various parts of the world, and probably 200 million people are infected with different filariae in the tropical and subtropical countries of Africa, Asia, Pacific Islands, and Central and South America. Several studies have recently shown a clear association between filariasis and glomerular disease (Langhammer et al. 1997; Pakasa et al. 1997). This association is often difficult to establish due to frequent coinfections (hepatitis B and malaria). Except for an occasional report on acute glomerulonephritis (Date et al. 1979), most reports in the literature describe mesangioproliferative or membranoproliferative glomerulonephritis (Ngu et al. 1985). Glomerular disease associated with filariasis is thought by most authors to be immune complex. The most common clinical findings are those related to "elephantiasis." The urinary tract may be involved with resultant chyluria, which is the passage of lymphatic fluid in urine associated with lymphatic abnormalities. Chyluria may be either tropical or nontropical in nature. The tropical form is by far the most common and is almost always due to *Wuchereria bancrofti* infection. Nontropical filarial parasites (*loa*, *dipetalonema*, *dirofilaria*, and *mansonella* species) rarely have urogenital manifestations, but *Onchocerca volvulus*, the agent of African river blindness, is known to cause massive inguinal lymphadenopathy and scrotal elephantiasis (Amaral et al. 1994). Filariasis results when the larvae of *W. bancrofti* are transmitted to the human by mosquitoes, after which they migrate in the lymphatics and nodes, where they mature. The pathological findings depend on the cycle of filariae and are due to the presence of living or dead larvae or adult worms in the lymphatics. The living worms cause lymphadenitis and lymphangitis with edema, eosinophilic infiltration, and fibroblastic reaction. When the disease becomes more chronic and the death of the worm occurs, there is thickening of the walls of the lymphatics and a marked granulomatous reaction in the vascular and lymphatic walls takes place (Chen 1971). The chronic complications of filariasis occur 5–20 years after the primary infection and include elephantiasis, chyluria, chylous ascites and effusion. Elephantiasis is not only due to fibrosis and obliteration of the lymphatics and lymph nodes, but is also due to a reaction in the small blood vessels, particularly the veins. Enlargement of the penis, scrotum, and breasts may be spectacular, in addition to the gross enlargement of one or more extremities.

A histologic finding of adult worms is a diagnostically definitive but insensitive technique. The presence of *Brugia* or *Wuchereria* microfilariae in peripheral blood, chylous urine, or hydrocele fluid is also diagnostic.

Plain radiography of the soft tissues shows gross thickening with loss or blurring of the fat planes. Intravenous urography is usually normal, but pyelolymphatic reflux may be noted. Dilated renal lymphatics may be clearly demonstrated, particularly when ureteric pressure is applied. Contrast medium may remain within the intrarenal lymphatics for a long time. These features can also be identified on retrograde pyelography (Fig. 6.1). Lymphangiography may show an increase in the number of small lymphatic channels, which have a redundant and tortuous course. Occasionally, contrast materials will flow from the lymphatics into the kidney and outline the calyces, infundibulae, renal pelves, and even the urinary bladder (Fig. 6.2). Although lymphoscintigraphy is a good diagnostic tool in patients with suspected lymphedema of filarial origin by demonstrating multiple dilated and tortuous lymphatic channels with dermal backflow (Shelley et al. 2006), it proved to be not useful in the demonstration of pyelolymphatic connections in one patient with chyluria described by Haddad et al. (1994); indeed, the pyelolymphatic connections were adequately demonstrated by a conventional bipedal lymphangiography in the same patient (Fig. 6.2). Whereas the lymphatics normally empty in a few hours, there may be a marked delay in the emptying of these vessels for several days in patients with filariasis (Dalela et al. 1992; Koga et al. 1992). Mild scrotal edema is not unusual during early infection or with established hydrocele. Penile edema is unusual, and the monstrous elephantine enlargements of the scrotum or penis depicted in textbooks occur largely in populations without access to medical care. Elephantiasis of the limbs poses the difficult differential diagnosis between filarial and other causes, but genital elephantiasis is rarely due to other causes, such as malignancy, lymph node surgery, or radiation.

In endemic areas, differentiation between filarial and idiopathic hydroceles is difficult on either clinical or laboratory grounds. Microfilariae or adult worms are rarely detected in hydrocele fluid, but a milky or sediment-rich hydrocele fluid suggests a filarial origin. Hydrocele accompanied by nodules in the cord or epididymis and a history of travel to or residence in an endemic area favors filariasis. Discovery of the thick, fibrous tunica, especially with cholesterol or calcium deposits, should prompt a diagnosis of filariasis; indeed, tunical calcification is so rare in idiopathic hydrocele.

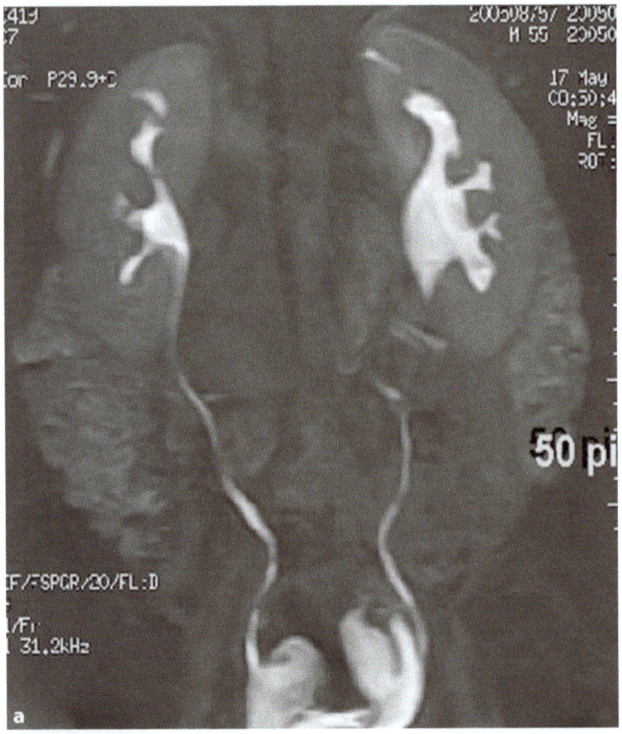

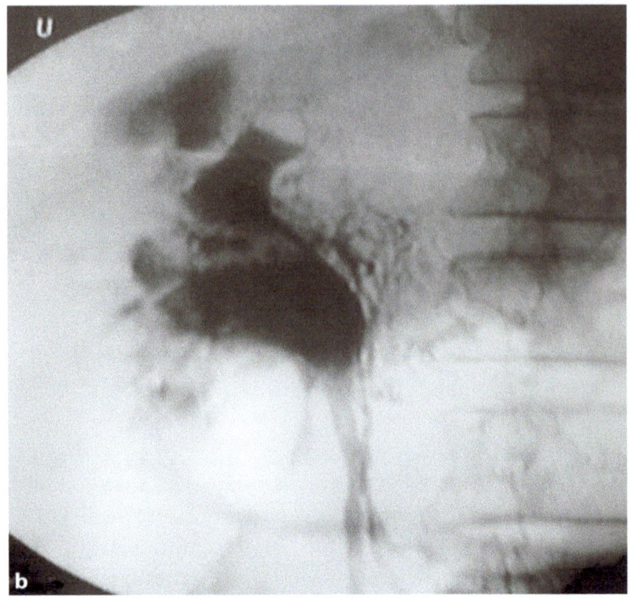

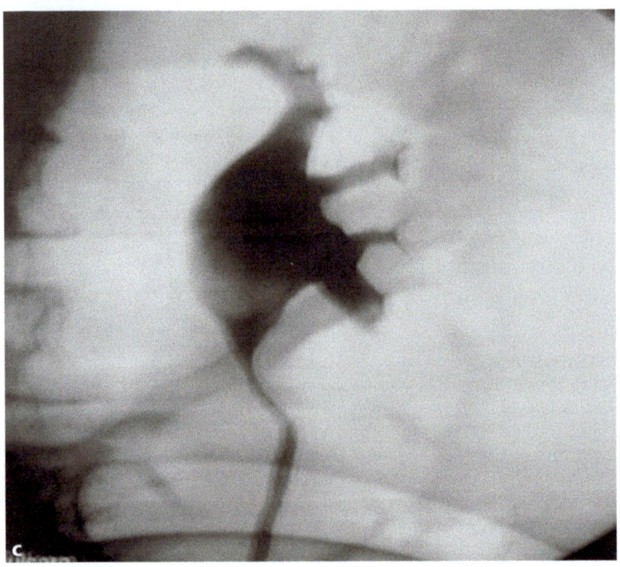

Fig. 6.1 A 56-year-old man presented with persistently milky urine. Turbid milky efflux from the right ureteric orifice was visualized on cystoscopy. **a** Contrast-enhanced T1-weighted MR urography (MRU) demonstrated a normal upper urinary tract. Bilateral retrograde pyelography showed **b** right pyelolymphatic backflow, and **c** a normal left pyelogram

Most symptomatic cases of filarial funiculoepididymitis appear before patients' fourth decade. The attack may be isolated, with remission, or may be repetitive and progressive. Local pain, often radiating to the testis or simulating ureteral colic, may be accompanied by systemic symptoms. Any palpable lumpy or cord-like swelling may mimic an intrascrotal tumor or torsion of the cord and may be accompanied by hydrocele or soft tissue edema. Varicocele or thrombosis of the pampiniform plexus may complicate inflammation (Kazura et al. 1995; Michael et al. 1996).

In patients with scrotal filarial lymphangiectasia ultrasound is capable of detecting worm movement, the so-called "filarial dance sign" within dilated intrascrotal lymphatic vessels containing living filarial worms (Noroes et al. 1996; Dreyer et al. 1998; Faris et al. 1998). In patients with scrotal elephantiasis, ultrasound shows marked thickening of the subcutaneous tissue and skin secondary to lymphedema (De Cassio Saito et al. 2004).

Magnetic resonance imaging and CT scans are also capable of demonstrating dilated retroperitoneal lymphatic channels and thoracic duct in patients with *W. bancrofti* filariasis (Mount and Thong 2006; Ahn et al. 2005).

Filarial loiasis caused by *Loa loa* is endemic in Central Africa. The microfilariae can migrate into the renal capillaries, causing vascular damage with secondary de-

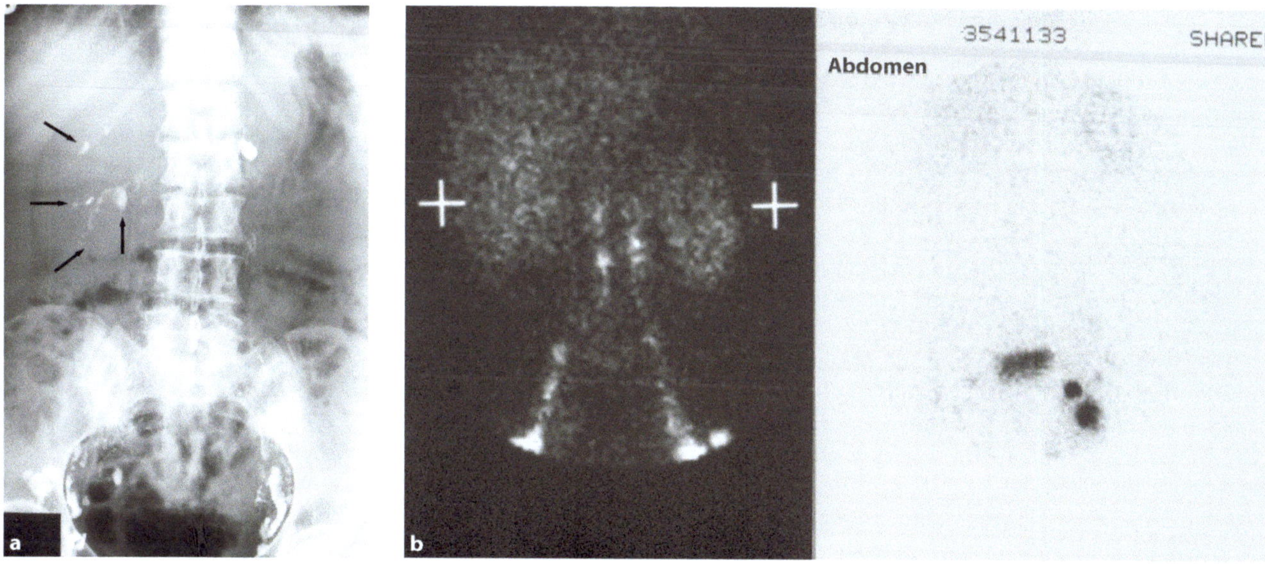

Fig. 6.2 Chyluria. **a** Bipedal lymphangiogram showing reflux of contrast material into the pelvicalyceal system (*arrows*) of the right kidney. **b** Radiocolloid lymphoscintigraphy images of abdomen failed to detect the abnormal pyelolymphatic connections

velopment of a nephrotic syndrome, glomerulopathy, and eventually renal failure (Hall et al. 2001; Katner et al. 1984; Pakasa et al. 1997).

Onchocerciasis is another filarial disease caused by the *Onchocerca volvulus* filarial worm, which affects the subcutaneous tissues. It can also migrate into the kidneys causing glomerular disease (Duvic et al. 1999).

The microfilariae are usually identified at urine examination.

6.3.2 Dioctophymiasis

The giant kidney worm *Dioctophyma renale* infects mammals worldwide, particularly dogs and minks. About 20 human infections have been reported, acquired by eating raw fish or frogs or less commonly, by drinking contaminated water. Many other fish-eating mammals can be infected, so the potential for human infection is significant. The clinical and imaging findings are nonspecific. On imaging, hyperdense renal cystic lesions mimicking hemorrhagic cysts, and solid renal masses with calcifications mimicking renal cancer, have been described on ultrasound, CT, and MR imaging (Sun et al. 1986; Ignjatovic et al. 2003; Narvaez et al. 1994).

6.3.3 Toxocariasis

Human infection is sporadic; it occurs in dirt-eating young children who ingest *Toxocara canis* or *T. catis* from soil or sand contaminated with animal feces. In humans, hatched larvae are unable to mature, but continue to migrate through the tissues producing "visceral larva migrans," and become lodged in various organs, mainly the lungs, liver, and less often the brain, myocardium, and other tissues, causing an eosinophilic granulomatous inflammatory reaction. Toxocariasis as a cause of renal disease was described in children of the Sharkia Governorate of Egypt (Nada et al. 1996).

6.3.4 Strongyloidiasis

Strongyloides stercoralis is an intestinal parasite; however, a hyperinfection with diffusion of the organism in various organs may occur in immunosuppressed patients or those taking corticosteroids, causing disseminated strongyloidiasis with a nephrotic syndrome and eosinophilia (Mori et al. 1998; Moritmoto et al. 2002).

6.3.5 Trichinosis

Trichinosis is an infection of humans and other mammals by *Trichinella spiralis*. This disease is characterized by diarrhea, myositis, fever, periorbital edema, and myocarditis or encephalitis. A few cases of membranoproliferative glomerulonephritis associated with trichinosis have been described (Kociecka et al. 1987).

6.4 Helminths – Cestodes (Tapeworms)

6.4.1 Hydatid Disease (Echinococcosis)

Hydatid disease (HD) is a unique parasitic disease that is endemic in many parts of the world; it can occur almost anywhere in the body and demonstrates a variety of imaging features that vary according to growth stage, associated complications, and affected tissues. Radiologic findings range from purely cystic lesions to a completely solid appearance. Calcification is more common in HD of the liver, spleen, and kidney. It can be quite large in compressible organs and can be solitary or multiple (Polat et al. 2003).

The liver is the most common organ involved with the kidney cysts seen in 2–4% of patients with HD in most series (Polat et al. 2003; Angulo et al. 1997).

Two species can affect the urinary tract, *Echinococcus granulosus* and *E. multilocularis*, although the latter very rarely does, and primarily involve the liver. The adult tapeworms are found in the intestine of dogs, the primary host; their eggs are excreted in the feces and then ingested by humans, sheep, cattle, or pigs, which act as intermediate hosts. The eggs hatch in the duodenum and migrate through the intestinal mucosa into the portal system, mesenteric venules, and lymphatics, from where they can spread to any part of the body. The cyst consists of three layers:

1. An adventitial layer caused by the compressed host tissues
2. The ectocyst, which is an outer laminated acellular membrane
3. The endocyst or inner germinal layer responsible for growth of the cyst and development of scolices

Daughter cysts develop within the mother cyst and finally the cysts die and frequently calcify (Angulo et al. 1997).

Involvement of the kidney is rare and usually located in the upper or lower poles. Hydatid cysts are frequently solitary, located in the cortex, and may reach 10 cm in diameter before any clinical symptoms are noted (Polat et al. 2003).

The renal hydatid cyst may grow outward and rupture into the retroperitoneum or may rupture into the renal pelvis with portions of the cyst contents present in the urine, compatible with hydatiduria. Eighteen percent of renal hydatid cysts can rupture into the collecting system (Hertz et al. 1984). Secondary infection of the renal hydatid cyst may occur. Escribano et al. (1997), in their study of 52 patients with renal and retroperitoneal echinococcosis, found that the lesion was solitary in 85% and bilateral in 6% of cases. Extrarenal disease was present in 16 patients, 13 had involvement of the psoas and quadratus lumborum muscles, and 3 were in the pararenal space (Escribano et al. 1997).

Plain film of the abdomen shows a localized bulge of the renal contour with calcifications, which may be curvi-

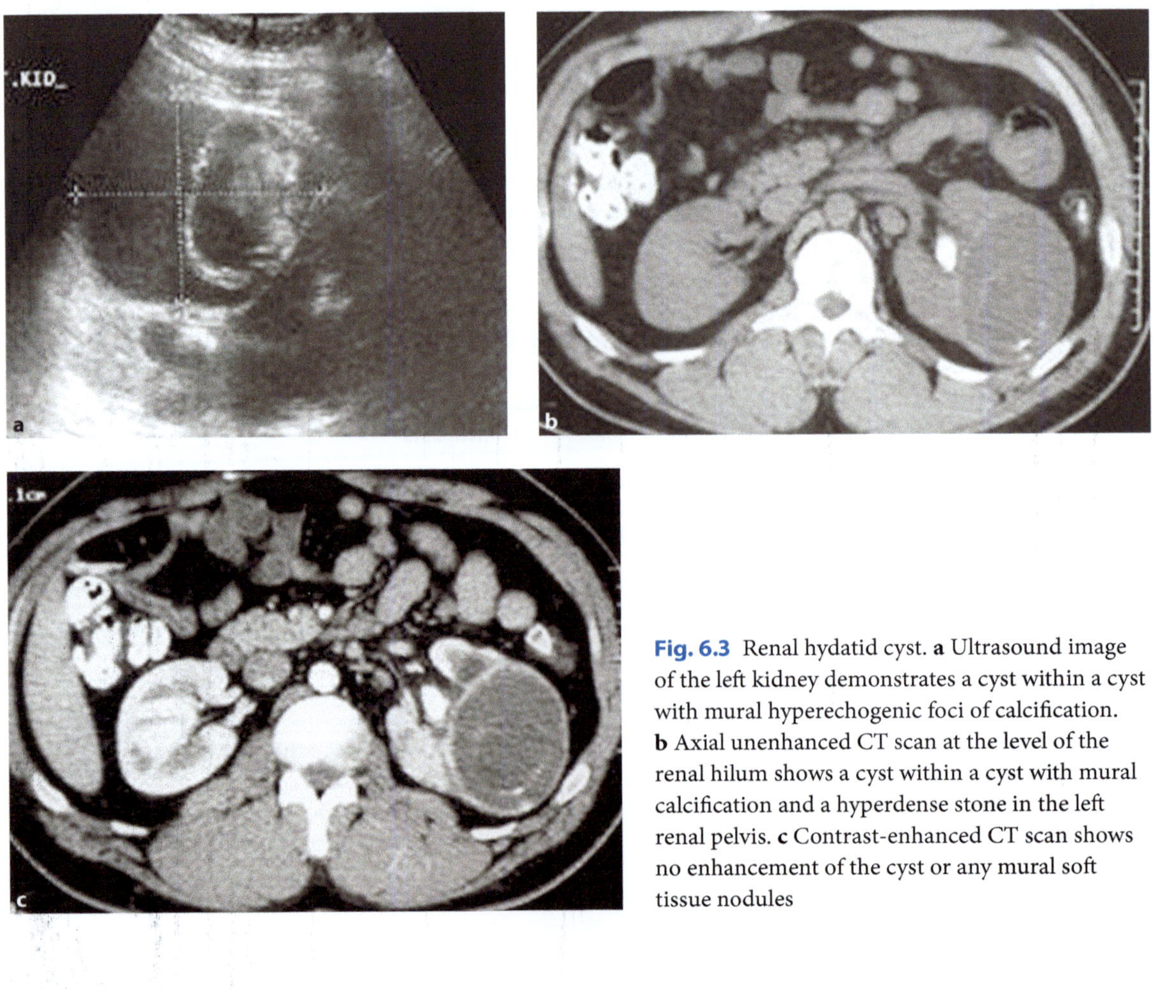

Fig. 6.3 Renal hydatid cyst. **a** Ultrasound image of the left kidney demonstrates a cyst within a cyst with mural hyperechogenic foci of calcification. **b** Axial unenhanced CT scan at the level of the renal hilum shows a cyst within a cyst with mural calcification and a hyperdense stone in the left renal pelvis. **c** Contrast-enhanced CT scan shows no enhancement of the cyst or any mural soft tissue nodules

linear, eggshell or reticular in shape. Multiple ring-shaped calcifications within a large calcified lesion suggest the presence of daughter cysts. Crushed eggshell calcifications also suggest a ruptured cyst (Von Sinner et al. 1993).

Intravenous urography may show elongation, stretching or splaying of the calyces in a similar fashion to other renal masses. When the cyst has ruptured, contrast media fill the cyst, simulating a renal abscess, or tuberculosis cavity with usually an identifiable neck of communication between the cyst and calyces (Von Sinner et al. 1993; Gilsanz et al. 1980).

Angiography plays a limited role as the cysts do not produce any neovascularity or vascular abnormalities other than displacement of the renal vessels, simulating other avascular masses, simple cysts or tumors (Baltaxe and Fleming 1970).

Ultrasound (US) and CT scans are very accurate at demonstrating renal hydatid cysts that may be unilocular, similar to simple cysts, but with thicker walls, or a multilocular structure with curvilinear septae (Figs. 6.3, 6.4). US and CT can easily detect the calcifications even if minor or faint. If scolices are present, the wall usually shows marked irregularities. Daughter cysts are usually arranged peripherally within the mother cyst. Ring enhancement on contrast-enhanced CT scan or the presence of air bubbles within the lesion is suggestive of secondary infection and abscess formation. However, in some cases, hydatid cysts may have a complex nature and cannot be differentiated from other atypical renal cystic masses (Karabekios et al. 1989; King 1989).

Magnetic resonance imaging (MRI) is not as accurate at detecting calcifications as unenhanced CT or ul-

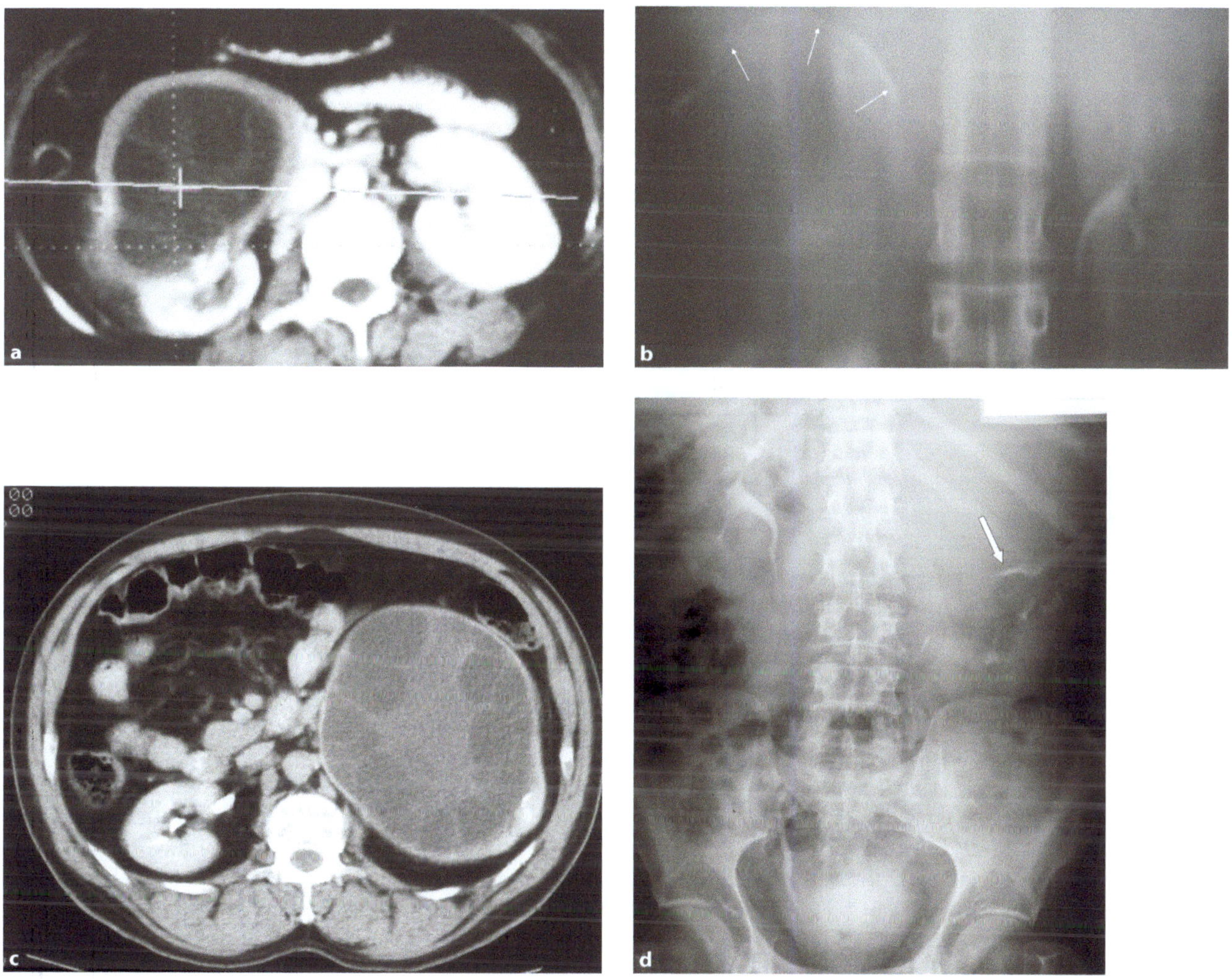

Fig. 6.4 Renal hydatid cysts. **a** Contrast-enhanced CT scan shows a large multilocular cyst displacing the right kidney posteriorly. Uniform mural thickening and enhancement are identified with calcification at the lateral wall. **b** Intravenous urography with tomography delineates mural calcification (*arrows*) and displacement of the right pelvicalyceal system inferiorly. **c** Contrast-enhanced CT scan showing a large type CE2 left renal hydatid cyst containing peripheral internal daughter cysts. **d** Intravenous urography showing inferior displacement of the left pelvicalyceal system (*arrow*) by the large hydatid cyst seen in **c**

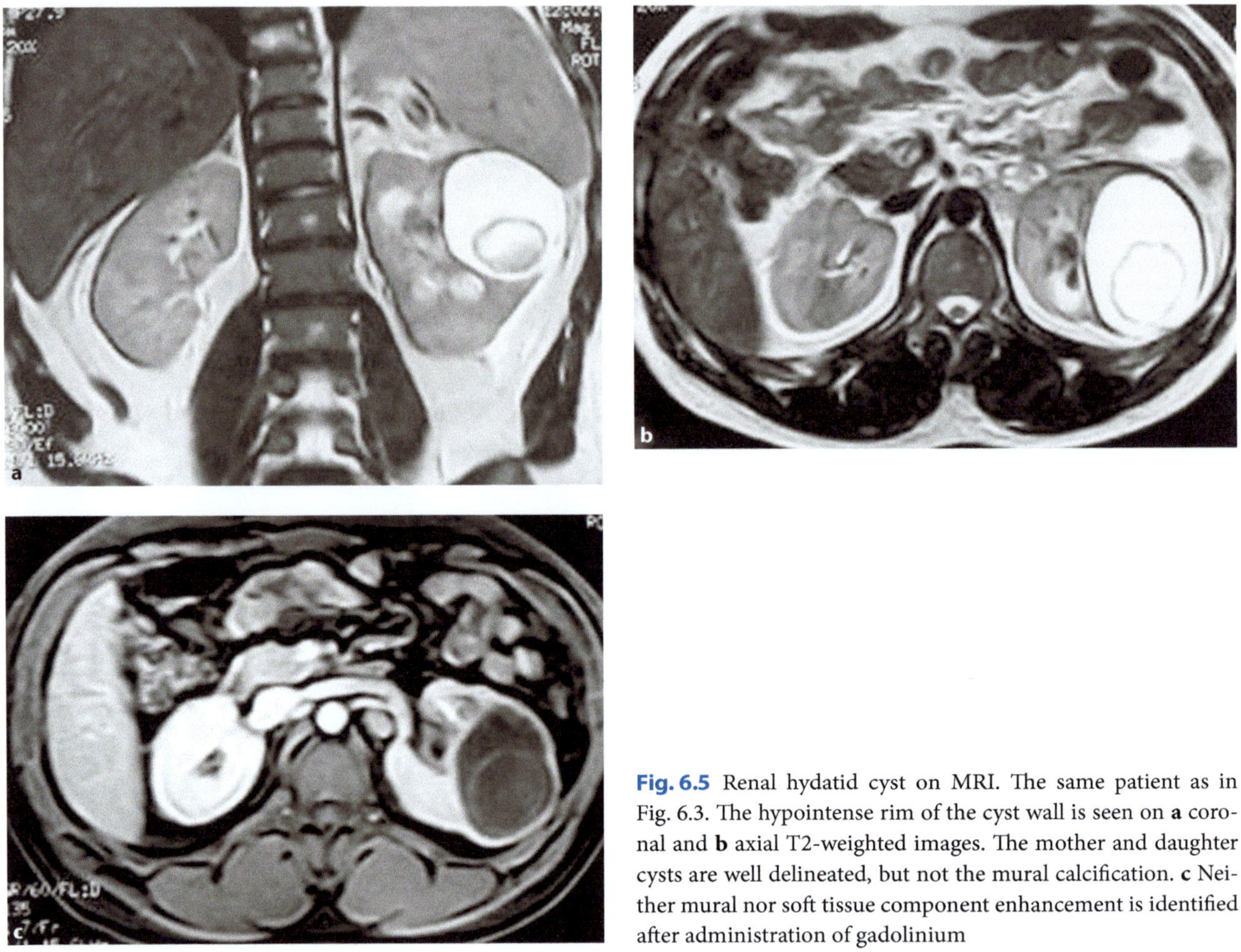

Fig. 6.5 Renal hydatid cyst on MRI. The same patient as in Fig. 6.3. The hypointense rim of the cyst wall is seen on **a** coronal and **b** axial T2-weighted images. The mother and daughter cysts are well delineated, but not the mural calcification. **c** Neither mural nor soft tissue component enhancement is identified after administration of gadolinium

trasound. A low-intensity rim on a T2-weighted image (Fig. 6.5) is suggestive, but not pathognomonic of a hydatid cyst (Marani et al. 1990).

Renal-sparing surgery, cystectomy plus pericystectomy, is possible in most cases (75%). Radical nephrectomy (25% of cases) must be reserved for destroyed kidneys resulting from aged cysts opening into the excretory cavities and complicated by renal infection (Zmerli et al. 2001). When surgery is contraindicated, chemotherapy with benzimidazoles (albendazole, mebendazole) allows for control of the disease. Delay in diagnosis may lead to serious complications or death (Von Sinner 1997).

Urinary bladder involvement can occur secondary to kidney hydatid disease, following rupture of a renal lesion into the collecting system with secondary spread into the ureter or bladder. However, primary hydatid disease of these structures is extremely rare (Hertz et al. 1984). Polat et al. (2003), in their series, found only one case of bladder echinococcosis in a 53-year-old woman who had suffered from liver and peritoneal hydatids for several years and had previously undergone repeated surgeries. There were three hydatids at different growth stages in the bladder and no lesions in the kidneys. One of the cysts originated from the anterior wall of the bladder, and the other two cysts were located in the posterolateral wall and protruded into the lumen of the bladder. One demonstrated dense circumferential calcification, whereas the other demonstrated stippled calcifications within the lesions. The anterior wall bladder lesion mimicked pseudodiverticulum formation, the other two simulated bladder carcinoma.

Scrotal hydatid disease is extremely rare with only a few case reports of hydatid of the testis reported in the literature (Kumar and Jahanshahi 1987). Sonography revealed anechoic fluid collection in the left side of the scrotum and freely floating isoechoic serpentine structures. These findings raised the suspicion of hydatid disease and when other organs were evaluated, multiple hydatids in the liver and peritoneal cavity were detected.

6.4.2 Sparganosis

Sparganosis was the cause of eosinophilic cystitis and granulomatous eosinophilic epididymo-orchitis in two cases reported in the literature (Oh et al. 1993; Sakamoto et al. 2003).

6.5 Helminths – Trematodes (Flukes)

6.5.1 Schistosomiasis/Bilharziasis

Bilharziasis is the most common parasitic infection in the world, affecting over 200 million people. *Schistosoma hematobium* is the form most likely to cause urinary tract symptoms, and is found throughout tropical and subtropical Africa and the African Islands, in most of the Middle East, and in parts of southern America, and it has now spread to India (Palmer and Reeder 2000). The infective agents of bilharziasis are the cercariae, which, after shedding their tails, pierce the human skin and reach the general circulation either directly by going through the superficial venules, or indirectly by way of the lymphatics. They are carried to the lungs and then to the left ventricle from which they are pumped to all parts of the body. Only those that reach the hepato-portal system live and grow. Under ordinary circumstances, the rest of the cercariae are destroyed in the other tissues. The liver may be regarded as the bilharzial incubator since in it most, if not all, of the stages of development of cercariae into worms take place. All schistosomes depend on a lifecycle involving fresh water and snails. This cycle starts when free-swimming cercariae penetrate the skin and eventually reach the liver. Access from the portal into the systemic venous system in the case of *S. hematobium* is probably through the hemorrhoidal plexus. The lifecycle is perpetuated by the passage of egg-containing urine into fresh-water localities where the intermediate snail host resides. Miracidia, which are released when the egg hatches, penetrate the snail; there, they eventually develop into cercariae, completing the cycle (Palmer and Reeder 2000; Alvarez 1972). The histopathological changes and clinical symptoms are almost entirely due to the dead egg. Schistosomiasis is thus primarily an infection of the vascular system and the underlying pathological process is the formation of granulomas and obliterative (embolic) endarteritis. Although in schistosomiasis from *S. hematobium*, the ureter and bladder are chiefly affected, granulomas may also be found in the testes, seminal vesicles, and not infrequently in the female genitalia such as the cervix, ovary, fallopian tubes, and endometrium (Palmer and Reeder 2000).

The clinical presentation of patients with schistosomiasis is typically with hematuria. In the initial stages, the bladder mucosa is edematous and hemorrhagic. Later, the bladder becomes fibrotic with reduced volume and calcified walls. Cystoscopic examination is mandatory to exclude squamous cell carcinoma of the bladder. Biopsy may be necessary to distinguish bilharzioma from carcinoma, although carcinoma usually presents as a latter complication. Schistosomiasis rarely affects the kidneys or collecting systems, except by obstruction due to bladder disease or involvement of the distal ureter (Farrell and Martinez 1995).

Patients may complain of dysuria and difficult micturition. At first, a little difficulty and a feeling of discomfort and perineal heaviness at the termination of micturition are reported by the patient secondary to congestive retention of urine. The subsequent development of bilharzial papillomata may create a little difficulty on micturition by hampering the bladder muscles in their proper contractions. Hemospermia is a frequent complaint of patients suffering from the early hyperemic stage of bilharzial prostatitis.

The most serious complication of urinary tract schistosomiasis is an increased incidence of squamous cell carcinoma of the bladder. Additional complications include urolithiasis, ascending tract infection, urethral and ureteral stricture with subsequent hydronephrosis, and renal failure. In Egypt there is a syndrome called "bladder neck obstruction." The trigone is most affected and hypertrophies to form a prominent bulging into the vesical lumen between the ureteral orifices. Eventually, this fibroses and atrophies, leaving the mucosa and muscularis as a mass, which is pushed forward over the internal ureteral orifice (Girges 1966; Shokier 1972). The prostate gland may occasionally be enlarged due to bilharzial prostatitis. Calcification may be seen in the seminal vesicles and may rarely be found in the spermatic cord. The fallopian tubes may be infected and blocked and also calcified as a result of egg deposition.

Schistosomiasis of the cervix uteri is not uncommon and is easily confused with carcinoma of the cervix, with which it may coexist. Schistosomal lesions of the vagina and cervix may predispose to the acquisition of HIV infection and AIDS (Feldmeier et al. 1994; Poggensee et al. 2000; Poggensee and Feldmeier 2001).

Urinary bladder wall calcification has relatively few etiologies. In a series of 19 patients with radiographically visible bladder wall calcification encompassing most of the known causes, 8 patients had schistosomiasis, 6 patients had primary carcinoma of the bladder, 2 patients had encrustation cystitis, and 3 patients had amyloidosis, cyclophosphamide induced cystitis, and tuberculosis respectively. While a correct diagnosis is often not possible solely on the basis of the appearance of the calcification, such a diagnosis can usually be obtained from a combination of history, clinical examination, appropriate laboratory studies, and radiographic evaluation of the bladder and remaining urinary tract. Cystoscopy with biopsy of the involved tissues is almost always necessary, however, for confirmation and to rule out bladder neoplasia (Pollack 1981).

Schistosomiasis can be imaged by radiography or sonography and, in the later stages, by CT scanning or MRI. Plain film radiography of the abdomen is not helpful until calcification has developed. The classic presentation of a calcified bladder, which looks like a fetal head in the pelvis, is pathognomonic of chronic urinary schistosomiasis (Fig. 6.6). The seminal vesicles,

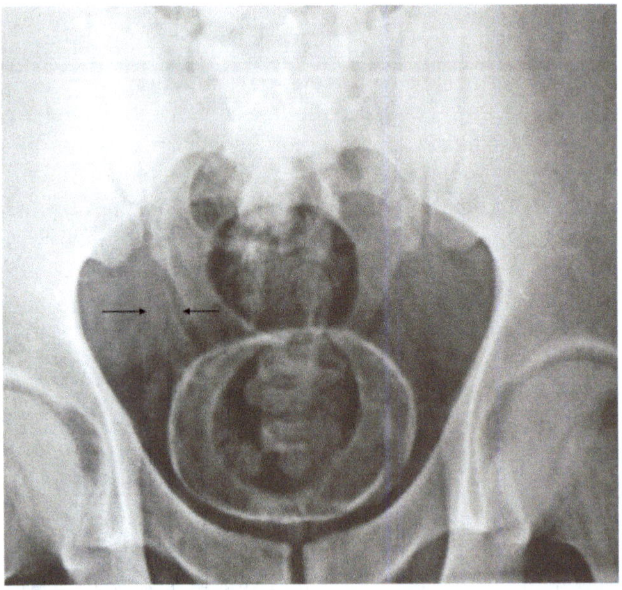

Fig. 6.6 Plain radiography of the pelvis demonstrates a ring of calcification overlying the region of the urinary bladder that looks like a fetal head. Note calcification of the pelvic segment of the right ureter (*arrows*)

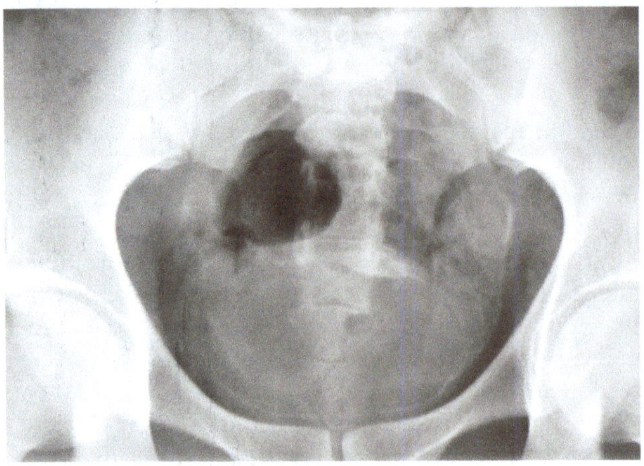

Fig. 6.7 Plain radiography of the pelvis shows the calcified wall of the urinary bladder and the pelvic segments of both ureters in a patient with chronic urinary schistosomiasis

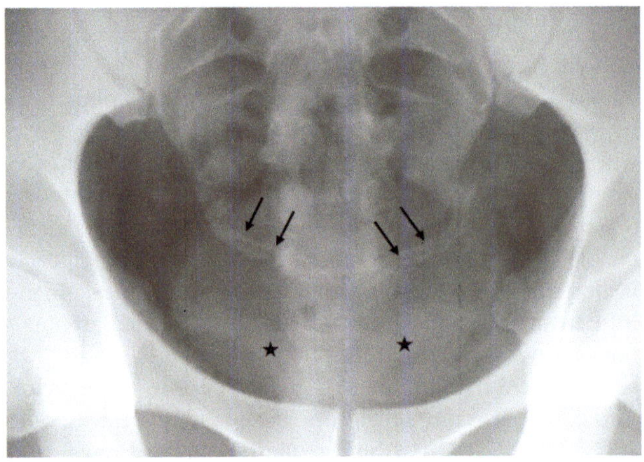

Fig. 6.8 Plain radiography of the pelvis in another patient with chronic urinary schistosomiasis shows calcified vas deferens (*arrows*) and faint calcification of both seminal vesicles (*stars*)

prostate, prostatic urethra, and distal ureters may be calcified (Figs. 6.7, 6.8), or striated renal pelves and ureters may be observed (Hugosson 1987). With intravenous urography, the earliest changes are seen in the ureters, with persistent filling of the lower segments throughout the urogram (Fig. 6.9). At this stage the ureters are not always dilated, but this develops next. At first, it results from dysfunction rather than tissue damage. The dilatation will be asymmetrical and may be slight or severe, sometimes without visible stenosis. Later, ureteric constriction will occur, initially within the bladder wall. As the disease progresses, the lower ureters become beaded in appearance, secondary to bilharzial granulomas in the submucosa of the ureter. Mucosal ureteric edema may result in luminal narrowing and striations in the ureter (Hugosson 1987). Air bubble-like filling defects are seen in uretero-pyelograms and are suggestive of ureteritis and pyelitis cystica (Figs. 6.10, 6.11). The common causes of ureteric dilatation are vesicoureteric reflux, stenosis of the ureter, or an edematous ureteral wall that causes deficient peristalsis (Fig. 6.12). The bladder may show mucosal edema, calcified wall, reduced capacity, and eventually tumor growth (Fig. 6.13) (Al-Ghorab et al. 1978; Sewcz 1985). The use of the voiding cystourethrogram allows the demonstration of vesicoureteral reflux, which is a useful method for the detection of focal thickening of the bladder wall, large polypoidal lesions of the urinary tracts, hydroureter, and hydronephrosis

(Fig. 6.14) (Hanafy et al. 1975). CT scanning delineates to a better advantage the extent of the calcification, thickness and dilation of the ureteral wall, hydronephrosis, as well as the bladder tumors (Figs. 6.15–6.17) (Jorulf and Lindstedt 1985). A heavily calcified area in the bladder has an estimated 500,000 to 1 million eggs per gram, but for calcification to be seen on plain radiography, it is necessary to have 100,000 eggs per cubic centimeter. The presence of *Schistosoma* eggs has been reported in 50% of postmortem studies of the prostate and seminal vesicles performed in endemic areas. Transrectal sonography shows prostatic calcification, increased prostatic size, calcification of the seminal vesicles, as well as dilatation of the ejaculatory ducts (Figs. 6.18, 6.19). Prostatic and seminal vesicle calcifications should alert physicians to the possibility of *Schistosoma* infection when they are found in young patients who have been in endemic areas (Vilana et al. 1997). Testicular schistosomal granuloma appears on ultrasound as a solid testicular mass with a heterogeneous or hypoechoic echotexture and increased vascularity on color Doppler blood flow examination, identical to that of most testicular malignancies (Richens 2004; Soans and Abel 1999; Woodward et al. 2003).

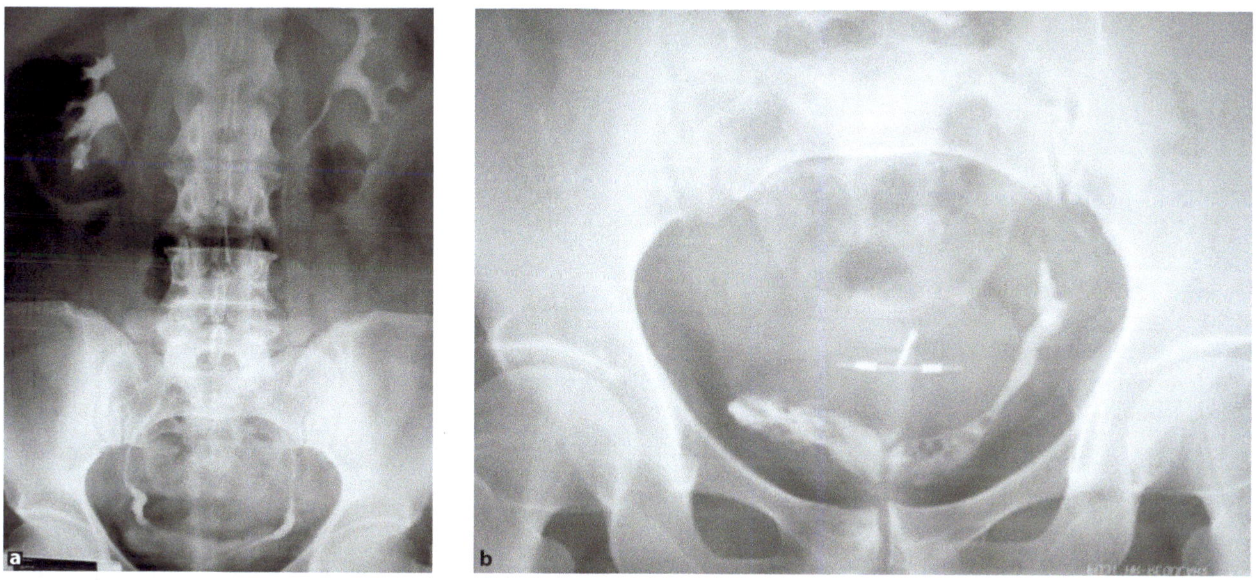

Fig. 6.9 **a** The earliest changes of urinary bilharziasis are seen in the ureters as persistent filling of the lower segments ("pelvic spindle") on intravenous urography. **b** Intravenous urography of another patient demonstrates mild dilatation of the left pelvic spindle with multiple filling defects of ureteritis cystica at its lower end

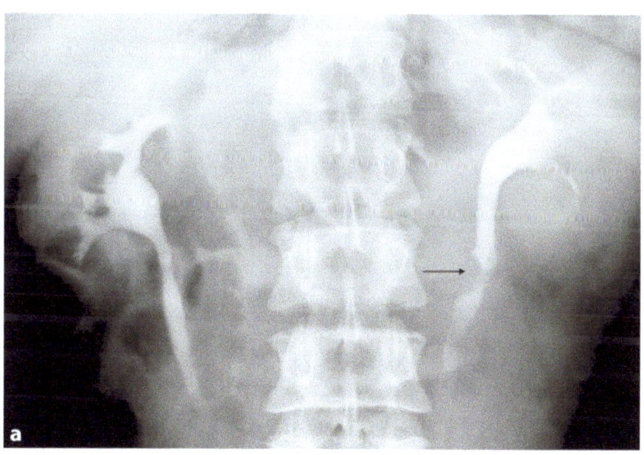

Fig. 6.10 Bilateral ureteritis cystica on intravenous urography. **a** A well-circumscribed filling defect (*arrow*) at the lumbar segment of the left ureter. **b,c** *see next page*

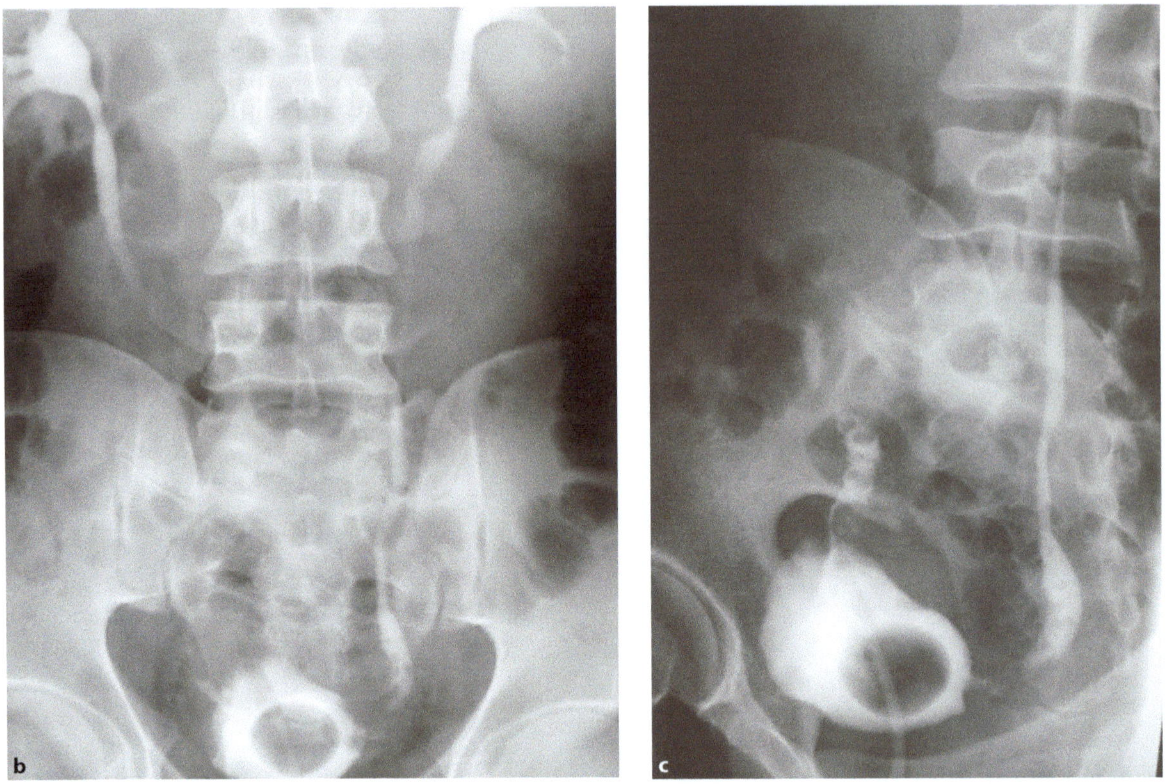

Fig. 6.10 Bilateral ureteritis cystica on intravenous urography. **b** The full-length film demonstrates multiple smaller filling defects at the pelvic segment of the left ureter. **c** Similar filling defects are also identified at the pelvic segment of the right ureter on the oblique view

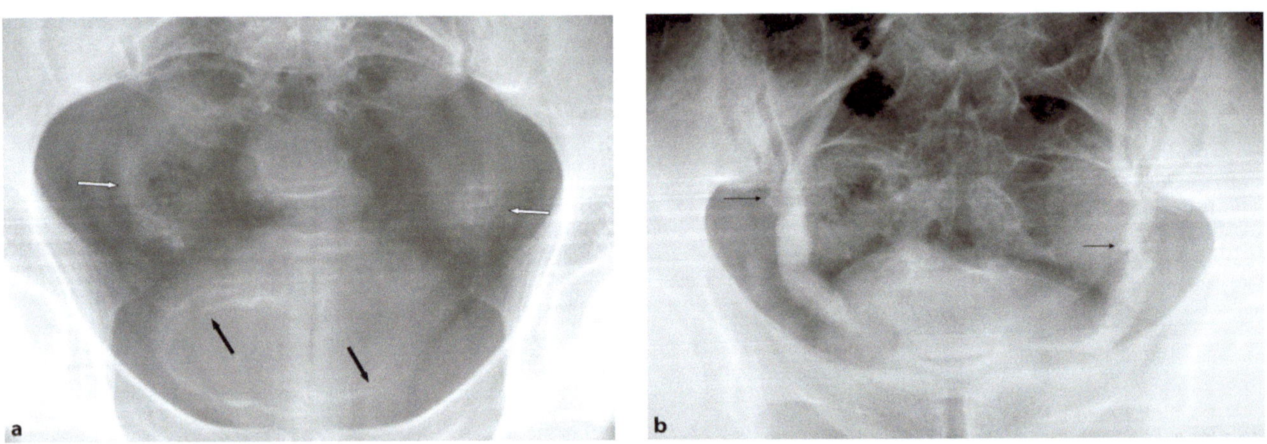

Fig. 6.11 Bilateral ureteritis, cystica calcinosa. **a** Plain radiograph shows linear calcification in the region of the urinary bladder (*black arrows*) and multiple calcific foci (*white arrows*) along the course of the pelvic segments of both ureters. **b** Intravenous urography shows bilateral persistent filling with contrast of the lower segments of the ureters. The calcific foci (*arrows*) are identified in the mural filling defects

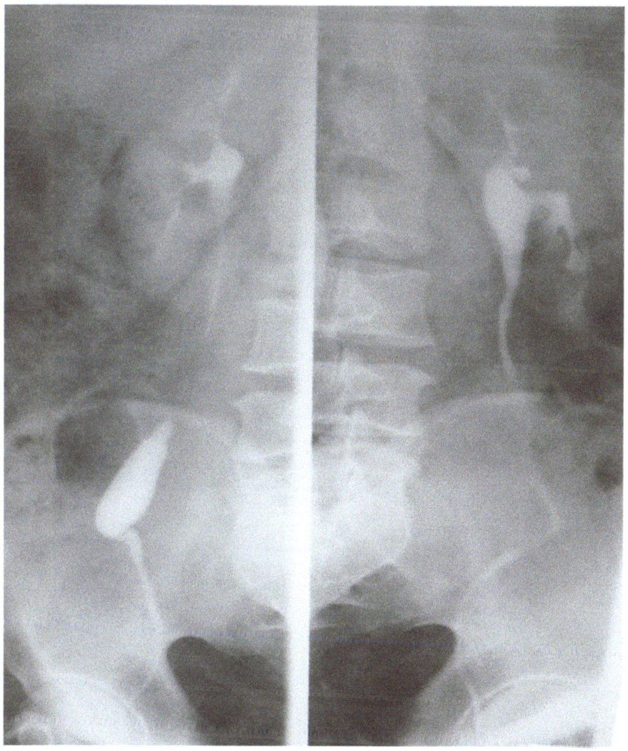

Fig. 6.12 Intravenous urography in a patient with urinary schistosomiasis demonstrates reduced ureteric peristalsis on oblique views. Persistent dilatation of the midureteric segment is noted on the right side

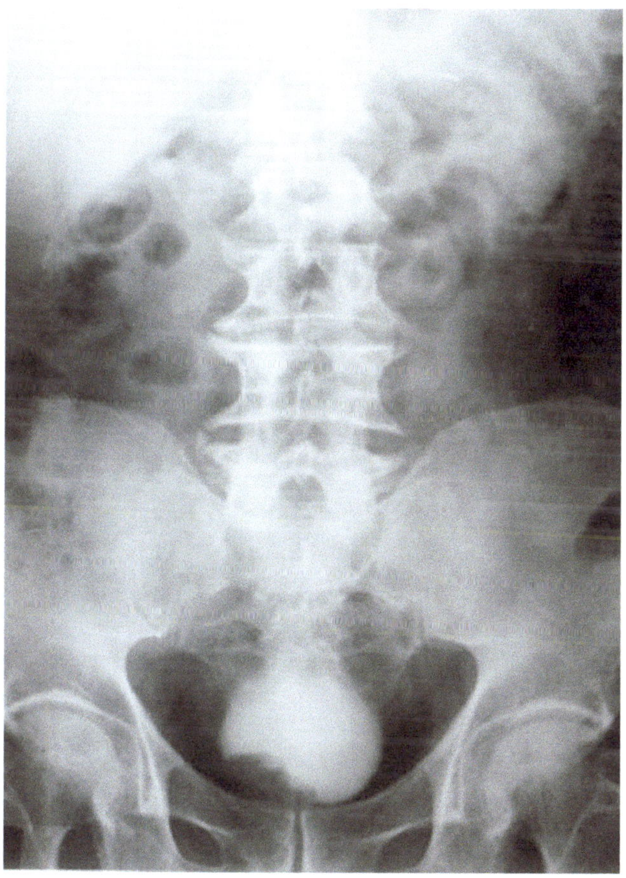

Fig. 6.13 Intravenous urography in a 53-year-old man with a history of hematuria and chronic urinary schistosomiasis. Reduced bladder capacity is seen on full-bladder film with a filling defect on the right side of the bladder base. Histopathological diagnosis was squamous cell carcinoma with bilharziasis

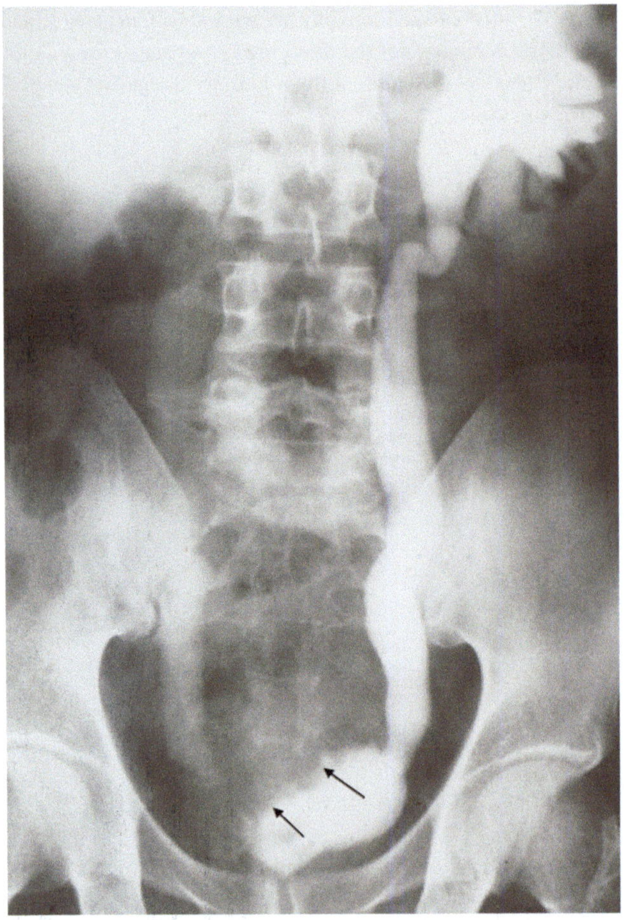

Fig. 6.14 Cystogram showing bilateral hydroureteronephrosis due to vesico-ureteric reflux, more advanced on the right side. A large filling defect (*arrows*) of the bladder cancer is also seen in the contrast-filled bladder

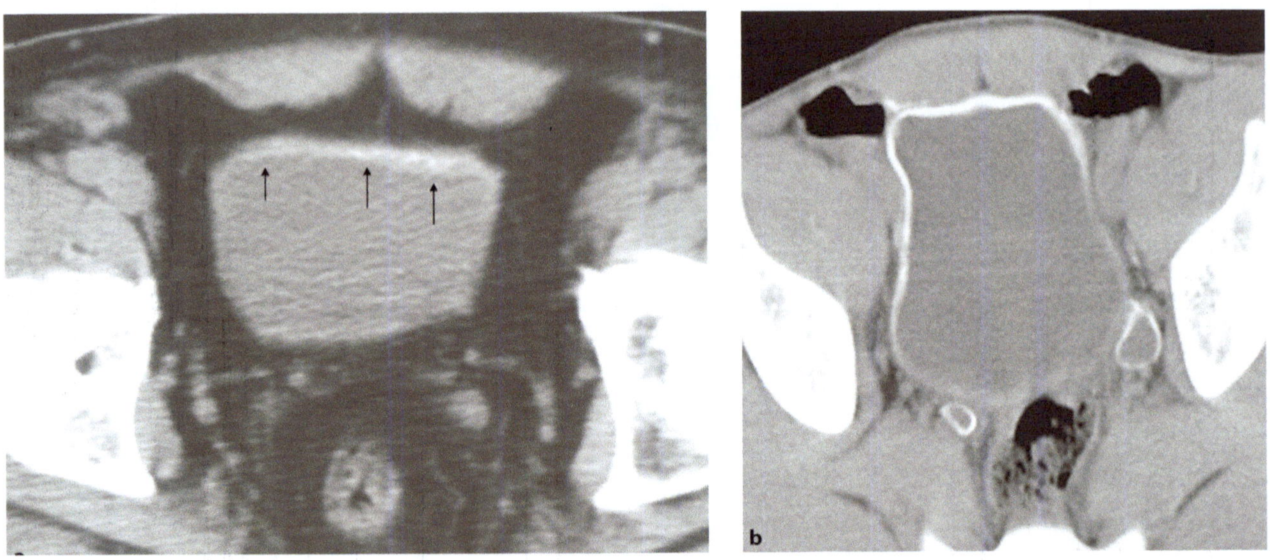

Fig. 6.15 **a** Axial unenhanced CT scan of the pelvis shows calcification (*arrows*) of the anterior wall of the bladder, which was not identified on plain radiography. **b** Axial unenhanced CT scan of the pelvis in another patient with chronic urinary schistosomiasis clearly demonstrates bladder and bilateral ureteric wall calcification. Ureteric dilatation, particularly on the left side, is also identified

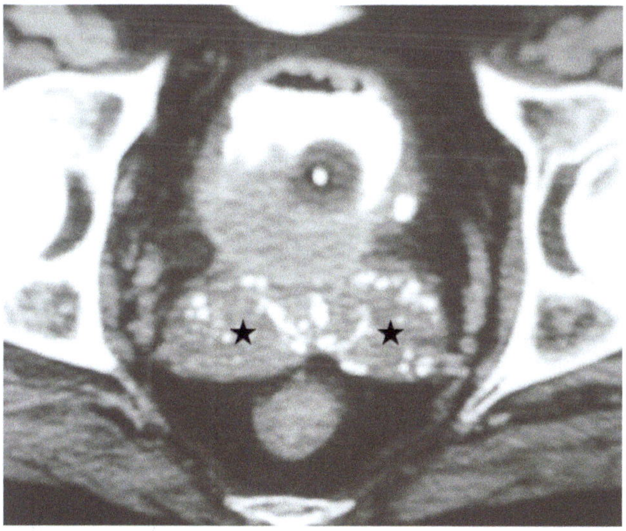

Fig. 6.16 Axial contrast-enhanced CT scan image at the lower pelvis clearly demonstrates calcifications of both seminal vesicles (*stars*

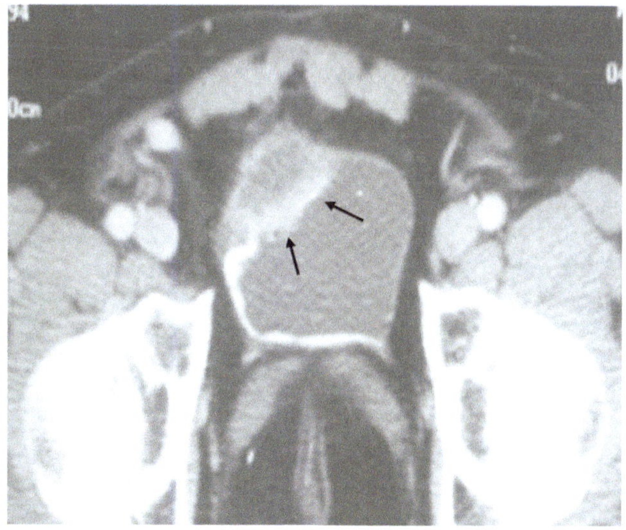

Fig. 6.17 Axial contrast-enhanced CT scan of the urinary bladder shows mural calcification at the posterior and right lateral wall with enhancing tumor (*arrows*) at the anterior wall, which was a transitional cell carcinoma proven by biopsy

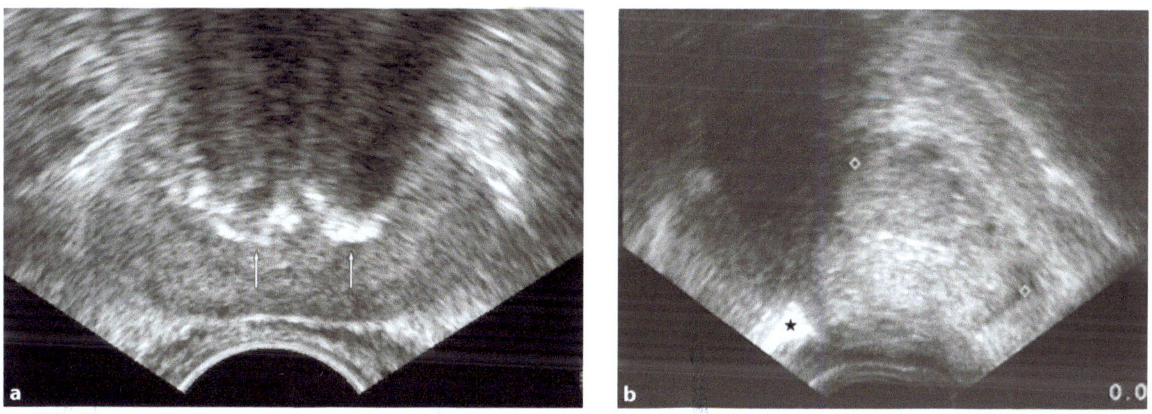

Fig. 6.18 **a** Transrectal ultrasound (TRUS) of the prostate shows increased prostatic size and multiple calcific foci (*arrows*) casting anterior acoustic shadows. **b** Transverse scan of TRUS in another patient with chronic genitourinary schistosomiasis shows calcification of the right seminal vesicle (*star*)

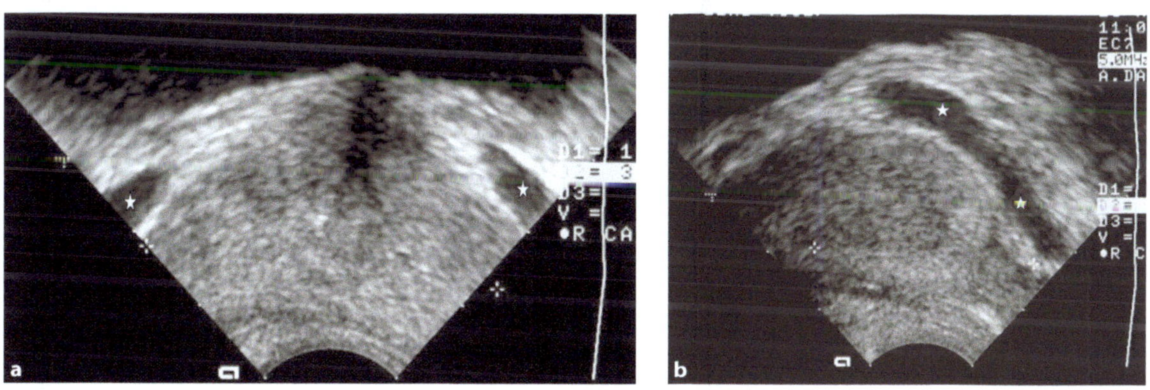

Fig. 6.19 Dilatation of the ejaculatory ducts on TRUS. **a** Transverse scan shows dilatation of both ejaculatory ducts (*stars*). **b** Longitudinal scan delineates the dilated right ejaculatory duct (*stars*)

6.5.2 Fascioliasis

Fasciola hepatica primarily involves the peritoneum and the liver; however, in some exceptional situations other organs such as subcutaneous tissue, heart, lungs, pleura, abdominal wall, brain, cecum, epididymis, and stomach can be involved. The first case involving the pancreas, spleen, and kidney was described by Zali et al. (2004) from Iran. The ectopic involvement is either a result of parasite migration or perhaps eosinophilic reaction.

6.6 Arthropods

6.6.1 Genitourinary Myiasis

Urogenital myiasis is almost always subsequent to conditions of poor personal hygiene. Human urinary myiasis caused by housefly (*Fannia canicularis*) larvae was described in an Algerian woman living in a village near Sidi Bel Abbes. The diagnosis of urinary myiasis was confirmed by repeated urinary emissions of *F. canicularis* larvae for a period of 2 weeks, following 6 days' treatment with cefotaxime for urinary tract infection (Perez-Eid and Mouffok 1999). Another case of genitourinary myiasis (maggot infestation) involving the perineum, legs, scrotum, and penile urethra was described by Makarov et al. (2006). Areas of crepitus, induration, and ulceration were observed in the perineal region and scrotal skin. Urogenital myiasis due to *Piophila casei* was also described in Egypt (Saleh and el Sibae 1993), and in the Netherlands caused by scuttle fly larvae (*Diptera: Phoridae*) (Meinhardt and Disney 1989).

6.7 Eosinophilia and Urinary Pathology

Renal pathology with blood eosinophilia may be associated with several pathologies including eosinophilic helminthic infection, drug-induced reactions, immunoallergic responses, malignancies, and hypereosinophilic syndrome (HES), i.e., an eosinophilic state with no identifiable cause. In HES, renal involvement has been attributed to the deleterious effects of eosinophil granulomas and possibly micro-emboli from the heart in patients presenting with eosinophilic myocarditis. Eosinophiluria may be observed in any clinical setting, but the prognostic value of this finding and its mechanism remain unclear (Giudicelli et al. 1998). Eosinophilic cystitis may simulate a bladder tumor (Fig. 6.20).

6.8 Conclusion

The genitourinary system is rarely affected by parasites. Of particular interest to radiologists are parasitic diseases that induce radiologic changes in the urinary tract such as schistosomiasis, filariasis, and echinococcosis. Other parasites, including scabies, rarely affect the kidneys, leading to parasitic nephropathy and renal failure secondary to complex immunologic reactions (Pakasa et al. 1997; Van Velthuysen 1996; Bourée 2005; Takiguchi et al. 1987).

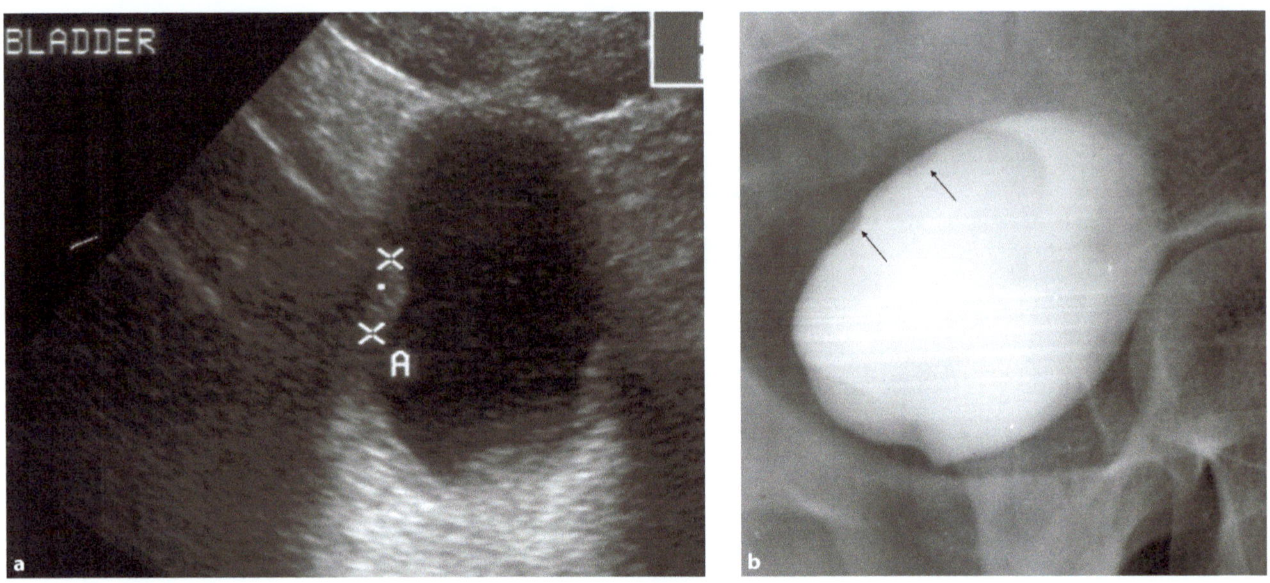

Fig. 6.20 Eosinophilic cystitis. **a** Ultrasound examination of the bladder showing a thickened bladder wall and a small polypoid lesion (*cursors*) of the right bladder wall. **b** Intravenous urogram film of the bladder in a left posterior oblique projection outlining a filling defect (*arrows*) in the bladder. Cystoscopy and biopsy revealed eosinophilic cystitis at histopathologic examination

References

Ahn PJ, Bertagnolli R, Fraser SL, Freeman JH (2005) Distended thoracic duct and diffuse lymphangiectasia caused by bancroftian filariasis. AJR Am J Roentgenol 185:1011–1014

Al-Ghorab MM, Rahman MA, El-Rifaie M, et al. (1978) Radiologic findings of bilharzial (schistosomal) contracted bladder. Urology 11(3):303–305

Alvarez SA (1972) Urogenital bilharziasis (a propos of 28 cases). J Trop Med Hyg 48:154–181

Amaral F, Dreyer G, Figueredo Silva J, et al. (1994) Live adult worms detected by ultrasonography in human bancroftian filariasis. Am J Trop Med Hyg 50:753–757

Angulo JC, Sanchez-Chapado M, Diego A, et al. (1997) Renal echinococcosis: clinical study of 34 cases. J Urol 157:787

Antony SJ, Lopez-Po P (1999) Genital amebiasis: historical perspective of an unusual disease presentation. Urology 54:952–955

Baltaxe HA, Fleming RJ (1970) The angiographic appearance of hydatid disease. Radiology 97:559–604

Becker K, Jablonowski H, Haussinger D (1996) Sulfadiazine-associated nephrotoxicity in patients with the acquired immunodeficiency syndrome. Medicine (Baltimore) 75(4):185–194

Bellinghieri G, Santoro D, Mallamace A, Ioli A, LoGiudice L, Venniro G, Savica V (2002) The discovery of nephrouroameba: was it real or not? Am J Nephrol 22(2–3):266–270

Besnier JM, Verdier M, Cotty F, Fetissof F, Besancenez A, Choutet P (1995) Toxoplasmosis of the bladder in a patient with AIDS. Clin Infect Dis 21:452–454

Blickstein I, Dgani R, Lifschitz-Mercer B (1993) Cutaneous leishmaniasis of the vulva. Int J Gynaecol Obstet 42:46–47

Bourée P (2005) Urinary parasitosis. Ann Urol 39:232–246

Brasseur P, Gorenflot A (1992) Human babesiosis in Europe. Mem Inst Oswaldo Cruz 87 [Suppl 3]:131–132

Cabello I, Caraballo A, Millan Y (2002) Leishmaniasis in the genital area. Rev Inst Med Trop Sao Paolo 44:105–107

Calore EE, Calore NM, Cavaliere MJ (2002) Salpingitis due to *Entamoeba histolytica*. Braz J Infect Dis 6:97–99

Caravaca F, Munoz A, Pizarro JL, Saez de Santamaria J, Fernandez-Alonso J (1991) Acute renal failure in visceral leishmaniasis. Am J Nephrol 11(4):350–352

Castro-Coto A, Hidalgo-Hidalgo H, Solano Aguilar F, et al. (1987) Leishmaniasis of the genital organs. Med Cutan Ibero Lat Am 15:145–150

Chemlal K, Delmas V, Toublanc M, Carbon C, Yeni P (1996) Toxoplasmosis localized to the bladder is diagnostic of human immunodeficiency virus infection: case report. Clin Infect Dis 22:740–741

Chen KC (1971) Lymphatic abnormalities in patients with chyluria. J Urol 106:111–114

Costa RS, Monteiro RC, Lehuen A, et al. (1991) Immune complex-mediated glomerulopathy in experimental Chagas disease. Clin Immunopathol 58:102–114

Dalela D, Kumar A, Ahlawat R, et al. (1992) Routine radio-imaging in filarial chyluria: is it necessary in developing countries? Br J Urol 69:291–293

Date A, Gunasekaran V, Kirubakaran MG, Shastry JC (1979) Acute eosinophilic glomerulonephritis with Bancroftian filariasis. Postgrad Med J 55(654):905–907

De Cassio Saito O, de Barros N, Chammas MC, Oliveira IRS, Cerri GG (2004) Ultrasound of tropical and infectious diseases that affect the scrotum. Ultrasound Q 20(1):12–18

De Sequera P, Albalate M, Hernandez J, Vasquez A, Abad J, Ramiro E, Fernandez Guerrero M, Caramelo C, Casado S, Ortiz A (1996) Acute renal failure due to sulphadiazine crystalluria in AIDS patients. Postgrad Med J 72(851):557–558

Dreyer G, Santos A, Noroes J, Amaral F, Addiss D (1998) Ultrasonographic detection of living adult *Wuchereria bancrofti* using a 3.5 MHz transducer. Am J Trop Med Hyg 59:399–403

Dutra M, Martinelli R, de Carvalho EM, et al. (1985) Renal involvement in visceral leishmaniasis. Am J Kidney Dis 6:22–27

Duvic C, Nedelec G, Debord T, Herody M, Didelot F (1999) Important parasitic nephropathies: update from the recent literature. Nephrologie 20(2):65–74

Eiam-Ong S (2003) Malarial nephropathy. Semin Nephrol 23(1):21–33

Escribano J, Angulo JC, Rueda O (1997) Imaging of renal and retroperitoneal echinococcosis: a study of 52 cases. Exhibit at the Radiological Society of North America Annual Meeting, Chicago

Faris R, Hussain O, El Setouhy M, Ramzy RMR, Weil GJ (1998) Bancroftian filariasis in Egypt: visualization of adult worms and subclinical lymphatic pathology by scrotal ultrasound. Am J Trop Med Hyg 59(6):864–867

Farrell B, Martinez R (1995) Urinary schistosomiasis: literature review and case presentation. Appl Radiol 24:19

Feldmeier H, Krantz I, Poggensee G (1994) Female genital schistosomiasis as a risk-factor for the transmission of HIV. Int J STD AIDS 5:368

Gilsanz V, Lozano G, Jiminez J (1980) Renal hydatid cysts communicating with collecting system. AJR Am J Roentgenol 135:357

Ginsburg BE, Wasserman J, Huldt G, Bergstrand A (1974) Case of glomerulonephritis associated with acute toxoplasmosis. Br Med J 3(5932):664–665

Girges MR (1966) The syndrome of bladder-neck obstruction and ureteric fibrosis in schistosoma haematobium infection. J Trop Med Hyg 69:187–188

Giudicelli CP, Didelot F, Duvic C, Desrame J, Herody M, Nedelec G (1998) Eosinophilia and renal pathology. Med Trop (Mars) 58 [4 Suppl]:477–481

Haddad MC, Al Shahed MS, Sharif HS, Miola UJ (1994) Case report: investigation of chyluria. Clin Radiol 49:137–139

Hall CL, Stephens L, Peat D, Chiodini PL (2001) Nephrotic syndrome due to loiasis following a tropical adventure holiday: a case report and review of the literature. Clin Nephrol 56(3):247–250

Hanafy HM, Youssef TK, Saad SM (1975) Radiologic aspects of bilharzial (schistosomal) urethra. Urology 6:118

Hatcher JC, Greenberg PD, Antique J, Jimenez-Lucho VE (2001) Severe babesiosis in Long Island: review of 34 cases and their complications. Clin Infect Dis 32:1117–1125

Hertz M, Zissin R, Dresnik Z, Morag B, Itzchak Y, Jonas P (1984) Echinococcus of the urinary tract: radiologic findings. Urol Radiol 6:175–181

Holch A, Opravil M, Moradpour D, Siegenthaler W, Schneider J, Luthy R (1993) Disseminated toxoplasmosis in AIDS. Dtsch Med Wochenschr 118(22):814–819

Hugosson CO (1987) Striation of renal pelvis and ureter in bilharziasis. Clin Radiol 38:407

Ignjatovic I, Stojkovic I, Kutlesic C, Tasic S (2003) Infestation of the human kidney with *Dioctophyma renale*. Urol Int 70:70–73

Jorulf H, Lindstedt E (1985) Urogenital schistosomiasis: CT evaluation. Radiology 157:745–749

Kane D, Murphy JM, Keating S, Wilson GF, Mulcahy FM (1996) Renal ultrasonic findings in sulphadiazine-induced renal failure. Br J Radiol 69(826):925–928

Karabekios S, Gouliamos A, Kalovidouris A, et al. (1989) Features of computed tomography in hydatid cysts of the urinary tract. Br J Urol 64(6):575–578

Katner H, Beyt BE Jr, Krotoski WA (1984) Loiasis and renal failure. South Med J 77(7):907–908

Kazura J, Bockarie M, Alexander N (1995) Risk factors for acute morbidity in bancroftian filiariasis. Am J Trop Med Hyg 53:100

Kibukamusoke JW, Hutt MS, Wilks NE (1967) The nephrotic syndrome in Uganda and its association with quartan malaria. Q J Med 36:393–408

King DL (1989) Ultrasonography of echinococcal cyst. J Clin Ultrasound 1:64–67

Kociecka W, Gabryel P, Leszyk A, Gustowska L (1987) A case of fatal trichinosis with early renal failure and involvement of the central nervous system. Wiad Parazytol 33:545–551

Koga S, Nagata Y, Arakaki Y (1992) Lymphangiography of filarial chyluria: injections via right and left feet at different times. Br J Urol 69:318

Kumar PV, Jahanshahi S (1987) Hydatid cyst of testis: a case report. J Urol 137:511–512

Langhammer J, Birk HW, Zahner H (1997) Renal disease in lymphatic filariasis: evidence of tubular and glomerular disorders at various stages of the infection. Trop Med Int Health 2:875–884

Lecuit M, Martinez F, Deray G, Beaufils H, Gubler MC, Nozais JP, Bricaire F, Jacobs C (1997) Clinical and pathophysiological aspects of immune complex glomerulonephritis associated with *Entamœba histolytica* abscess of the liver. Clin Infect Dis 25(2):335–336

Makarov DV, Bagga H, Gonzalgo ML (2006) Genitourinary myiasis (maggot infestation). Urology 68:889

Marani SA, Canossi GC, Nicoli FA, et al. (1990) Hydatid disease: MR imaging study. Radiology 175:701–706

Margolis J, Arganaras E, Margolis R (1971) *Entamœba histolytica* associated with chronic glomerulonephritis: case report. J Am Geriatr Soc 19(7):646–648

Mehta KS, Halankar AR, Makwana PD, Torane PP, Satija PS, Shah VB (2001) Severe acute renal failure in malaria. J Postgrad Med 47(1):24–26

Meinhardt W, Disney RH (1989) Urogenital myiasis caused by scuttle fly larvae (*Diptera: Phoridae*). Br J Urol 64(5):547–548

Michael E, Bundy DA, Grenfell BT (1996) Re-assessing in global prevalence and distribution of lymphatic filariasis. Parasitology 112:409

Mori S, Konishi T, Matsuska K, Deguchi M, Ohta M, Mizuno O, Veno T, Ikinaka T, Nishimura Y, Ito N, Nakano T (1998) Strongyloidiasis associated with nephrotic syndrome. Intern Med 37(7):606–610

Morimoto J, Kaneska H, Sasatomi Y, Sato YN, Murata T, Ogahara S, Sakata N, Takebayashi S, Naito S, Saito T (2002) Disseminated strongyloidiasis in nephrotic syndrome. Clin Nephrol 57(5):398–401

Mount P, Thong M (2006) Perirenal lymphatic filariasis presenting as chyluria during pregnancy. Kidney International 69:2115

Nada SM, Abazza BE, Mahmoud LA, Habeeb YS, Hussein HF, Amer OT (1996) Toxocariasis as a cause of renal disease in children in Sharkia Governorate, Egypt. J Egypt Soc Parasitol 26(3):709–717

Narvaez JA, Turell LP, Serra J, Hidalgo F (1994) Hyperdense renal cystic lesions caused by *Dioctophyma renale*. AJR Am J Roentgenol 163:997–998

Ngu JL, Chatelanat F, Leke R, Ndumbe P, Youmbissi J (1985) Nephropathy in Cameroon: evidence for filarial derived immune-complex pathogenesis in some cases. Clin Nephrol 24:128–134

Noroes J, Addis D, Santos A (1996) Ultrasonographic evidence of abnormal lymphatic vessels in young men with adult *Wuchereria bancrofti* infection in the scrotal area. J Urol 156:409–412

Oh SJ, Chi JG, Lee SE (1993) Eosinophilic cystitis caused by vesical sparganosis: a case report. J Urol 149:581–582

Othman NH, Ismail AN (1993) Endometrial amoebiasis. Eur J Obstet Gynecol Reprod Biol 52:135–137

Pakasa NM, Nseka NM, Nyimi LM (1997) Secondary collapsing glomerulopathy associated with *Loa loa* filariasis. Am J Kidney Dis 30:836–839

Palmer PE, Reeder MM (2000) Parasitic diseases involving the urinary tract. In: Pollack HM, McClennan BL (eds) Clinical urography, vol 1. Saunders, Philadelphia, pp 1167–1991

Perez-Eid C, Mouffok N (1999) Human urinary myiasis caused by *Fannia canicularis* (Diptera, Muscidae) larvae in Algeria. Presse Med 28(11):580–581

Poggensee G, Feldmeier H (2001) Female genital schistosomiasis: facts and hypotheses. Acta Trop 79:193

Poggensee G, Kiwelu I, Weger V, et al. (2000) Female genital schistosomiasis of the lower genital tract: prevalence and disease-associated morbidity in northern Tanzania. J Infect Dis 181:1210–1213

Polat P, Kantarci M, Alper F, Suma S, Koruyucu MB, Okur A (2003) Hydatid disease from head to toe. Radiographics 23:475–494

Pollack HM (1981) Diagnostic considerations in urinary bladder wall calcification. AJR Am J Roentgenol 136:791–797

Richens J (2004) Genital manifestations of tropical diseases. Sex Transm Infect 80:12–17

Roussel B, Pinon JM, Birembaut P, Rullier J, Pennaforte F (1987) Congenital nephrotic syndrome associated with congenital toxoplasmosis. Arch Fr Pediatr 44(9):795–797

Saggie JL, Dwomoa A (1988) Nephrotic syndrome in tropics. In: Cameron JS, Glassock RJ (eds) The nephrotic syndrome. Dekker, New York, pp 635–695

Sakamoto T, Gutierrez C, Rodriguez A, Santo S (2003) Testicular sparganosis in a child from Uruguay. Acta Trop 88:83–86

Saleh MS, el Sibae MM (1993) Uro-genital myiasis due to *Piophila casei*. J Egypt Soc Parasitol 23(3):737–739

Sartori A, De Oliveira AV, Roque-Barreira MC, Rossi MA, Campos-Neto A (1987) Immune complex glomerulonephritis in experimental kala-azar. Parasite Immunol 9(1):93–103

Sewcz C (1985) X-ray findings in urogenital bilharziosis. Radiol Diagn 26:213–219

Shahin B, Papadopoulou ZL, Jenis EH (1974) Congenital nephrotic syndrome associated with congenital toxoplasmosis. J Pediatr 85(3):366–370

Shelley S, Manokaran G, Indirani M, Gokhale S, Anirudhan N (2006) Lymphoscintigraphy as a diagnostic tool in patients with lymphedema of filarial origin-an Indian study. Lymphology 39:69–75

Shokier AA (1972) Urinary bilharziasis in upper Egypt (I and II). East Afr Med J 49:298–326

Soans B, Abel C (1999) Ultrasound appearance of schistosomiasis of the testis. Australas Radiol 43:385–387

Sun T, Turnbull A, Lieberman PH, Sternberg SS (1986) Giant kidney worm (*Dioctophyma renale*) infection mimicking retroperitoneal neoplasm. Am J Surg Pathol 10(7):508–512

Takiguchi Y, Kusama K, Nagao S, Iijima S (1987) A case of scabies complicated by acute glomerulonephritis. J Dermatol 14(2):163–166

Van Velthuysen ML (1996) Glomerulopathy associated with parasitic infections. Parasitol Today 12(3):102–107

Vilana R, Corachan M, Gascon J, Valls E, Bru C (1997) Schistosomiasis of the male genital tract: transrectal sonography findings. J Urol 158:1491–1493

Von Sinner W, Hellstrom M, Kagevi I, et al. (1993) Hydatid disease of the urinary tract. J Urol 149:577–580

Von Sinner WN (1997) Advanced medical imaging and treatment of human cystic echinococcosis. Semin Roentgenol 32:267–290

Westendorp RG, Doorenbos CJ, Thompson J, Von Es LA, Von Furth R (1990) Immune complex glomerulonephritis associated with an amoebic liver abscess. Trans R Soc Trop Med Hyg 84(3):385–386

Woodward PJ, Schwab CM, Sesterhenn IA (2003) From the archives of the AFIP: extratesticular scrotal masses: radiologic-pathologic correlation. Radiographics 23:215–240

Yachnis AT, Berg J, Martinez-Salazar A, Bender BS, Diaz L, Rojiani AM, Eskin TA, Orenstein JM (1996) Disseminated microsporidiosis especially infecting the brain, heart and kidneys. Report of a newly recognized pansporoblastic species in two symptomatic AIDS patients. Am J Clin Pathol 106(4):535–553

Zali MR, Ghaziani T, Shahraz S, Hekmatdoost A, Radmehr A (2004) Liver, spleen, pancreas and kidney involvement by human fascioliasis: imaging findings. BMC Gastroenterol 4:15–17

Zmerli S, Ayed M, Horchani A, Chami I, El Ouakdi M, Ben Slama MR (2001) Hydatid cyst of the kidney: diagnosis and treatment. World J Surg 25:68–74

Chapter

Imaging of Parasitic Diseases of the Musculoskeletal System and Soft Tissues

7

Mohamed E. Abd El Bagi

Contents

7.1 Introduction

Musculoskeletal parasites (MSKP) are usually encountered in tropical areas. However, there have recently been reports from western countries, e.g., Germany (Kienast et al. 2007), France (Ansart et al. 2007; Bouchaud et al. 2000), and Canada (Ancelle et al. 2005; Davies et al. 1993). The relation of the musculoskeletal system (MSK) to parasites has its own peculiarity. The large surface area of the overlying skin is an open entrance gate, particularly during swimming in polluted ponds and swamps. The exposure of farmers to parasites is compulsory in agricultural irrigation canals. Sleeping on the bare ground provides a fast track into the human body. Soil-transmitted parasites are a major health problem in many countries, particularly in children (Xu et al. 1995). Temporarily, the subcutaneous tissues provide a medium for local wandering movement as in cutaneous larva migrans (Jelinek et al. 1994). The MSK may act as a graveyard for those parasites that do not complete their life cycle and finally lodge in muscles or bones. Unlike the gastrointestinal tract (GIT), there is no continuous supply of soluble nourishment and no room for delivery of offspring or reproduction because of bone tissue compactness, muscle movements, and contractions. Lactic acid production in the muscles is hostile to parasites. This is why musculoskeletal parasites are of rare occurrence, even in hyperendemic areas. Intradermal parasites are amenable to direct clinical inspection and do not require radiologic investigation. MSKP can be detected incidentally as calcified dead worms (Box 7.1) or present with bizarre lesions like elephantiasis.

According to Professor Woodruff's book, one in ten inhabitants of Great Britain and of many other non-tropical countries, visit the tropics or subtropics each year (Woodruff 1984). He himself has spent some time at Juba University in southern Sudan. Currently, it is a two-way passage. Tourists, adventurers, businessmen seeking cheap labor communities, expatriates providing their expertise to developing countries, and Western forces deployed into tropical locations are reciprocated by an influx of refugees, adopted children, and asylum seekers. The enthusiasm of the volunteers of the humanitarian relief organizations may render them closely exposed to parasites in countries affected by war or famine.

Parasitic infestation afflicts a considerable proportion of the world's population. Many parasites are able to bypass the host's immune system leading to chronic asymptomatic carrier state (McGill 1995). The objective of this chapter is to describe the radiologic manifestations of the commonest MSKP. These include hydatid disease, cutaneous larva migrans, Guinea worm, filariasis, and cysticercosis. Ectoparasites and cutaneous predators like scabies, lice, myiasis ("Old World screw worm"), cutaneous leishmaniasis, and several other parasitic dermatosis are excluded (Ansart et al. 2007).

Box 7.1 Calcified parasites in soft tissues

Parasite	Calcifications
Cysticerci	Muscles
Guinea worm	Subcutaneous tissues
Loa loa	Subcutaneous tissues
Armillifer armillatus	Muscles

7.2 Pathways into the Musculoskeletal System

7.2.1 Direct Skin Penetration

This is the entrance route for many MSK and GIT parasites. There is, however, less emphasis on this route in daily clinical practices. Cutaneous larva migrans, or the creeping eruption, is the best example (Jelinek et al. 1994).

7.2.2 Oral Route

The oral route is the classic and well-known access of parasites into the human body. Ingested forms may hatch in the stomach or small intestine. They might migrate to distant organs, e.g., hydatid oncospheres usually pass into the portal system and lodge in the liver and less commonly reach the lungs. Rarely, they escape through the liver and lung filters to reach the circulation and thereby the bones and muscles.

7.2.3 Lymphatic Route

This follows either the transcutaneous or transoral entry of the parasite into the human body. Parasites that pass into the lymphatics readily reach the lungs, muscles or bones (Lewall 1998).

7.3 Impact of Musculoskeletal Parasites

The damage caused by parasites has been well described (Thomas 1986). Production of toxins enables the parasites to disrupt the integrity of tissue barriers. Deprivation of the host of nutrients and metabolites is not a major problem with MSKP unlike in the GIT. The introduction of pathogenic organisms is important with transcutaneous invaders because of soil and water contamination. MSKP are notorious for causing aggressive tissue reaction, inflammation, and fibrosis, which may lead to gigantism. Immunologic responses are provoked if a cyst ruptures or an adult worm is cut, which can cause severe anaphylaxis. The native African tribes have learned to avoid pulling out Guinea worms forcibly, but instead allow them to roll themselves gradually onto tiny wood sticks. There is no direct evidence of carcinogenic effect from MSKP. However, what is called chronic tropical ulcer is precancerous if neglected for decades (Fig. 7.1) (Holcombe and Hassan 1991). These chronic ulcers could be provoked or secondarily infested by parasites or by parasite-borne bacteria. Filariasis is not well-known for being precancerous. However, it has been reported that chronic lymphedema of other causes predisposes to lymphangiosarcoma (Szuba and Rockson 1998). There has recently been controversy as to whether geoparasites would predispose to or protect the human body from allergic reactions (Zeyrek and Zeyrek 2006).

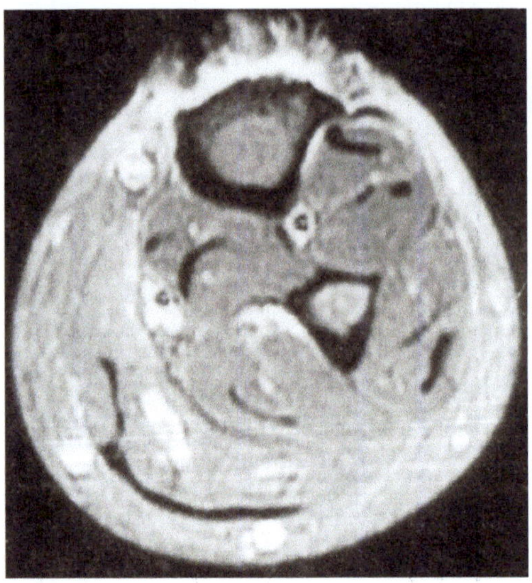

Fig. 7.1 Axial T2-weighted MR image of the calf of a 68-year-old man who has had a chronic tropical ulcer for over 10 years. There are polypoid and "hair-on-end" soft tissue budding within the ulcer crater due to squamous cell carcinoma. There is inflammation and edema of the surrounding soft tissue planes, small bone erosions, sclerosis, and cortical thickening. The original cause of the ulcer could not be identified (whether parasitic or not) (Abd El Bagi et al. 1999)

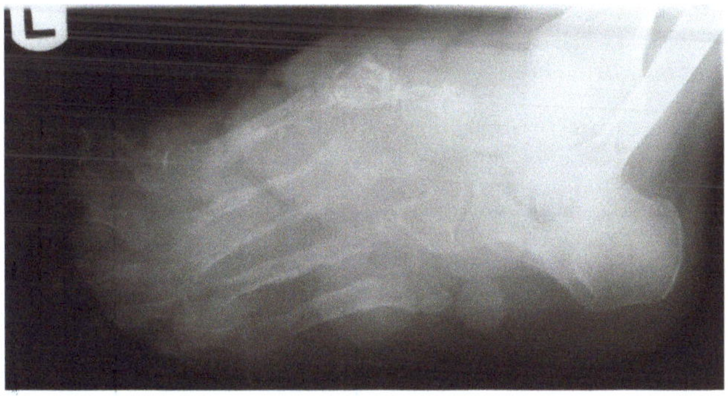

Fig. 7.2 Radiograph of the foot of an adult man who presented with long-standing soft tissue swelling. There are numerous rounded soft tissue nodules associated with multiple bone erosions and the slimming and separation of the metatarsal bones. Appearances are typical of pedal mycetoma, which is not a parasite, but due to either bacteria (actinomycetoma) or fungi (maduromycetoma)

7.4 Clinical Presentation

1. Soft tissue swelling
2. Pain
3. Itching
4. Papules
5. Ulcers
6. Bone cysts
7. Pathological fractures
8. Gigantism
9. Soft tissue calcification
10. Myalgia
11. Rheumatism
12. Larva migrans (cutaneous and subcutaneous)

Soft tissue swellings are of variable sizes and shapes. They could be tiny papules, small nodules, intermediate-sized swellings or large pseudotumors. It is important to remember that mycetoma, which is a sinister tropical disease, should not be confused with MSKP (Fig 7.2). It is peculiarly caused by either bacteria or fungi and may present with soft tissue swelling and sinuses (Abd El Bagi et al. 1999).

7.5 Parasitic Rheumatism

Parasites are often ignored as a cause of rheumatism and not mentioned in the differential diagnosis of rheumatic disease presentation (Peng 2002; Pinals 1994). Parasitic rheumatism encompasses a wide spectrum of disease presentations caused by a large variety of parasites (Box 7.2). There are three mechanisms for developing arthritic symptoms in patients with MSKP. If the parasite enters a joint, it would provoke inflammatory reaction or arthritis. Pyogenic arthritis could be due to the bacterial cargo on a worm or due to opportunistic microbes that might enter the joints through the burrowed tunnels. Schistosomes have been identified in the synovium of inflamed knees (Adebajo 1996). Articular invasion by parasites may progress to marked derangement of the affected joint, e.g., "Ibadan knee" (Greenwood 1968). The second mechanism is an inflammatory reaction secondary to periarticular deposition of a parasite. The third and most common mechanism is immunologic arthritis in response to the presence of a parasite in other organs (Doury 1990). This can be monoarticular, pauciarticular or polyarticular, and does not respond to antirheumatic drugs until the parasite is eradicated (Doury et al. 1977). Other forms of parasitic rheumatism include enthesitis, myositis and vasculitis (McGill 1995). Achilles tendonitis and plantar fasciitis were described in patients infected with urinary schistosomiasis (Bassiouni and Kamel 1984). The diagnosis of parasitic rheumatism is supported by a poor response to anti-inflammatory drugs and improvement following anti-parasitic treatment (McGill 1995). In tropical settings there are other local nonparasitic diseases that can cause rheumatism like dengue (virus), tuberculosis and leprosy (mycobacteria), rheumatic fever, and *Brucella* (bacteria).

Box 7.2 What is the spectrum of parasitic rheumatism? (Peng 2002; McGill 1995)

Infective arthritis	Amoeba
Reactive arthritis	Tapeworms, schistosomiasis, hydatid
Rheumatoid-like	Malaria
Juvenile arthritis	*Giardia*
Polymyositis	Malaria, sarcocystosis, microsporidiosis
Reiter's-like disease	*Strongyloides*, coccidia
Polyarteritis nodosa-like	Trichinosis
Destructive arthritis	*Dracunculus*
Dermatomyositis	Toxoplasmosis
Chylous arthritis	Filariasis

7.6 Helminths (Nematodes)

7.6.1 Geohelminths

Geohelminths or soil-transmitted parasites are intestinal nematodes, part of the development of which takes place outside the body in the soil (Table 7.1) (Gilles 1995). In type 1, the eggs, which are passed with stools, hatch and are carried directly from the anal margin to the mouth

Table 7.1 Types of geohelminths according to their life cycle

Type 1 Direct ano-oral, do not reach the soil	Threadworm (*Enterobius*), whipworm (*Trichuris*)
Type 2 Modified in soil, but hatches in man	Roundworm (*Ascaris*)
Type 3 Larva hatch in soil, then penetrate skin	Hookworm (*Ancylostoma*), strongyloidiasis

Table 7.2 Comparison of the prevalence of common nematodes on three continents

	China (Xu et al. 1995)	Indonesia (Widjana and Sutisna 2000)	Nigeria (Asaolu et al. 1992)	Afghanistan (Gabrielli et al. 2005)	Bolivia (Flores et al. 2001)	Ecuador (Andrade et al. 2001)
n	1,477,742	2,394	–	1,001	2,723	151
Ascaris	47%	73%	61–72%	41%	1–28%	63%
Trichuris	19%	62%	65–74%	10%	0–24%	10%
Hookworms	17%	24%	52–63%	0.7%	Very rare	1.4%

Table 7.3 Soft tissue nematodes

Filariasis	*W. bancrofti*	Elephantiasis
	B. malayi	
Loiasis	*Loa loa*	Eye worm, Calabar swelling
Onchocerciasis	*Onchocerca volvulus*	River blindness
Guinea worm	*Dracunculus medinensis*	Subcutaneous calcifications
Trichinosis	*Trichinella spiralis*	Embedded in muscles
Larva migrans	*Toxocara canis*	In liver, eye, and brain

within a few hours. In type 2, the eggs reach the soil where they undergo some development, but they only hatch after being ingested into the stomach of the patient. In type 3, eggs are passed onto the soil where they hatch into larvae that enter the body via the skin. Geohelminths have a worldwide prevalence of variable intensity. They are less prevalent in the highlands of endemic regions (Table 7.2) (Flores et al. 2001).

7.6.2 Prevalence of Nematodes

The prevalence of common nematodes is widespread. The locations are summarized in (Table 7.3). Nearly all nematodes have a soft tissue phase.

7.6.3 Cutaneous Larva Migrans

The syndrome of cutaneous larva migrans develops when certain skin-penetrating larvae migrate into the dermis and cause cutaneous parasitism (**Box 7.3**). It is characterized by serpiginous or tunnel-like migrating erythema and pruritis, known as creeping eruptions (Jelinek et al. 1994). Secretion of hyaluronidase renders movement of larva possible (Hotez et al. 1992). The typical erythema occur 3–4 cm away from the penetration site and the larva itself is 1–2 cm ahead of the creeping eruption (Jelinek et al. 1994). Cutaneous larva migrans is caused by dog and cat hookworms namely *Ancylostoma braziliense* (Davies et al. 1993). The disease is prevalent in the tropics, but is seen in 7–25% of patients attending travel-related disease

Box 7.3 What are the causes of larva migrans?

Visceral larva migrans (Sakai et al. 2006)	Cutaneous larva migrans (Jelinek et al. 1994)	Ocular larva migrans (Jaksche et al. 2004)
In tropical regions: all metazoan helminthic infections during parasitic migration (see also page 64) *In nontropical regions:* *Ascaris suum* *Toxocara canis*	1. *Ancylostoma* sp. Human hookworms Dog and cat hookworms 2. *Bunostomum* sp. Cattle hookworm 3. *Gnathostoma* sp. Cat and pig roundworm 4. *Capillaria* sp. Rodents and poultry whipworm 5. *Strongyloides* Mammals 6. Myiasis Old World screw worm 7. Others see page 5	*Loa loa* *Baylisascaris procyonis* *Toxoplasma gondi* *Toxocara* *Onchocerca volvulus* *Trypanosoma* *Taenia solium* *Trichinella spiralis*

clinics in Germany and France (Bouchaud et al. 2000). Differential diagnosis includes larva currens, cutaneous myiasis, scabies, and lyme disease (Elliot et al. 1985). Human beings are incidental hosts in which the larva cannot complete the life cycle and remain blocked in the dermis (Elliot et al. 1985).

Of the causes of subcutaneous larva migrans, gnathostomiasis and sparganosis should be considered, especially in international travelers and persons eating exotic diets (Gillespie 2004; Moore et al. 2003). Patients present with painful or painless subcutaneous lumps. On imaging, the majority of the lesions in soft tissue are confined to the subcutaneous layer, but may extend deep into the underlying muscles. Sonography reveals hypoechoic serpiginous tubular tracts, and MRI shows serpiginous tubular tracts with peripheral rim enhancement and perilesional soft tissue edema. Pathologically, the lesion consists of a larva surrounded by layers of inflammation (Moore et al. 2003; Cho et al. 2000; Kim and Lee 2001; Pampiglione et al. 2003). Other causes of subcutaneous parasitism such as dirofilariasis, dracunculiasis, loiasis, and muscular parasitism, such as cysticercosis and pentastomiasis, are discussed separately.

7.6.4 Trichinellosis

Trichinellosis is one of the intestinal helminths with a significant tissue phase. It is common where swine are fed undercooked garbage and slaughterhouse scraps. It is also prevalent in black bears, foxes, and seals. It has been recently reported in Canadian hunters (Ancelle et al. 2005). The disease is also prevalent in the Far East (Kaewpitoon et al. 2006). The parasite provokes tissue reaction, vasculitis, and muscle destruction. The disease was very common in the United States in the first half of the last century when undercooked pork was eaten, before appropriate legislation was passed (Markell et al. 1992).

7.6.5 Filariasis

Filariae are thread-like nematodes that inhabit the lymphatic system and the subcutaneous tissues. They are transported to human beings by mosquito insects. The commonest type of filaria is *Wuchereria bancrofti.* The disease is common in central Africa, the Far East, and Brazil. As many as 80 million cases were prevalent worldwide 20 years ago (WHO 1984). The African type of filariasis is commoner and more severe than the Malayan type. Ulcerations are common in the latter. *Brugia timoria* is prevalent on Timor Island. An exceedingly rare form of non-filarial elephantiasis was described in East Africa (Markell et al. 1992).

7.6.5.1 Life Cycle of Filaria

After the mosquito sucks blood from an infected patient, the microfilaria develops within the insect into infective larvae to enter into another human victim with the next mosquito bite. The worms settle in the lymph nodes. The males and females mate to produce microfilariae, which circulate in the blood (and much more so at night time). The parasite can live in the body for a few years.

7.6.5.2 Clinical Presentation

This includes fever, lymphadenitis, and lymphangitis, which may involve the extremities, breast or scrotum. Abscesses may form. Filariasis is the commonest cause of lymphedema (Szuba and Rockson 1998). Chyluria occurs when a lymphatic ruptures into the urinary tract. Hydroceles are seen in 5% of cases. Chylous arthritis is a common complication (McGill 1995). Elephantiasis is a famous but relatively uncommon end result, even in endemic areas. Chronic lymphedema provokes intense tissue reaction leading to woody indurations, verrucous skin, and elephantiasis. Tropical pulmonary eosinophilia (TPE) is common particularly in the Far East.

7.6.5.3 Radiological Features

In endemic areas, diagnosis is easy by symptoms and limb enlargement, and is confirmed by microscopic examination of a night-time blood film. However, in countries that have suddenly come out of hardship and moved into prosperity, the few residual cases are missed or confused with lipedema or phlebedema. Radiology is of paramount importance in differentiating among the three entities, whether they are causing unilateral or bilateral limb swelling (Fig. 7.3). The CT signs of filarial lymphedema include soft tissue and skin thickening, lines perpendicular and parallel to the skin, and perimuscular edema (Fig. 7.4) (Marotel et al. 1998). CT of the abdomen and pelvis would exclude intra-abdominal masses causing lymphatic obstruction. On MRI of lipedema, fat is hyperintense on T1- and T2-weighted images (WI) (Fig. 7.5). In cases of lymphedema, the inflammatory fluid excess is hyperintense on T2-WI, but hypointense on T1-WI, unlike lipedema (Fig. 7.6). A characteristic honeycomb appearance of the engorged lymphatics is seen on the various MRI sequences, including T1-WI, T2-WI, and STIR, and in various MRI planes including axial, coronal, and sagittal (Fig. 7.6a–c) (Duewell et al. 1992). In the past, conventional lymphangiograms were used for demonstrating lymphatic obstruction. This was an invasive, tedious procedure (Case et al. 1992). Lymphoscintigraphy is a good method for the assessment of lymphatic flow and the evaluation of lymphangiectasis and lymphedema, whether due to mild stasis or in severe cases with total obstruction (Fig. 7.7a–c) (Shelly et al. 2006). The combination of MRI and lymphangioscintigraphy is complementary, pending the development of a supermagnetic MR lymphangionodal contrast agent (Case et al. 1992). Recently, the movement of adult worms ("filarial dance") within a breast lesion was seen by real-time ultrasound (Rathi et al. 2006).

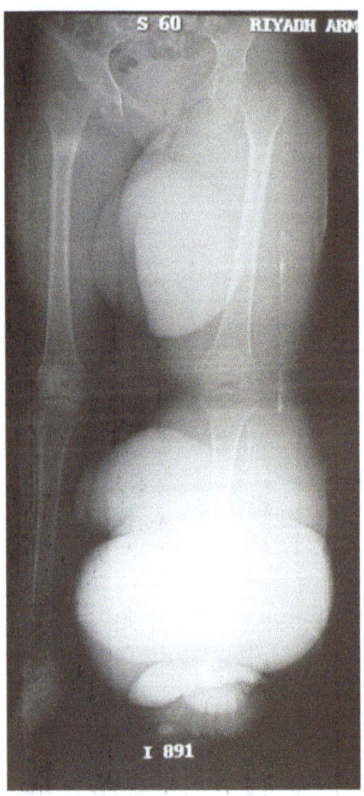

Fig. 7.3 Computed tomographic scanogram of an adult woman who presented for the first time with a unilaterally swollen limb showing marked elephantiasis due to filariasis; the differential diagnosis includes other causes of lymphedema, lipedema, and phlebedema

7.6.6 Dirofilariasis

Dirofilariasis is a zoonotic disease sporadically affecting humans. Subcutaneous nodular disease caused by *Dirofilaria repens* is the most frequently reported manifestation of human dirofilariasis, compared with the human pulmonary dirofilariasis caused by *Dirofilaria immitis*. The endemic areas for *D. repens* infection have been identified in South Asia, and in some parts of Eastern and Southern Europe including the Mediterranean regions. Humans acquire the infection by a mosquito bite containing infective larvae; these larvae fail to reach maturity in humans, the latter being their unnatural hosts. The incompletely matured worm dies localized in subcutaneous sites, which initiates the typical host immune tissue reaction. The biopsy specimen examination of symptomatic nodules remains the mainstay of diagnosis, depicting the worm in a chronic abscess. The first documented case of subcutaneous dirofilariasis in the Arabian region was reported from Kuwait (Hira et al. 1994), and the second case from Saudi Arabia (Chopra et al. 2004).

7.6.7 Onchocerciasis

Human onchocerciasis is a severe, disabling disease endemic in 28 African countries, six Latin American countries, and Yemen (Thylefors and Alleman 2006). The disease is caused by *Onchocerca volvulus*. The adult female worm measures 35–70 cm long, while the male measures only 2–4 cm. Fortunately, onchocerciasis has shown a good response to ivermectin mass therapy. The disease

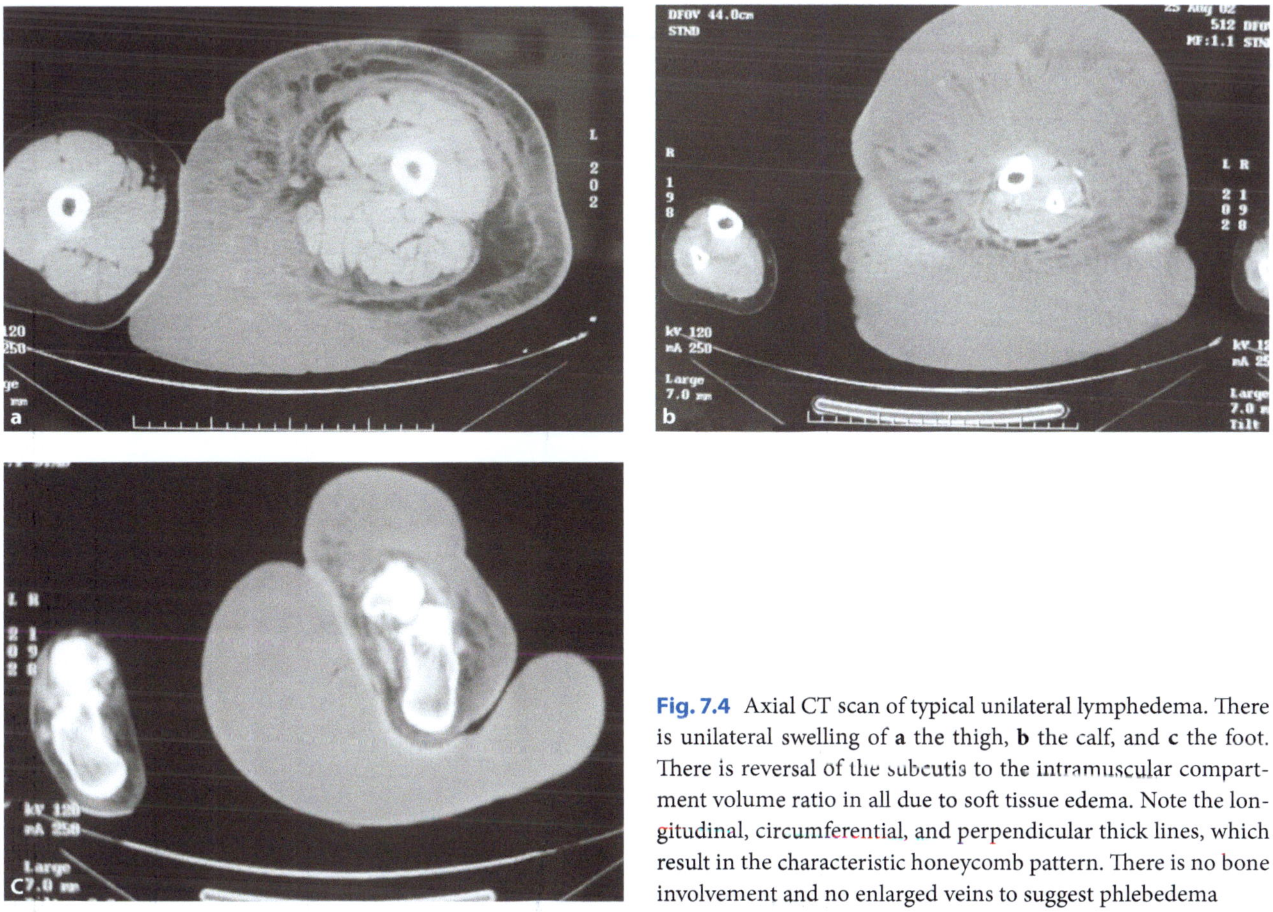

Fig. 7.4 Axial CT scan of typical unilateral lymphedema. There is unilateral swelling of **a** the thigh, **b** the calf, and **c** the foot. There is reversal of the subcutis to the intramuscular compartment volume ratio in all due to soft tissue edema. Note the longitudinal, circumferential, and perpendicular thick lines, which result in the characteristic honeycomb pattern. There is no bone involvement and no enlarged veins to suggest phlebedema

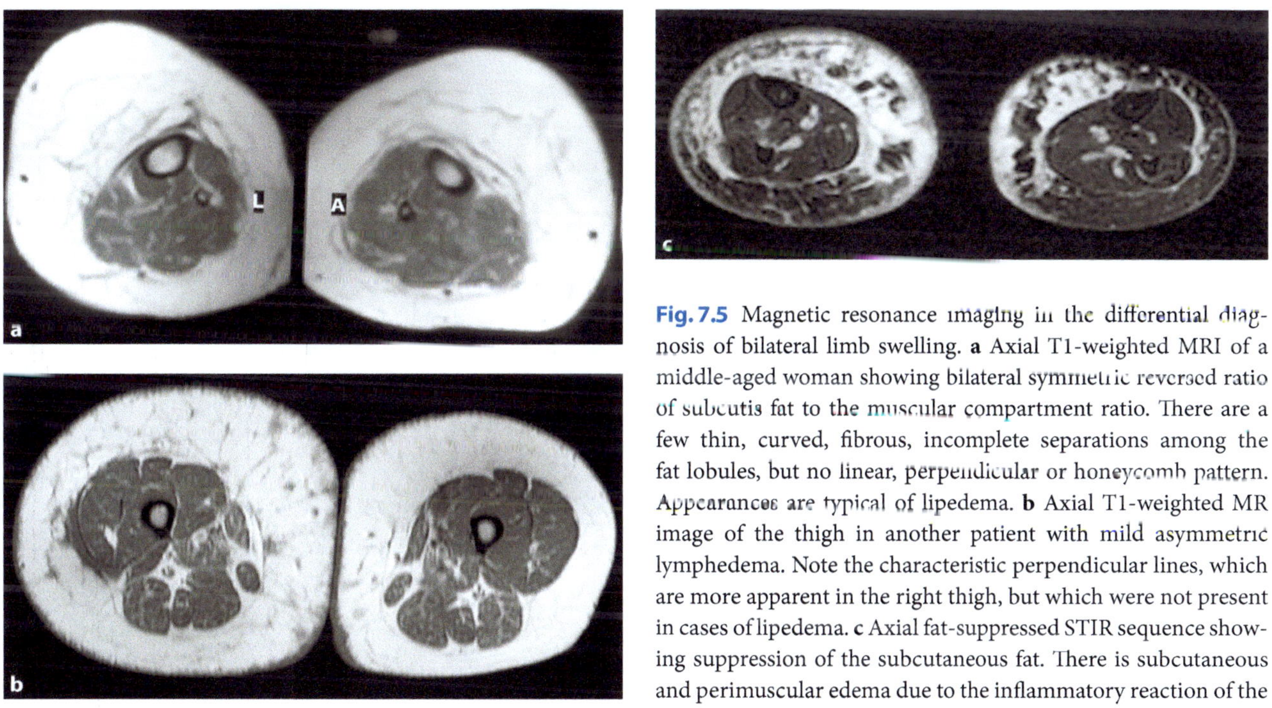

Fig. 7.5 Magnetic resonance imaging in the differential diagnosis of bilateral limb swelling. **a** Axial T1-weighted MRI of a middle-aged woman showing bilateral symmetric reversed ratio of subcutis fat to the muscular compartment ratio. There are a few thin, curved, fibrous, incomplete separations among the fat lobules, but no linear, perpendicular or honeycomb pattern. Appearances are typical of lipedema. **b** Axial T1-weighted MR image of the thigh in another patient with mild asymmetric lymphedema. Note the characteristic perpendicular lines, which are more apparent in the right thigh, but which were not present in cases of lipedema. **c** Axial fat-suppressed STIR sequence showing suppression of the subcutaneous fat. There is subcutaneous and perimuscular edema due to the inflammatory reaction of the body to its own trapped proteins within the stagnant lymphatics

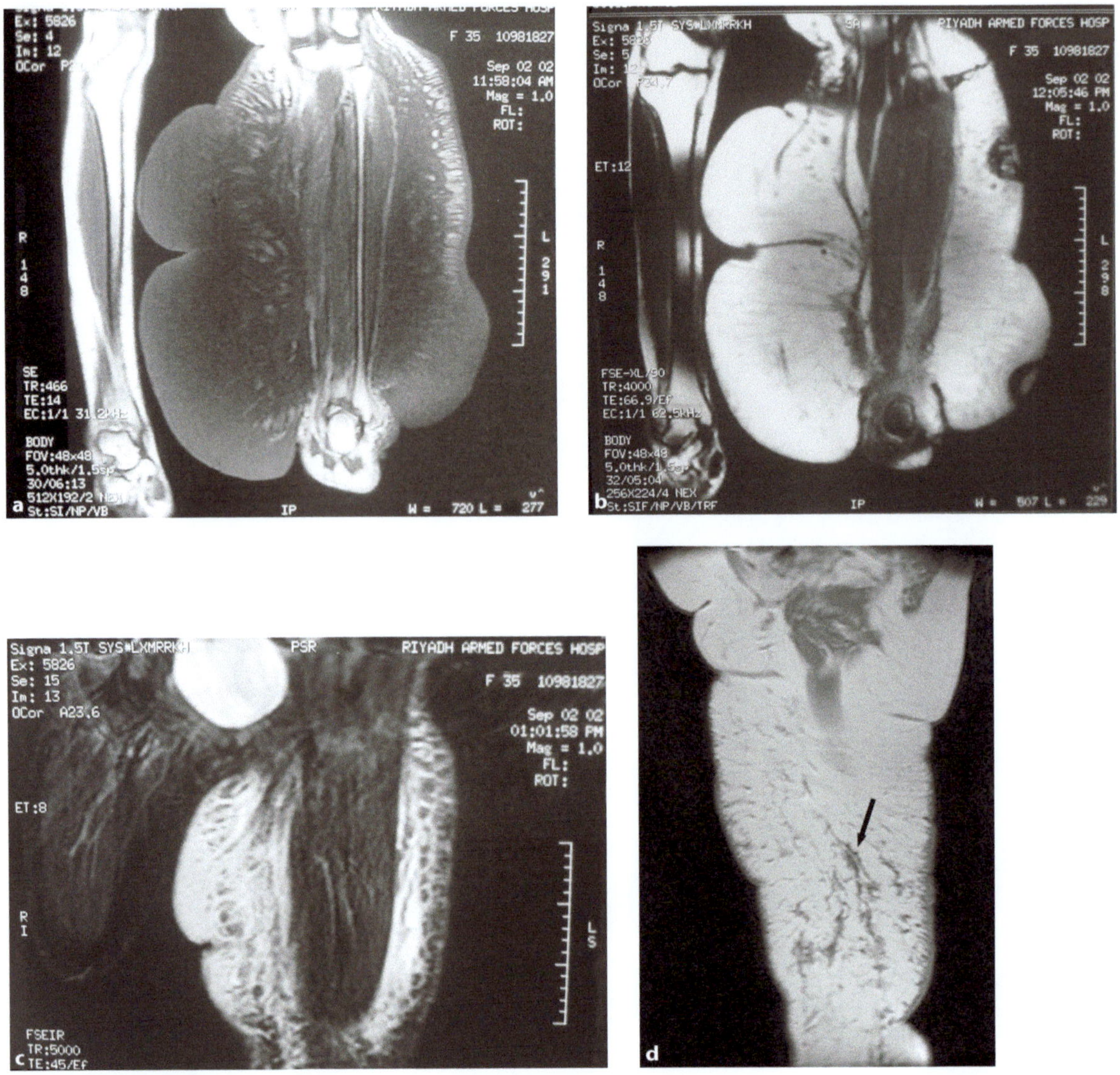

Fig. 7.6 Typical MRI findings in filarial lymphedema. **a** Coronal T1-weighted MRI of elephantiasis in the calf and leg. Characteristic perpendicular and honeycomb appearance of lymphatics surrounded by low signal massive soft tissue edema. Note the lobulation and redundancy of the contours. **b** Coronal T2-weighted MRI of the leg and calf in elephantiasis showing hyperintense subcutaneous edema traversed by perpendicular lymphatics. There are no giant veins or intramuscular engorgement to suggest phlebedema. **c** Coronal fat-suppressed STIR MR image of the thigh in elephantiasis confirming the absence of lipedema and showing the extent of subcutaneous edema with a honeycomb pattern. **d** Sagittal T1-weighted MRI of the thigh in a patient with a short history of moderate thigh swelling due to lymphedema, showing the engorged serpiginous lymphatics (*arrow*). There is no marked soft tissue edema at this stage

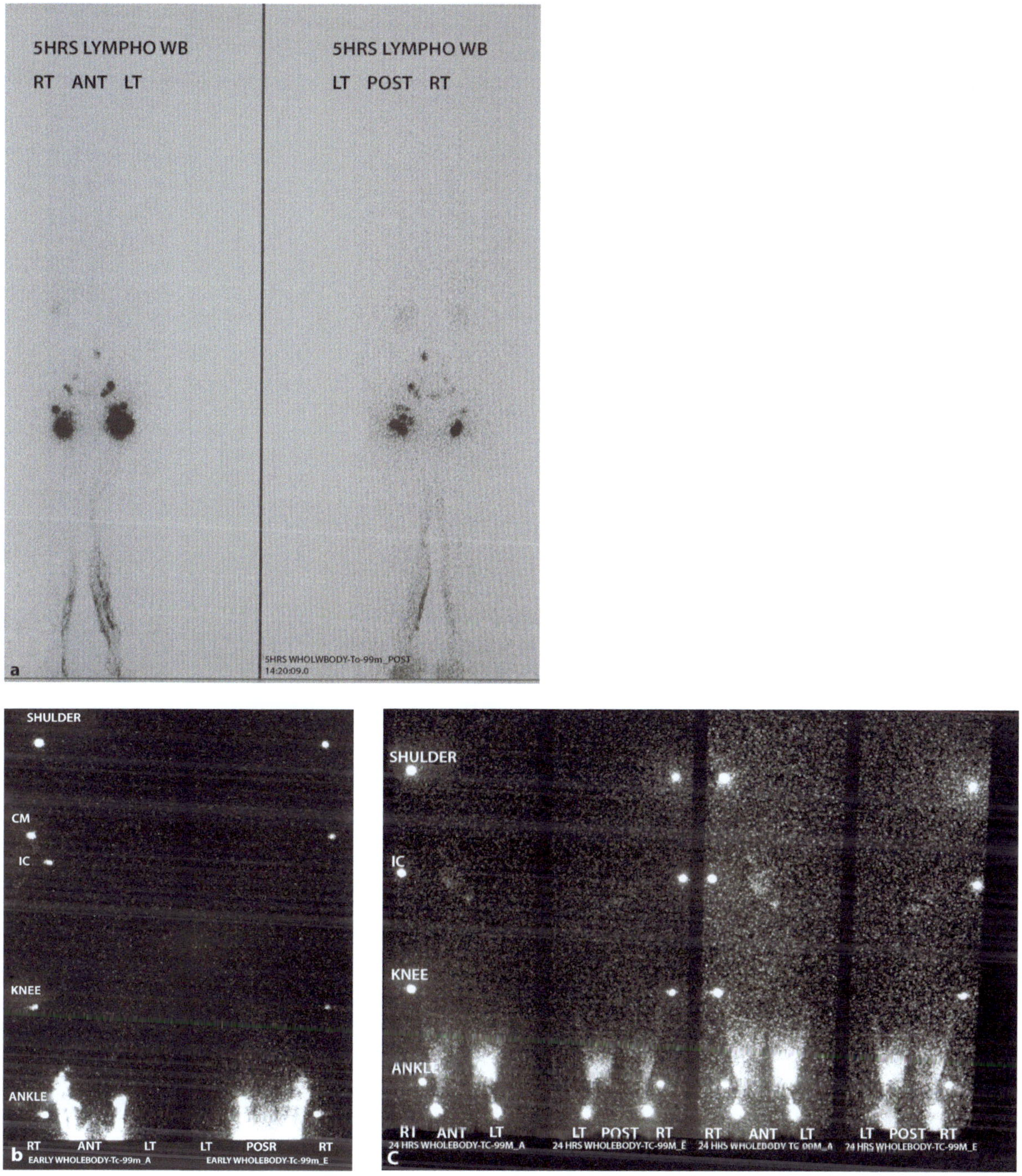

Fig. 7.7 Lymphoscintigraphy for diagnosis of lymphatic stasis or total obstruction. **a** Five-hour delayed lymphoscintigram images showing the tracer reaching the inguinal, pelvic, and para-aortic lymph nodes. There is, however, prominence of the lymphatic channels in the left leg compared with the right, with soft tissue traces due to localized stasis and earliest traces of leakage. **b** Early lymphoscintigram images showing engorged ankle lymphatic channels with abrupt bilateral hold-up due to complete proximal occlusions. **c** Twenty-four-hour delayed lymphoscintigram images of the patient in **b** showing failure of ascent, absence of groin or retroperitoneal node uptake, and leakage of the isotope traces in the feet and ankles due to total obstruction above the ankles (Courtesy of Dr. J. Nabulsi, Riyadh Military Hospital, Riyadh, Saudi Arabia)

may present with skin nodules over bony prominences like the occiput or iliac crest. More seriously, patients may present with loss of vision "river blindness" (Mukhtar et al. 1998). Another form is endemic in southern Saudi Arabia and Yemen and is characterized by hyperpigmented, lichenified, papular lesions with severe localized pruritis, called "sowda" (Siddiqui and al-Khawajah 1991; Helmy and Al Mathal 2003).

7.6.8 Dracunculiasis (Guinea Worm)

Guinea worms are not a true filarial disease. They are caused by *Dracunculus medinensis*. The female may reach 1 m in length, while the male is only 2 cm in length. The gravid female worm eventually settles under the skin. It may be expelled or calcify in situ. Dracunculiasis is acquired by drinking water containing crustacea infected with larvae (McGill 1995). It is said to affect only 3 million people and is an index for the poorest 10 countries. The disease is limited to remote rural villages in sub-Saharan Africa (Greenway 2004). Guinea worm provides an example of eradication programs being successful, causing a 98% reduction in the disease over 20 years (Greenway 2004). Calcified dracunculiasis is another example of disease remnants in rapidly developing countries in which the people are no longer living in poverty. We frequently see cases of calcified Guinea worm in Saudi Arabia in various parts of the body (Fig. 7.8). In African countries like Ghana nearly everyone carries a specimen around with them (McGill 1995). The disease commonly affects lower limb joints, particularly the knee, either by direct invasion, reactive or septic arthritis gaining access to the joint via sinuses created by the worm (McGill 1995). Aggressive joint derangement may end in what is called "Ibadan knee" (Greenwood 1968; Peng 2002).

7.6.9 Loiasis

Loiasis affects millions of individuals living in the rain forests of the savannah regions of central Africa (Boussinesq 2006). It could present with ocular swelling or parasitic rheumatism. The African eye worm of *Loa loa* is prevalent in the rain forests of Sudan and West Africa and is transmitted by the mango fly. The worm may be seen migrating through the conjunctiva or as "Calabar swellings," which are patches of subcutaneous edema (Markell et al. 1992).

7.7 Helminths (Cestodes)

7.7.1 Echinococcosis (Hydatid Disease)

Hydatid disease is caused by the larvae of cestodes of the genus *Echinococcus*. The exact worldwide prevalence of hydatid disease is yet to be determined, although it is seen in most countries in relation to sheep-raising. The frequency of hydatid disease in Tunisia was estimated to affect 5.33% of the general population (Ben M'Rads et al. 1998). Cattle, horses, and camels can act as reservoirs or intermediate hosts (Sadjjadi 2006). Peculiarly, cats are exempt. The highest prevalence is around the Mediterranean, South America, and Australia (Beggs 1985). A lot of the published work has come from Tunisia (Gharbi 1981), Turkey (Polat et al. 2003), and Saudi Arabia (Lewall 1998). The highest rate in the world of hyda-

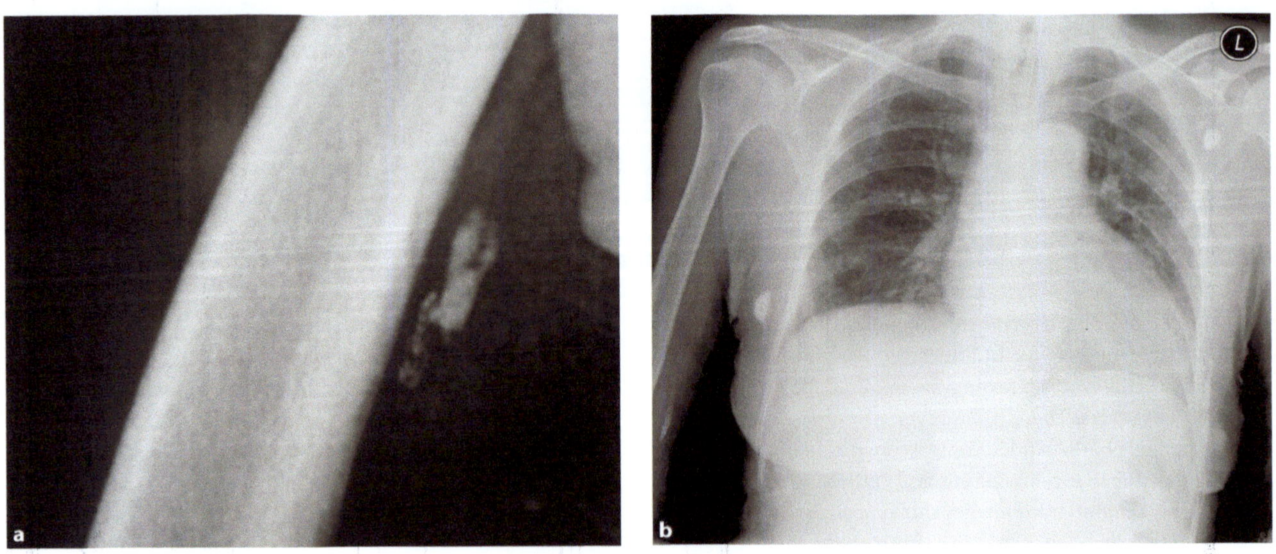

Fig. 7.8 Calcified Guinea worms in various part of the body. **a** Right groin of an adult man showing calcified worm. **b,c** Chest radiographs of an adult woman showing multiple subcutaneous calcified worms in the right breast, left lower lateral chest wall, right lower arm medially, and left elbow. **c–f** *see next page*

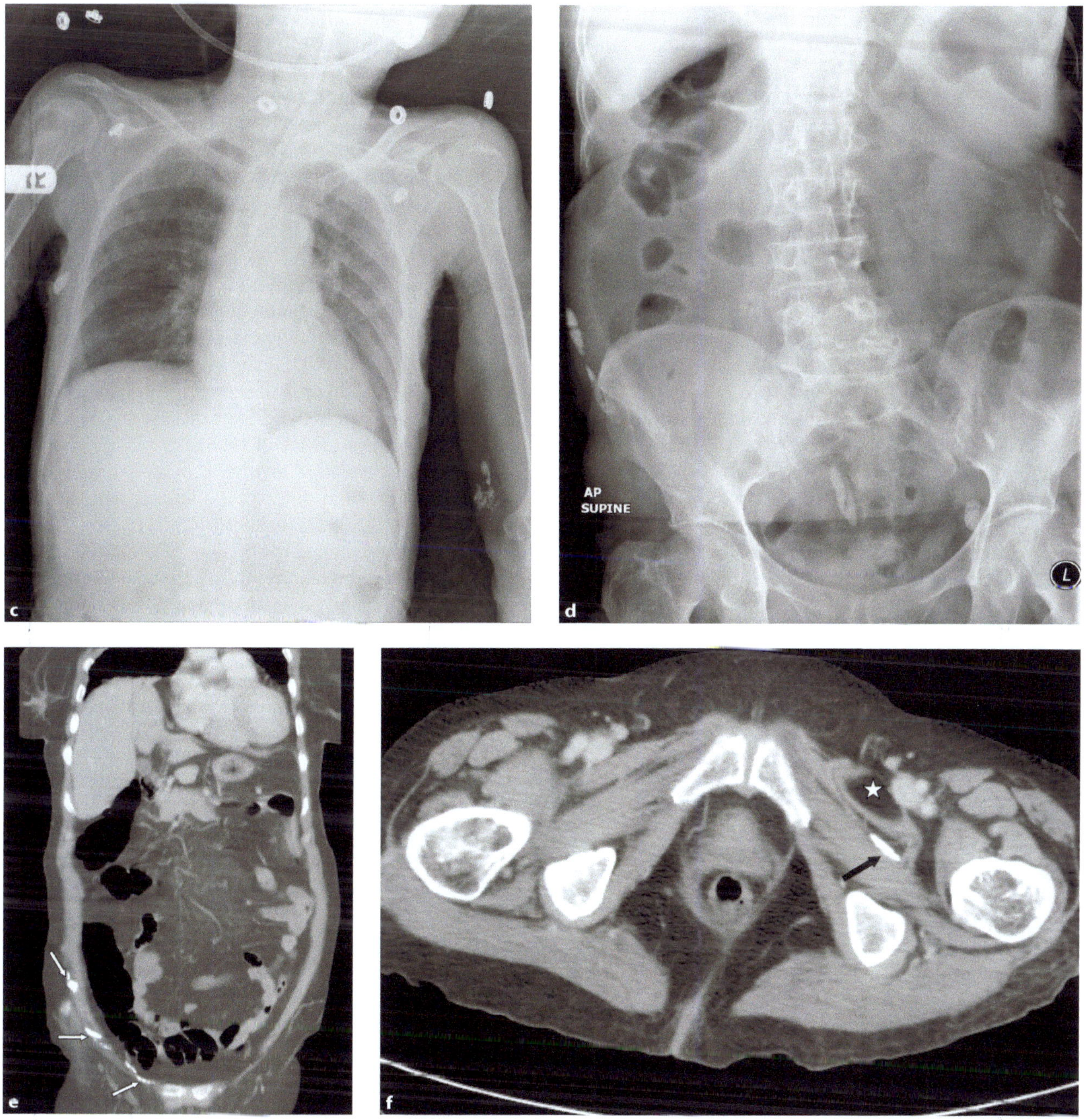

Fig. 7.8 *(continued)* Calcified Guinea worms in various part of the body. **d** Abdominal radiograph of an adult woman showing multiple calcified worms in the left loin, the lateral wall of the right iliac fossa, left buttock, and two more worms overlapping the pelvis. **e** Coronal reconstruction of a CT scan of the abdomen showing long, but interrupted Guinea worm calcification (*arrows*) over the right inguinal ligament. **f** Axial CT scan of an adult man who had a lipoma seen on ultrasound, but a radiograph demonstrated overlying calcification. This raised some suspicion. CT scan demonstrated the intramuscular location of benign lipoma (*star*) within the adductor brevis muscle with a separate calcified Guinea worm (*arrow*) in the adductor magnus muscle sheath (Courtesy of Dr. M. El Mutairi, Riyadh Military Hospital, Riyadh, Saudi Arabia)

tid disease was reported from the Turkana at the border junction between Kenya, Ethiopia, and Sudan (Nelson 1990). The relative incidence of soft tissue hydatid disease varied from 0.8 to 2.3% of cases and bone hydatid varied from 0.8 to 4% of cases (Pedrosa et al. 2000; Polat et al. 2003). Hydatid cysts are uncommon in muscles, even in endemic zones (Mseddi et al. 2005). The spine is involved in 1% of all cases of hydatid disease, but is the main bone in the body that is involved (Kahilogullari et al. 2005).

Hydatid muscle disease carries a better outcome, while bone lesions are likely to recur postoperatively (Arazi et al. 2005). The disease is usually solitary, but multiple bone involvement has been reported (Karray et al. 1992). Bone and soft tissue hydatid are initially asymptomatic (Kalinova et al. 2005). Patients may present at an advanced stage. Hydatid disease can mimic other bone cysts, tuberculosis, fibrous dysplasia, osteochondroma or other neoplastic conditions (Fig. 7.9a–d). In endemic regions, hydatid cyst should be excluded if a tumor is detected in any part of the body (Kazakos et al. 2005).

Sites of bone involvement are summarized in (Table 7.4). As mentioned above, the spine is the commonest site. Diagnosis of spinal hydatid is challenging. Surgical excision is difficult as it tends to recur. Mortality and morbidity are high (Prabhakar et al. 2005). Hydatid bone cysts may not be spherical like liver cysts for two reasons. First, bone is rigid, and second, there is no pericyst formation (Fig. 7.10). This allows proliferation along the lines of least resistance. With time the parasites destroy the bone trabeculae and cortex (Pedrosa et al. 2000). Intraosseous hydatid cysts do not usually calcify. The disease tends to spare the intervertebral discs, which helps differentiation from tuberculosis (Fig. 7.10a). In long bones a cyst may be seen on radiographs. A honeycomb shape is common, but not pathognomonic and could be due to a variety of lesions (Fig. 7.9a). Pathologic fracture may be the first presentation (Fig. 7.10b). Healing may end with deformities (Fig. 7.10c). Indirect inflammatory polyarthritis has been described with hydatid liver disease in the absence of bone or joint cysts (McGill 1995).

Hydatid disease may involve the skull bones. Plain skull radiographs may show cystic lesions with sclerotic margins (Fig. 7.11a). CT is useful for assessing the size and extent of bone expansion (Fig. 7.11b). MRI depicts cyst contents and the relation to soft tissue planes, neurovascular bundles, and adjacent organs (Fig. 7.11c).

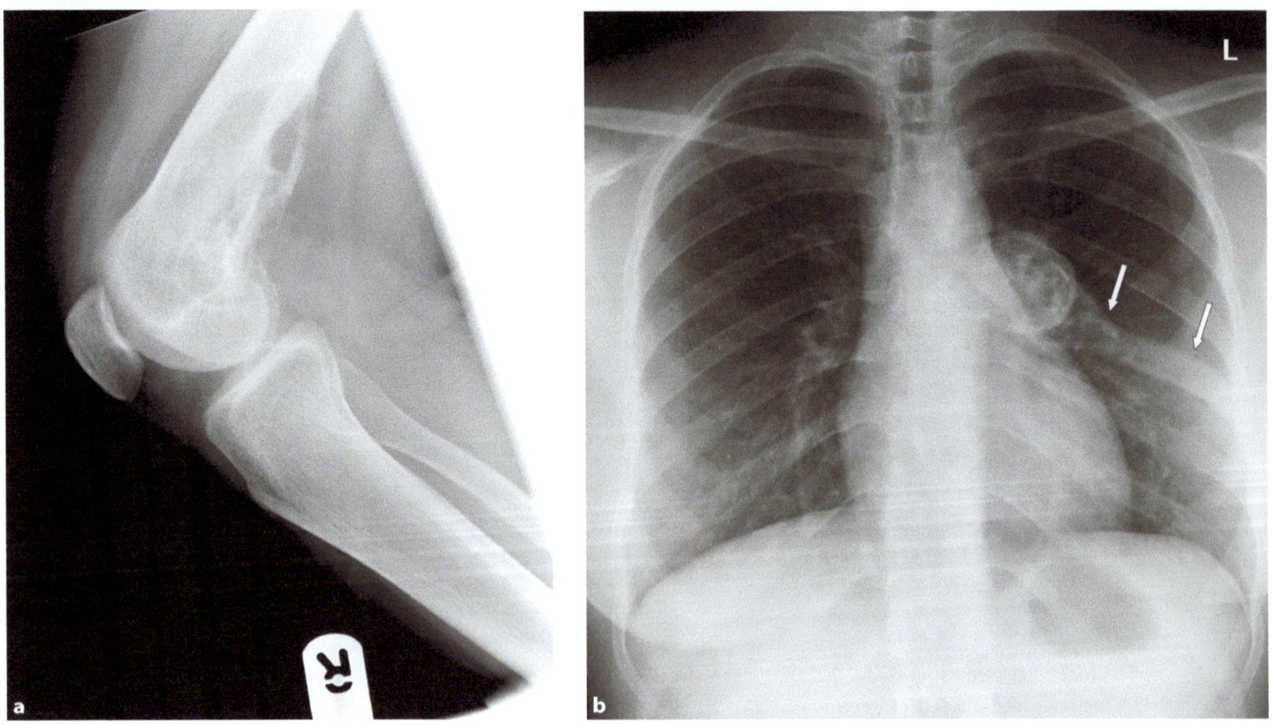

Fig. 7.9 Differential diagnosis of hydatid bone disease. **a** Plain radiograph of a honeycomb cystic bone lesion in the lower femur of a young man due to hydatid disease. The differential diagnosis includes fibrous dysplasia, aneurysmal bone cyst, brown tumors, other benign tumors and cysts, and expansile bone metastasis from renal cell carcinoma. **b** Frontal chest radiograph of an adult woman showing a round, dense, cyst-like calcified lesion. Lung hydatid cysts do not calcify except for faintly in the compressed surrounding lung tissue. This lesion was actually in the rib and the transverse process of a dorsal vertebra. Note: sclerosis of the posterior end of the left seventh rib (*arrows*). **c–f** *see next page*

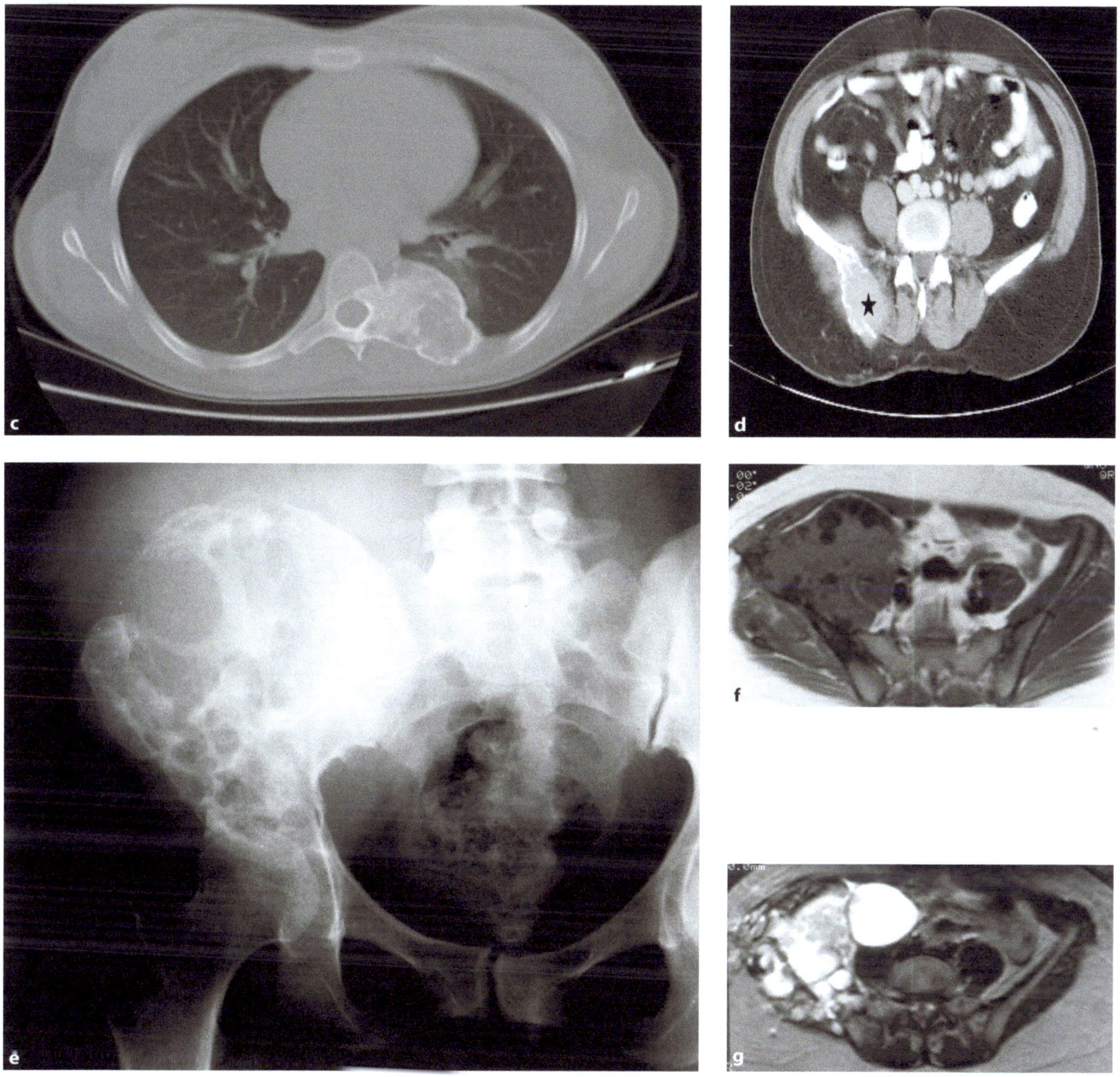

Fig. 7.9 *(continued)* Differential diagnosis of hydatid bone disease. **c** Bone setting of axial CT scan for the patient in **b** showing expansile costotransverse cystic lesion. Besides hydatid disease, the possibilities include osteochondroma and fibrous dysplasia. **d** Axial CT scan of an adult man showing an expansile cystic lesion (*star*) in the right iliac crest causing pressure erosion of the inner cortex. Besides hydatid cyst, the differential diagnosis should include hemophilic pseudotumor, plasmacytoma, and metastasis. **e–g** Plain radiograph of the pelvis (**e**) and MRI of the pelvis, T1-weighted (**f**) and T2-weighted (**g**) images of a large hydatid involving the right iliac bone. Note the advantage of MRI in the demonstration of the cystic nature of the lesion and the true extent of the intrapelvic soft tissue component of the hydatid cyst

Table 7.4 Sites of bone involvement in hydatid disease (Polat et al. 2003)

Site	Percentage
Spine	35
Pelvis	21
Femur	16
Tibia	10
Ribs	6
Skull	4
Scapula	4
Humerus	2
Fibula	2

7.7.2 Cysticercosis

Cysticercosis is the larval stage of the pork tapeworm, which was initially thought to be a separate parasite. Cysticercosis is transmitted to humans via the fecal–oral route (Evans et al. 2000). Usually, humans acquire the disease by eating infected undercooked pork meat. However, even strict vegetarians, Muslims, and orthodox Jews can acquire the infection by consuming vegetables or water contaminated with human feces containing the eggs of *Taenia solium* (Horton 1996). Humans can act as a definitive host when they eat undercooked pork meat or as an intermediate host when they ingest water or vegetables contaminated by feces containing eggs. The disease is endemic in Mexico, India, and South Africa. In swine it lodges in voluntary muscles, while in humans it tends to lodge in the central nervous system and to a lesser extent in the muscles and eyes. Other rare sites include the

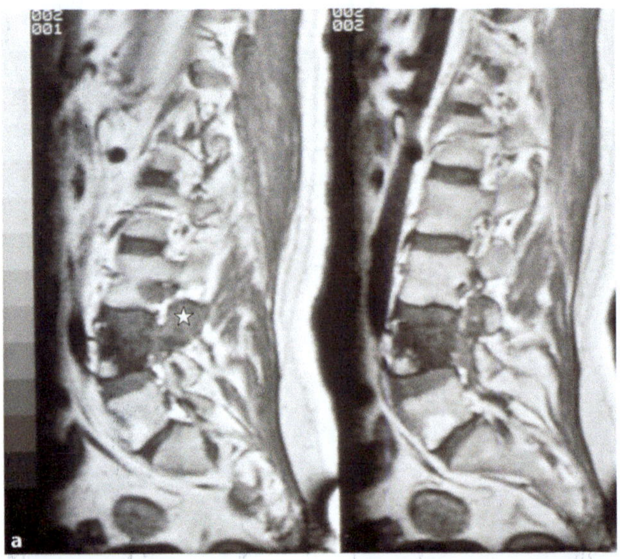

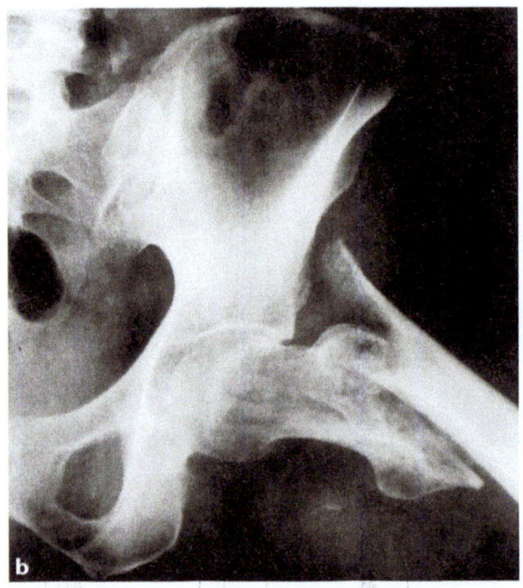

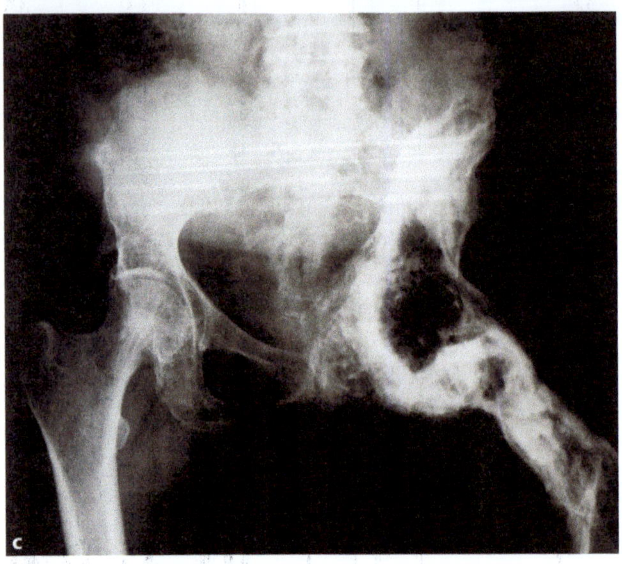

Fig. 7.10 Hydatid bone disease (Abd El Bagi et al. 1999). **a** Sagittal T1-weighted MR images of hydatid disease of the lumbar spine showing involvement of the L4 vertebral body extending into the appendages (*star*), but the disc is spared. This excludes causes of infective spondylitis like tuberculosis and *Brucella*. Note the lack of calcification or sharp demarcation, unlike hydatid disease of long bone. **b** Plain radiograph in a young man who presented with subtrochanteric pathologic fracture of the left femur due to underlying hydatid disease. **c** Hydatid disease of the left hemipelvis and left femur with distortion and deformity due to healed pathologic fractures, cysts, osteosclerosis and bony ankylosis across the left hip

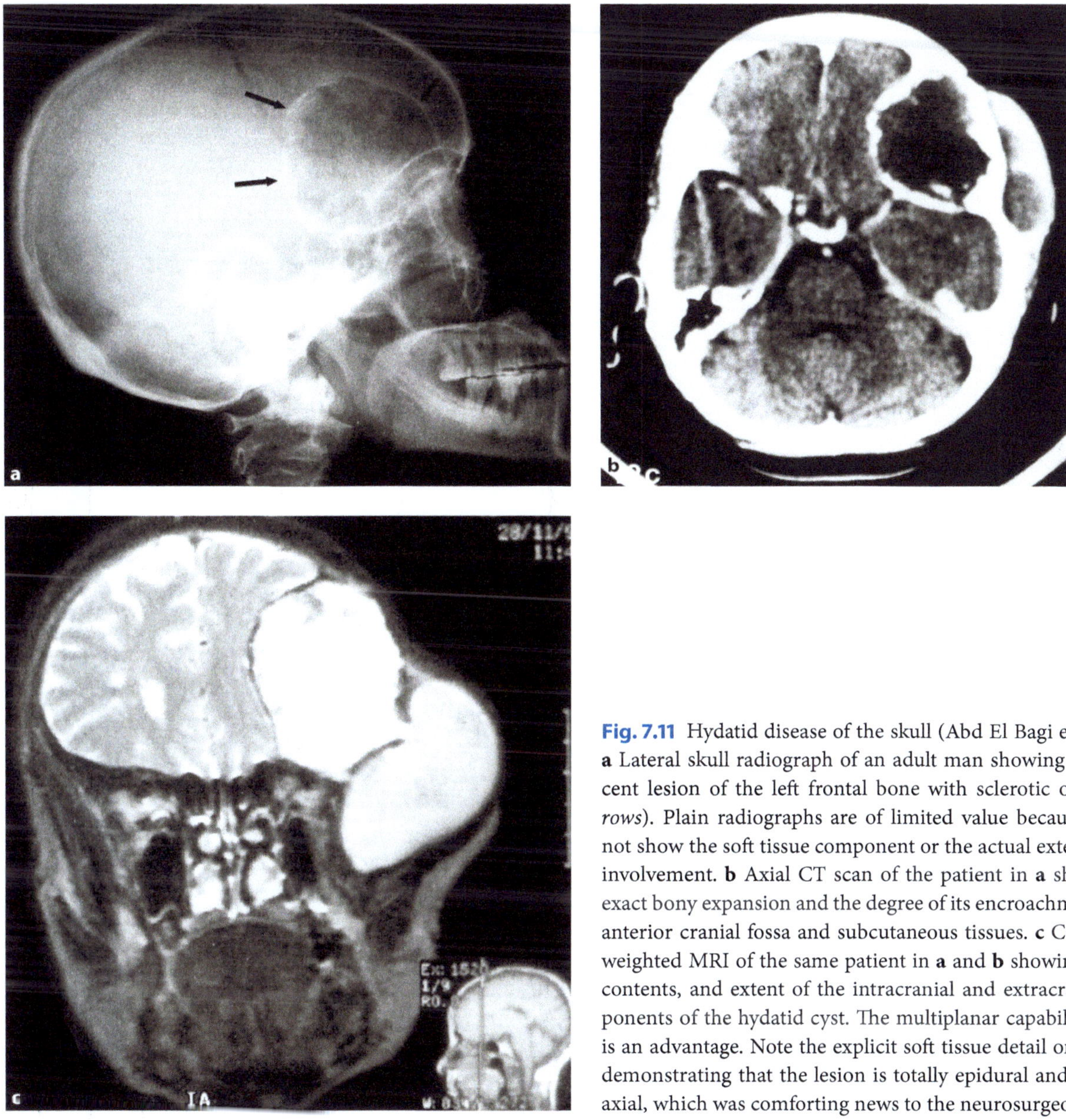

Fig. 7.11 Hydatid disease of the skull (Abd El Bagi et al. 1999). **a** Lateral skull radiograph of an adult man showing a large lucent lesion of the left frontal bone with sclerotic outline (*arrows*). Plain radiographs are of limited value because they do not show the soft tissue component or the actual extent of bone involvement. **b** Axial CT scan of the patient in **a** showing the exact bony expansion and the degree of its encroachment on the anterior cranial fossa and subcutaneous tissues. **c** Coronal T2-weighted MRI of the same patient in **a** and **b** showing the size, contents, and extent of the intracranial and extracranial components of the hydatid cyst. The multiplanar capability of MRI is an advantage. Note the explicit soft tissue detail on the MRI, demonstrating that the lesion is totally epidural and not intra-axial, which was comforting news to the neurosurgeon

tongue, lungs, heart, and breast (Ergen et al. 2005). It is the commonest parasite of the central nervous system and the eyes. Unlike strongyloidiasis, the disease is not more prevalent in patients with AIDS (Castillo 2004).

In the muscles, cysticerci may calcify (Fig. 7.12) and become asymptomatic, causing a diagnostic dilemma (Jankharia et al. 2005). Perhaps this is why the parasite is not commonly reported in the soft tissues (Mani et al. 2001). Concomitant cerebral and muscular locations of cysticercosis are nearly always simultaneous; therefore, a combined search by brain CT and limb radiography or even CT should be performed in either situation (Ky et al. 2000). Subcutaneous involvement was reported in 17–78.5% of cases of neurocysticercosis, depending on geographic location (Dixon and Lipscomb 1961). Cysticercosis may present in many forms (Rahalkar et al. 2000). Ultrasound can demonstrate an intramuscular or subcutaneous cyst or calcific nodule, which could be single or multiple with up to 1,000 per patient. The cyst represents the cysticercus vesicle containing the characteristic invaginated scolex (Fig. 7.13). The size of the cyst is about 10 mm. Identification of the scolex helps to differentiate the disease from gnathostomiasis and sparganosis in endemic areas. An inflammatory reaction could be demonstrated using color Doppler techniques (Mani et al. 2001). Peculiarly, the live cysticerci evade the immunoreaction of the body. However, during the death of the larva, the leakage of fluid from the cyst may trigger

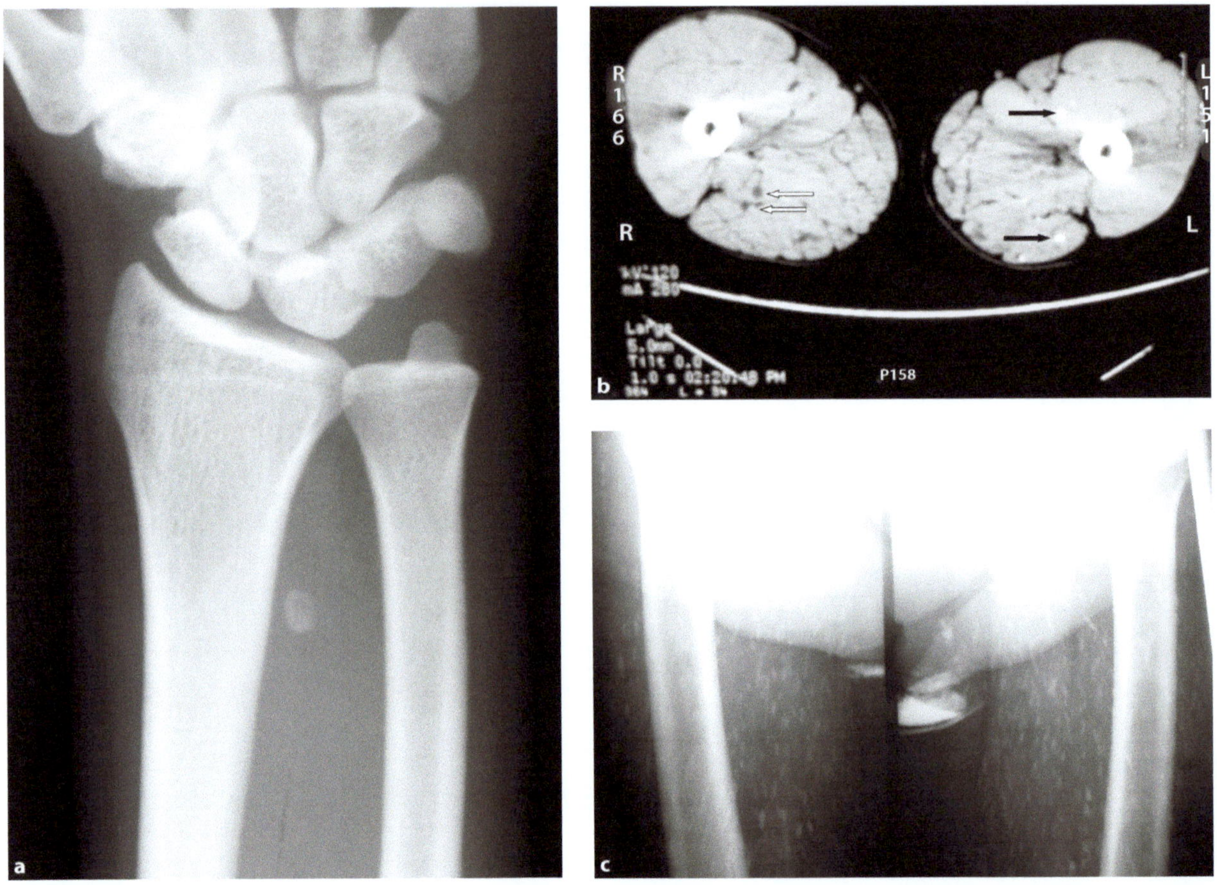

Fig. 7.12 Cysticercosis. **a** Plain radiograph of an adult patient showing solitary calcified cysticercosis larva in the muscles of the forearm. **b** Axial CT scan of the mid-thigh in an adult man showing multiple calcified cysticerci (*black arrows*) in the left thigh with bilateral intramuscular noncalcified cysticerci (*white arrows*) (Courtesy of Dr. F. El Zein, Department of Infectious Diseases, Riyadh Military Hospital, Riyadh, Saudi Arabia). **c** Cysticercosis of the lower limb muscles

an inflammatory response, leading to one of four clinical forms: the myalgic form, the myopathic form, the nodular mass-like lesion, or the pseudohypertrophic type (Evans et al. 2000; Mani et al. 2001). The finding of diffuse millet seed elliptical calcifications in the subcutaneous tissues and muscles is pathognomonic of cysticercosis. In the brain, CT or MRI shows small ring-enhancing active lesions or calcified inactive lesions. MRI can show the lesions and any surrounding edema or inflammatory reaction much more elaborately than CT (Ergen et al. 2005).

7.8 Helminths (Trematodes) – Schistosomiasis

Schistosomiasis can involve almost any organ; however, involvement of soft tissues is rare. Ectopic granulomatous schistosomiasis of the breast has been radiologically described on routine screening mammography. The disease appears to be difficult to discriminate from breast cancer before biopsy (Gorman et al. 1992).

7.9 Arthropods – Pentastomiasis/ Porocephalosis

Pentastomiasis is a rare zoonotic disease caused by *Armillifer armillatus*. It is almost always asymptomatic, and is detected incidentally on radiographs of the abdomen and localized in the hepatic area or peritoneum. The encysted dead parasites appear as comma-shaped or horseshoe-like calcifications. The disease is encountered in snake-eating Africans (Tiendrebeogo et al. 1982). Occasionally, it may be a cause of muscle parasitism.

7.10 Conclusion

Musculoskeletal parasites are rare compared with gastrointestinal parasites, which themselves may settle in one form inside the MSK system. In tropical areas they are relatively common. Global warming and the excess bidirectional movement of people increase the exposure to

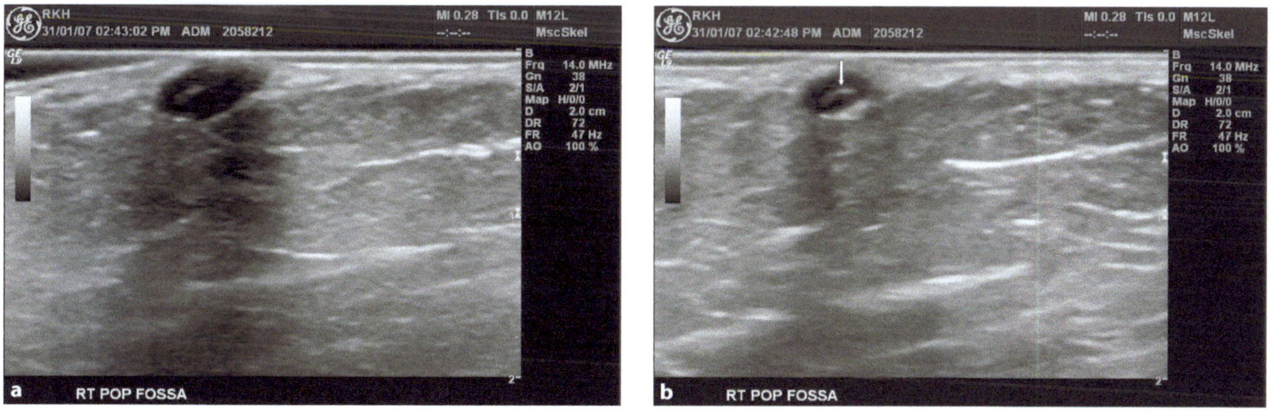

Fig. 7.13 Cysticercosis. **a** Ultrasound scan of the subcutaneous tissues of the right popliteal fossa in a woman showing an 8-mm oval hypoechoic lesion that is not transonic. This could be a larva in the process of impending calcification. **b** Visible intracystic structure (*small arrow*) suggestive of a dead scolex

and the spread of parasites in general. Studying MSKP demonstrates so many peculiarities. Parasitic rheumatism is an important clinical presentation of parasites that is often overlooked. MSKP should be considered in the differential diagnosis of any bone cyst or soft tissue tumor in tropical countries or immigrants. Eradication programs have proved successful and should be maintained and expanded to encompass all MSKP (Box 7.4). Plain radiographs, which are available where MSKP are prevalent, are of paramount importance in detecting MSKP. Ultrasound, CT, and MRI provide a confident diagnosis where available.

Box 7.4 The challenge of controlling musculoskeletal parasites (MSKP)

- Clean drinking water
- Health education
- C max Community participation
- Annual mass treatment
- Monitor evaluation
- Avoid sleeping on tropical ground
- Avoid infected beaches
- Wise intimacy with pets
- Avoid global warming

References

Abd El Bagi M, Sammak B, Al Shahed M, et al. (1999) Rare bone infections "excluding the spine". Eur Radiol 9:1078–1087

Adebajo A (1996) Rheumatic manifestations of tropical diseases. Curr Opin Rheumatol 8:85–89

Ancelle T, De Bruyne A, Poisson D, et al. (2005) Outbreak of trichinellosis due to consumption of bear meat from Canada and France. Euro Surveill 10(10):E051013.3

Andrade C, Alava T, De Palacio I, et al. (2001) Prevalence and intensity of soil-transmitted helminthiasis in the city Portoviejo (Ecuador). Mem Inst Oswaldo Cruz 96(8):1075–1079

Ansart S, Perez L, Jaureguiberry S, et al. (2007) Spectrum of dermatoses in 165 travelers returning from the tropics with skin diseases. Am J Trop Med Hyg 76(1):184–186

Arazi M, Erikoglu M, Odev K, et al. (2005) Primary echinococcus infestation of the bone and muscles. Clin Orthop Relat Res 432:234–24.

Asaolu S, Holland C, Jegede J, et al. (1992) The prevalence and intensity of soil-transmitted helminthiases in rural communities in Southern Nigeria. Ann Trop Med Parasitol 86(3):279–287

Bassiouni M, Kamel M (1984) Bilharzial arthropathy. Ann Rheum Dis 43:806–809

Beggs I (1985) The radiology of hydatid disease. AJR Am J Roentgenol 145:639–648

Ben M'Rad S, Mathlouthi A, Merai S, et al. (1998). Multiple hydatid cysts of the thigh: the role of magnetic resonance imaging. J Radiol 79(9):877–879

Bouchaud O, Houze S, Schiemann R, et al. (2000) Cutaneous larva migrans in travelers. A prospective study with assessment of therapy with ivermectin. Clin Infect Dis 31(2):493–498

Boussinesq M (2006) Loiasis. Ann Trop Med Parasitol 100(8):715–731

Case T, Witte C, Witte M, et al. (1992) Magnetic resonance imaging in human lymphedema: comparison with lymphangioscintigraphy. Magn Reson Imaging 10:549–558

Castillo M (2004) Imaging of neurocysticercosis. Semin Roentgenol 39(4):465–473

Cho J-H, Lee K-B, Yong T-S, Kim B-S, Park H-B, Ryn K-N, Park J-M, Lee S-Y, Suh J-S (2000) Subcutaneous and musculoskeletal sparganosis: imaging characteristics and pathologic correlation. Skelet Radiol 29:402–408

Chopra R, Panhotra B, Al-Marzooq Y, Al-Mulhim A (2004) Subcutaneous dirofilariasis caused by *Dirofilaria repens.* Saudi Med J 25(11):1694–1696

Davies H, Sakuls P, Keystone J, et al. (1993) Creeping eruption. Arch Dermatol 129:587–591

Dixon H, Lipscomb F (1961) Cysticercosis: an analysis and follow up of 450 cases. Medical Research Council Special Reports Series (London) 196(299):1

Doury P (1990) Is there a role for parasites in the etiology of inflammatory rheumatism? Bull Acad Natl Med 174(6):743–751

Doury P, Pattin S, Dienot B, et al. (1977) Parasitic rheumatism. Sem Hop 53(22–23):1359–1363

Duewell S, Hagspiel K, Zuber J (1992) Swollen lower extremity: role of MR imaging. Radiology 184(1):227–231

Elliot D, Tolle S, Goldberg L, et al. (1985) Pet-associated illness. N Engl J Med 313:985–995

Ergen F, Turkbey V, Kerimoglu U, et al. (2005) Solitary cysticercosis in the intermuscular area of the thigh. J Comput Assist Tomogr 29:260–263

Evans C, Garcia H, Gilman R (2000) Cysticercosis. In: Strickland G (ed) Hunter's tropical medicine, 8th edn. Saunders, Philadelphia, p 862

Flores A, Esteban J, Angles R, et al. (2001) Soil-transmitted helminth infections at very high altitude in Bolivia. Trans R Soc Trop Med Hyg 95(3):272–277

Gabrielli A, Ramsan M, Naumann C, et al. (2005) Soil-transmitted helminths and haemoglobin status among Afghan children in World Food Programme assisted schools. J Helminthol 79(4):381–384

Gharbi HA, Hassine W, Brauner MW, Dupuch K (1981) Ultrasound examination of the hydatic liver. Radiology 139:459–463

Gilles H (1995) Trichuriasis. In: Cook G (ed) Masons tropical diseases, 20th edn. Saunders, London, pp 1372–1374

Gillespie SH (2004) Cutaneous larva migrans. Curr Infect Dis Rep 6(1):50–53

Gorman JD, Champaign JL, Sumida FK, Canavan L (1992) Schistosomiasis involving the breast. Radiology 185(2):423–424

Greenaway C (2004) Dracunculiasis (guinea worm disease). CMAJ 170(4):495–500

Greenwood B (1968) Guinea worm arthritis of knee joint. Br Med J 1:314

Helmy MM, Al Mathal IM (2003) Human infection with *Onchocerca volvulus* in Asir District (Saudi Arabia). J Egypt Soc Parasitol 33(2):385–390

Hira PR, Madda JP, Al-Shamali MA, Eberhard ML (1994) Dirofilariasis in Kuwait: first report of human infection due to *Dirofilaria repens* in the Arabian Gulf. Am J Trop Med Hyg 51:590–592

Holcombe C, Hassan S (1991) Major limb amputation in Northern Nigeria. Br J Surg 68(7):885–886

Horton J (1996) Biology of tapeworm disease [letter]. Lancet 348:481

Hotez P, Narasimhan S, Haggerty J, et al. (1992) Hyaluronidase from infective Ancylostoma hookworm larvae and its possible function as a virulence factor in tissue invasion and in cutaneous larva migrans. Infect Immun 60:1018–1023

Jaksche A, Wessels L, Martin S, et al. (2004) Ocular involvement in systemic Loa-Loa filariasis. Case report and review of the literature. Ophthalmologe 101(9):931–934

Jankharia B, Chavhan G, Krishnan P, et al. (2005) MRI and ultrasound in solitary muscular and soft tissue cysticercosis. Skeletal Radiol 34(11):722–726

Jelinek T, Maiwald H, Norhdurft H, et al. (1994) Cutaneous larva migrans in travelers: synopsis of histories, symptoms and treatment of 98 patients. Clin Infect Dis 19:1062–1066

Kaewpitoon N, Kaewpitoon J, Philasri C, et al. (2006) Trichinosis: epidemiology in Thailand. World J Gastroenterol 12(40):6440–6445

Kahilogullari G, Tuna H, Aydin Z, et al. (2005) Primary intradural extramedullary hydatid cyst. Am J Med Sci 329(4):202–204

Kalinova K, Proichev V, Stefanova P, Tokmakova K, Poriazova E (2005) Hydatid bone disease: a case report and review of the literature. J Orthop Surg (Hong Kong) 13(3):323–325

Karray S, Zlitni M, Karray M, et al. (1993) Extensive vertebral hydatidosis. A study. Acta Orthop Belg 59(1):100–105

Kazakos C, Galanis V, Verettas D, et al. (2005) Primary hydatid disease in femoral muscles. J Int Med Res 33(6):703–706

Kienast A, Bialek R, Hoeger P (2007) Cutaneous larva migrans in northern Germany. Eur J Pediatr 10

Kim J-R, Lee J-M (2001) A case of intramuscular sparganosis in the sartorius muscle. J Korean Med Sci 16:378–380

Ky H, Van Chap N (2000) Radioclinical aspects of cerebral and muscular cysticercosis: 20 cases. J Neuroradiol 27(4):264–266

Lewall D (1998) Hydatid disease: biology, pathology, imaging and classification. Clin Radiol 53:863–874

McGill P (1995) Rheumatic syndromes associated with parasites. Baillieres Clin Rheumatol 9(1):201–213

Mani N, Kalra N, Jain M (2001) Sonographic diagnosis of a solitary intramuscular cysticercal cyst. J Clin Ultrasound 29(8):472–475

Markell E, Voge M, John D (1992) Medical parasitology, 7th edn. Saunders, Philadelphia

Marotel M, Cluzan R, Pascot M, et al. (1998) Computerized tomography of 150 cases of lymphedema of the leg. J Radiol 79(11):1373–1378

Moore DA, McCroddan J, Dekumyoy P, Chiodini PL (2003) Gnathostomiasis: an emerging imported disease. Emerg Infect Dis 9(6):647–650

Mseddi M, Mtaoumi M, Dahmene J, et al. (2005) Hydatid cysts in muscles: eleven cases. Rev Chir Orthop Reparatrice Appar Mot 91(3):267–271

Mukhtar M, Khier M, Baraka O, et al. (1998) The burden of Onchocerca volvulus in Sudan. Ann Trop Med Parasitol 92 [Suppl 1]:S129–S131

Nelson G (1990) Microepidemiology: the key to control of parasitic infections. Trans R Soc Trop Med Hyg 84:3–13

Pampiglione S, Fioravanti ML, Rivasi F (2003) Human sparganosis in Italy. APMIS 111:349–354

Pedrosa I, Saiz A, Arrazola J (2000) Hydatid disease: radiologic and pathologic features and complications. Radiographics 20:795–817

Peng S (2002) Rheumatic manifestations of parasitic disease. Semin Arthritis Rheum 31(4):228–247

Pinals R (1994) Polyarthritis and fever. N Eng J Med 330:769–774

Polat P, Kantarci M, Alper F (2003) Hydatid disease from head to toe. Radiographics 23:475–494

Prabhakar M, Acharya A, Modi D, et al. (2005) Spinal hydatid disease: a case series. J Spinal Cord Med 28(5):426–310

Rahalkar M, Shetty D, Kelkar A, et al. (2000) The many faces of cysticercosis. Clin Radiol 55:668–674

Rathi V, Bhargava S, Gupta A, et al. (2006) Filarial dance in a breast mass on colour Doppler imaging. Australas Radiol 50(2):183–185

Sadjjadi S (2006) Present situation of echinococcosis in the Middle East and Arabic North Africa. Parasitol Int 55: S197–S202

Sakai S, Shiday, Takahashi, et al. (2006) Pulmonary lesions associated with visceral larva migrans due to Ascaris suum or Toxocara canis: imaging of six cases. AJR Am J Roentgenol 186(6):1697–1702

Shelley S, Manokaran G, Indirani M, et al. (2006) Lymphoscintigraphy as a diagnostic tool in patients with lymphedema of filarial origin – an Indian Study. Lymphology 39(2):69–75

Siddiqui M, al-Khawajah M (1991) The black disease of Arabia, Sowda-onchocerciasis. New findings. Int J Dermatol 30(2):130–133

Szuba A, Rockson S (1998) Lymphedema: classification, diagnosis and therapy. Vasc Med 3(2):145–156

Thomas A (1986) Radiological manifestations of parasitic disease. Br J Hosp Med 35(5):303–311

Thylefors B, Alleman M (2006) Towards the elimination of onchocerciasis. Ann Trop Med Parasitol 100(8):733–746

Tiendrebeogo H, Levy D, Schmidt D (1982) Human pentastomiasis in Abidjan. A report on 29 cases. Rev Fr Mal Respir 10(5):351–358

WHO Expert Committee on Filariasis (1984) Fourth Report Lymphatic Filariasis. Technical report series 702. World Health Organization, Geneva

Widjana D, Sutisna P (2000) Prevalence of soil-transmitted helminth infections in the rural population of Bali, Indonesia. Southeast Asian J Trop Med Public Health 31(3):454–459

Woodruff A (1984) Tropical medicine, 2nd edn. Longman, White Plains

Xu L, Yu S, Jiang Z, et al. (1995) Soil-transmitted helminthiases: nationwide survey in China. Bull World Health Organ 73(4):507–513

Zeyrek F, Zeyrek C (2006) Allergic diseases and parasitosis. Turkie Parazitol Derg 30(2):135–140

Chapter 8

Conclusions

Maurice C. Haddad

Parasitic diseases are common worldwide. The term "tropical diseases" is a misnomer, because parasitoses are present in all parts of the world and are not only confined to tropical or subtropical areas. Zoonosis is another term that can be used to describe a disease of animals that may be transmitted to humans. Some of the parasitic diseases are prevalent in countries with endemic regions, and may not or only sporadically exist as isolated cases in other developed and developing non-endemic countries. Even in non-endemic regions the disease may be encountered in immigrants, but it can also be imported by civilian travelers and military individuals who have lived in or traveled to endemic areas. For example, during 1990–1991 and 2002–2004 the military operations "Desert shield/Desert storm" and "Operation Enduring Freedom" resulted in the deployment of US troops to the Persian Gulf, Afghanistan, and Iraq. After their return to the US, a number of soldiers developed viscerotropic or cutaneous leishmaniasis (McGill et al. 1993; Halsey et al. 2004; Elston and Miller 2004).

In general, zoonoses affect low socio-economic classes or debilitated individuals with poor sanitation or hygiene. They are usually accidentally acquired either by ingesting contaminated food or drinking water, or by skin bite with penetration to various organs in the body, so-called mouth and foot diseases. Intestinal parasitism is the commonest, but it has been on the decline over the past decades because of the liberal use of antiparasitic drugs in some countries. However, there is a worldwide resurgence of parasitic diseases in the increasing number of immunosuppressed individuals. Most infected people are asymptomatic, while a minority of patients with splenectomy, immunosuppression (AIDS, transplant, and cancer patients) or high worm load develop symptomatic clinical disease. Several parasites can cause multisystem involvement. A high index of clinical suspicion of parasitic disease should be raised in patients living in endemic areas or returning from travel to endemic regions, patients with a history of eating raw or undercooked food, and those presenting with fever and peripheral blood eosinophilia or anemia. The diagnosis may be difficult to establish because the parasite or its eggs are seldom present in the stool examination as egg production may be intermittent so repeated stool specimens are usually required. Combining disease-specific serologic tests increases the sensitivity for the serodiagnosis of parasitic diseases, and eliminates the problem of cross-reactivity. Some of the imaging features are characteristic and diagnostic; however, the imaging findings are often nonspecific and mistaken for other inflammatory or neoplastic diseases. Nevertheless, imaging plays an important role in the detection of atypical abnormalities and allows for an image-guided biopsy in the presence of other negative laboratory tests. The reaction of host tissue to parasitic injury is variable, manifesting by an inflammatory eosinophilic granulomatous reaction leading to granuloma formation or nodules with or without fibrosis, abscesses, or cyst formation. Parasitic diseases are often treatable and curable. Some important and relevant epidemiological, pathological, clinical, laboratory, and characteristic imaging findings are summarized in Tables 8.1–8.5.

References

Elston DM, Miller SD (2004) Leishmaniasis acquired in the Iraqi Theater Operations. Cutis 74(4):253–255

Halsey ES, Bryce LM, Wortmann GW, Weina PJ, Ryan JR, De Witt CC (2004) Visceral leishmaniasis in a soldier returning from Operation Enduring Freedom. Mil Med 169(9):699–701

Magill AJ, Grogl M, Gasser RA Jr, Sun W, Oster CN (1993) Visceral infection caused by *Leishmania tropica* in veterans of Operation Desert Storm. N Engl J Med 328(19):1383–1387

Table 8.1 Protozoa

Parasite species	Geographical distribution	Organs affected	Pathology	Clinical	Laboratory	Imaging	Diagnosis
Plasmodium falciparum *P. vivax* *P. ovale* *P. malariae*	Africa, South America, South Asia	Lungs Liver and spleen	ARDS Hepatitis/malarial hepatopathy	Fever HSM ± LNs	Anemia	ARDS HSM	Identification of parasite within RBCs on a thin blood smear
		Brain	Edema and infarct				
		Kidney		Kidney failure			
Entamoeba histolytica	Worldwide	Colon	Colitis	Dysentery		Thickened conical cecum	Cysts in stools
		Liver	Abscess	RUQ pain ± fever	Leukocytosis	Abscess	Serology FNA yield odorless reddish-brown pus, i.e., "anchovy paste" No growth on culture, i.e., sterile culture
		CNS	Meningoencephalitis or abscess	Granulomatous skin lesions preceding neurological symptoms Headache and fever		Punctate nodular or ring-enhancing lesions and edema	
Toxoplasma gondii	Worldwide	Eye and brain	Chorioretinitis Encephalitis	Congenital Acquired disseminated in immunosuppressed Fever ± cervical LNs		Microcephaly Hydrocephalus Periventricular calcifications Ring-enhancing microabscesses	Serology Identification of intracellular parasite in tissue biopsy
		Lungs Liver and spleen	Pneumonia Hepatitis	HSM		Nonspecific HSM	

ARDS acute respiratory distress syndrome, *HSM* hepatosplenomegaly, *LNs* lymph nodes, *RBCs* red blood cells, *RUQ* right upper quadrant, *FNA* fine needle aspiration, *CNS* central nervous system, *PCR* polymerase chain reaction, *RES* reticuloendothelial system

Table 8.1 *(continued)* Protozoa

Parasite species	Geographical distribution	Organs affected	Pathology	Clinical	Laboratory	Imaging	Diagnosis
Trypanosoma cruzi	Central and South America	Esophagus and colon	Destruction of myenteric nerve plexuses			"Chagasic achalasia," i.e., megaesophagus and megacolon	Detection of parasite or antibodies to the parasite in host blood Culture and xenodiagnosis PCR techniques
		Heart	Myocarditis			Cardiomegaly	
		Eye and brain	Meningoencephalitis	"Romana's sign," i.e., unilateral palpebral edema		Ring-enhancing lesions in the white matter	
T. gambiense *T. brucei rhodesiense*	Africa			"African sleeping sickness"		Edema, petechial hemorrhage	
Leishmania infantum *L. tropica* *L. donovani* *L. chagasi*	Mediterranean basin, Middle East, and South America	Liver and spleen RES	Hepatitis	Kala-azar, i.e., visceral leishmaniasis Fever, HSM, LNs	Neutropenia Thrombocytopenia	HSM LNs	Identification of intracellular amastigote in splenic or bone marrow aspirate
Giardia lamblia	Worldwide	Jejunum	Mucosal inflammation	Diarrhea	Macrocytic anemia	Malabsorption pattern Thickened mucosal folds and small nodularity	Identification of cysts or trophozoites in stools Serology Jejunal biopsy
Cryptosporidium parvum	Worldwide	Small and large bowel	Necrotizing and sclerosing inflammation	Immunosuppressed, i.e., AIDS and transplant patients Diarrhea		Pneumatosis coli	Isolation of organism from stool, bile, and biopsy specimen
		Biliary	AIDS-related cholangiopathy		Cholestatic jaundice	Acalculous cholecystitis Sclerosing cholangitis	

ARDS acute respiratory distress syndrome, *HSM* hepatosplenomegaly, *LNs* lymph nodes, *RBCs* red blood cells, *RUQ* right upper quadrant, *FNA* fine needle aspiration, *CNS* central nervous system, *PCR* polymerase chain reaction, *RES* reticuloendothelial system

Table 8.1 *(continued)* Protozoa

Parasite species	Geographical distribution	Organs affected	Pathology	Clinical	Laboratory	Imaging	Diagnosis
Babesia croti	North America and Europe	Liver	Hepatitis	Immunosuppressed and splenectomized patients Malaria-like symptoms, i.e., fever and anemia	Hemolytic anemia	Hepatomegaly	Identification of intraerythrocytic parasite on blood smear
Balantidium coli	Europe	Colon		Dysentery			Colonic endoscopy and biopsy
Trichomonas hominis and *T. vaginalis*	Worldwide	Genitalia	Urethritis	Urethral and vaginal discharge			Microscopy and culture of secretions

ARDS acute respiratory distress syndrome, *HSM* hepatosplenomegaly, *LNs* lymph nodes, *RBCs* red blood cells, *RUQ* right upper quadrant, *FNA* fine needle aspiration, *CNS* central nervous system, *PCR* polymerase chain reaction, *RES* reticuloendothelial system

Table 8.2 Nematodes

Parasite species	Geographical distribution	Organs Affected	Pathology	Clinical	Laboratory	Imaging	Diagnosis
Ascaris lumbricoides	Worldwide	Small bowel		Intestinal obstruction		Elongated filling defects on contrast studies of bowel and biliary tree	Imaging
		Biliary		Cholangitis Jaundice			Retrieval of parasite at ERCP
Ascaris suum	Northern Europe and Far East	Liver	Granulomatous eosinophilic inflammatory lesions	VLM, i.e., Loefler syndrome	Eosinophilia Elevated IgE	Hepatic focal nodular lesions mimicking metastases	Serology Liver biopsy: focal eosinophil necrosis or granulomas
Bayliascaris procyonis	Northern America and Europe	Eye	Chorioretinitis	Ocular larva migrans/blindness	Eosinophilia		Immunologic tests
		Brain	Encephalitis	Neural larva migrans Fever		Periventricular white matter lesions	Identification of larvae in brain biopsy
Toxocara catis *T. canis*	Worldwide	Eye and CNS	Eosinophilic meningoencephalitis/myelitis	Ocular and neural larva migrans	Eosinophilia	Cortical and subcortical white matter enhancing lesions	Serology
		Lungs and liver	Eosinophilic granulomatous inflammatory lesions	VLM		Numerous focal small nodular lesions	Tissue biopsy: focal eosinophil necrosis or granulomas
Strongyloides stercoralis	Worldwide	Small and large bowel	Submucosa and lamina propria inflammatory lesions		Eosinophilia	Loss of mucosal pattern	Serology Identification of alive rhabditiform larvae in intestinal aspirate or biopsy and stool examination
		Lungs and liver	Focal inflammatory eosinophilic lesions	Rare extraintestinal hyperinfection in immunosuppressed patients		Hepatomegaly with focal nodular lesions mimicking metastases Pneumonitis	

Table 8.2 (*continued*) Nematodes

Parasite species	Geographical distribution	Organs Affected	Pathology	Clinical	Laboratory	Imaging	Diagnosis
Gnathostoma spinigerum	Far East	Soft tissues	Subcutaneous inflammation	Creeping eruption	Eosinophilia		Retrieval of parasite from resection of skin swellings
		Abdomen		Acute abdomen			
		CNS	Myeloencephalitis			White matter lesions	
Anisakis marina	South East Asia and Europe	Gastrointestinal tract	Enterocolitis Stomach stricture or submucosal mass	Acute abdomen	Eosinophilia		Endoscopy and biopsy
Enterobius vermicularis	Worldwide	Cecum	Enterocolitis Appendicitis	Perianal itching Acute abdomen			Cellophane tape test
Angiostrongylus costaricensis	South America	Terminal ileum, cecum, appendix, and ascending colon	Bowel ischemia or necrosis	Acute abdomen		Bowel wall thickening with ulcerations Nodular granulomas	Serology Endoscopic biopsy or at surgery
Angiostrongylus cantonensis	South East Asia, Pacific islands	Meninges	Eosinophilic meningitis		Eosinophilia	No brain lesions	CSF examination
Ancylostoma duodenale and Necator americanus	Africa and Mediterranean, America	Small bowel			Anemia	Thickened mucosal folds	Capsule endoscopy and biopsy
		Lungs	Transient pneumonitis	Loeffler-like syndrome	Eosinophilia		Identification of parasite eggs in respiratory, gastric or duodenal secretions or stools
Trichuris trichiura		Cecum and rectum		Dysentery	Anemia	Granular mucosa and small coiled worms	

Table 8.2 (*continued*) Nematodes

Parasite species	Geographical distribution	Organs Affected	Pathology	Clinical	Laboratory	Imaging	Diagnosis
Capillaria philippinensis	South East Asia and Middle East	Small bowel		Diarrhea		Malabsorption pattern	Detection of eggs and larvae in stool samples
Capillaria hepatica	South East Asia and Europe	Liver	Granulomatous inflammation leading to fibrosis	Children with fever and hepatomegaly	Eosinophilia		Liver biopsy: presence of typical intracellular eggs
Trichinella spiralis	Worldwide	Muscles	Myositis	Fever			
		Brain	Infarct Vasculitis Encephalitis			Brain infarction Sinus venous thrombosis	Identify anti-*Trichinella* antibodies in CSF immunologic tests
Wuchereria bancrofti and Brugia malayi	Worldwide	Genitourinary tract	Granulomatous reaction in the lymphatic walls	Chyluria Elephantiasis Hydrocele		Demonstration of pyelolymphatic connections Scrotal "filarial dance" sign Lymphedema	Presence of microfilariae in peripheral blood, chylous urine or hydrocele fluid Serology
	India and South East Asia	Lungs	Eosinophilic pneumonia	Asthma-like syndrome (TPE)	Eosinophilia Elevated IgE serum levels	Reticulonodular infiltrates or military pattern	Lung biopsy: identification of microfilariae
Loa loa	Central Africa	Eye	Ocular swelling	"African eye worm," "Calabar swelling"			
		Subcutaneous tissues and joints		Parasitic rheumatism "Calabar swelling"		Thread-like coil calcifications in the subcutaneous tissues particularly in web spaces of the hand	Imaging

Table 8.2 (*continued*) Nematodes

Parasite species	Geographical distribution	Organs Affected	Pathology	Clinical	Laboratory	Imaging	Diagnosis
Dirofilaria immitis	North America	Lungs	Pulmonary infarct	Hemoptysis	Eosinophilia	Solitary pulmonary nodule, simulating malignancy, i.e., coin lesion	Biopsy: demonstration of fragments of the parasite
Dirofilaria repens	South Asia, Eastern and Southern Europe, and Mediterranean	Subcutaneous tissues	Chronic abscess	Subcutaneous nodule			Biopsy specimen depicting worm in a chronic abscess
Onchocerca volvulus	Africa Middle East South America	Skin	Hyperpigmented lichenified papular lesions	Skin nodules over bony prominences like occiput and iliac crest ("Sowda")			Biopsy of skin nodule
		Eye		"African river blindness"			
Dracunculus medinensis	Sub-Saharan Africa	Subcutaneous tissues and joints		Aggressive joint derangement ("Ibadan knee")		Irregular coiled calcification in subcutaneous tissues of lower limbs and trunk	Imaging
Dioctophyma renale	America, Europe, South East Asia	Kidney	Granulomatous inflammatory and necrotic tissue	Flank pain Worm passage from urethra Hematuria	Anemia	Hyperdense renal cystic lesions mimicking hemorrhagic cysts, and solid renal masses with calcifications mimicking renal cancer	Ring-like structures called Liesegang rings representing eggs of the parasite are identified in the cyst fluid or urine

VLM visceral larva migrans, *ERCP* endoscopic retrograde cholangiopancreatography, *CNS* central nervous system, *CSF* cerebrospinal fluid, *TPE* tropical pulmonary eosinophilia,

RUQ right upper quadrant

Table 8.3 Cestodes

Parasite species	Geographical distribution	Organs affected	Pathology	Clinical	Laboratory	Imaging	Diagnosis
Echinococcus granulosus	Worldwide Rural	All body organs	Cysts	Mass effect symptoms	Eosinophilia	Hepatic cyst with variable appearance depending on type of lesion	Serology and imaging Identification of viable scolices at cyst needle aspirate if serology is negative and imaging not diagnostic
E. multilocularis	Northern Europe and America					Pseudotumoral appearance ± calcifications	
Taenia solium	Africa, South America, and Far East	Muscles	Small cysts, i.e., cysticerci vesicles containing the invaginated scolex	Myopathy		Oval-shaped calcifications arranged in the direction of muscle fibers	Immunologic tests Muscle biopsy
		Brain		Seizures		Small nodular or ring-enhancing active lesions, or calcified inactive lesions depending on stage of disease	
Taenia saginata	Africa, South America, and Far East	Small and large bowel				Ribbon-like structure in the lumen of the bowel	
Taenia multiceps	Mediterranean	Brain	Coenuri cysts	Increased intracranial pressure		Cerebral cysts with a contrast-enhanced peripheral rim ± ventricular obstruction	

Table 8.3 (*continued*) Cestodes

Parasite species	Geographical distribution	Organs affected	Pathology	Clinical	Laboratory	Imaging	Diagnosis
Spirometra mansoni	Far East	Subcutaneous tissues	Larva surrounded by layers of inflammation	Subcutaneous lump		Subcutaneous serpiginous tubular tracts and perilesional edema	Excision biopsy
		Brain	Chronic granulomatous reaction	Seizures Headache		White matter lesions with adjacent cortical atrophy and ex-vacuo ventricular dilatation	Serology and imaging
Diphyllobothrium latum	Northern Europe and America	Small bowel		Intestinal obstruction	Anemia Vitamin B12 deficiency Eosinophilia		Parasite eggs in stools
Hymenolepis nana	Central Europe and South America	Small bowel		Intestinal obstruction	Eosinophilia		Parasite eggs in stools

Table 8.4 Trematodes

Parasite species	Geographical distribution	Organs affected	Pathology	Clinical	Laboratory	Imaging	Diagnosis
Schistosoma mansoni	Middle East, Africa, South America	Descending and sigmoid colon Liver	Acute granulomatous inflammation	Dysentery Pain Fever "Katayama syndrome"	Eosinophilia	Hepatomegaly with periportal inflammation or focal nodular granulomas mimicking metastases Colonic inflammatory changes	Serology Identification of eggs in stool specimens and on rectal or lesional biopsy
			Chronic inflammation "Symmer's periportal fibrosis"	Bloody stools Portal hypertension		Submucosal colonic calcified granulomas Prominent portal tracts due to periportal fibrosis Esophageal varices Splenomegaly Small contracted liver, but smooth regular surface contour	Liver biopsy is usually not needed
Schistosoma japonicum	Far East	Duodenum and jejunum					
		Liver	Septal fibrosis			Irregular surface outline of "turtle-back" liver ± capsular calcifications	

Table 8.4 (*continued*) Trematodes

Parasite species	Geographical distribution	Organs affected	Pathology	Clinical	Laboratory	Imaging	Diagnosis
Schistosoma hematobium	Middle East, Africa, South America	Urinary tract	Granulomatous inflammation	Bloody urine		Striated renal pelvis and ureter due to mucosal edema Submucosal filling defects due to granulomas Dilatation of ureters with deficient peristalsis Ureteral and bladder wall calcifications Squamous cell carcinoma Polypoid lesions	Cystoscopy and biopsy
Fasciola hepatica	Worldwide	Liver	Acute hepatic eosinophilic granulomatous phase, microabscesses, necrosis	RUQ pain and fever	Eosinophilia	Subcapsular lesions best visualized by CT or MR	Serology
		Biliary	Chronic biliary phase with hyperplasia and obstruction	Jaundice Cholangitis		Biliary parasite best visualized by US and ERCP	Identification of fluke eggs at duodenal or bile aspirates Retrieval of fluke at ERCP
Clonorchis sinensis	Far East	Biliary	Intrahepatic pigmented bilirubinate bile duct calculi and cholangitis Cholangiocarcinoma	RUQ pain and fever Recurrent pyogenic cholangitis	Eosinophilia	Intrahepatic bile duct calculi ± obstruction Small intraluminal filling defects due to the presence of flukes	Serology Identification of fluke eggs in duodenal or bile aspirates

Table 8.4 *(continued)* Trematodes

Parasite species	Geographical distribution	Organs affected	Pathology	Clinical	Laboratory	Imaging	Diagnosis
Opisthorchis viverrini	Far East	Biliary	Cystic or saccular intrahepatic biliary ductal dilatation Cholangiocarcinoma	RUQ pain and fever Recurrent pyogenic cholangitis	Eosinophilia	Intrahepatic cystic bile duct dilatation ± calculi	Serology Identification of fluke eggs in duodenal or bile aspirates
Dicrocoelium dendriticum	Worldwide	Biliary	Biliary obstruction	Cholangitis	Eosinophilia	Biliary sludge Gallstones Chronic cholecystitis	Serology Identification of ova in bile aspirates or in stool specimens
Paragonimus westermani	Far East	Lungs	Pleurisy or parenchymal lesions	Chest pain and fever, hemophysis Loeffler-like syndrome	Eosinophilia	Migratory consolidations Thin-walled cysts Calcified granulomas in the chronic stage	Serology Detection of parasite eggs in the sputum, pleural fluid or feces
		Brain	Abscess			Ring-enhancing abscesses surrounded by edema Calcified granulomas in the chronic stage	
Fasciolopsis buski *Metagonimus yokogawai* *Echinostoma ilocanum and E. lindoense*	South East Asia	Proximal small bowel	Ulcerations, necrosis, granulomas, fibrosis	Diarrhea	Anemia Eosinophilia		Identification of characteristic eggs on stool examination
Heterophyes heterophyes	Middle East, North Africa						

RUQ right upper quadrant, *CT* computed tomography, *MR* magnetic resonance, *US* ultrasound, *ERCP* endoscopic retrograde cholangiopancreatography

Table 8.5 Arthropods

Parasite species	Geographical distribution	Organs affected	Pathology	Clinical	Laboratory	Imaging	Diagnosis
Armillifer armillatus	Central and West Africa	Peritoneum	Peritoneal irritation and inflammation	Acute abdomen	Eosinophilia	Peritoneal inflammatory reaction or thickening	Identification of viable worms in the peritoneum at laparotomy for acute abdomen
		Liver	Granulomatous reaction leading to hepatic fibrosis with calcified granulomas	Incidental		Comma or C-shaped calcifications in liver, spleen, peritoneum, and muscles of the trunk not involving the limbs, unlike cysticerci, representing calcified dead larvae	Imaging
Linguatula serrata	Middle East, Southern Europe	Nasopharynx	Nasopharyngeal irritation	"Halzoun" "Marrara"			
		Liver	Abscess Granulomas	RUQ pain and fever	Leukocytosis	Abscess Calcified granuloma	No growth on culture Identification of encysted nymph within pathological specimen
Fannia canicularis	North Africa	Genitourinary tract	Urinary tract infection				Repeated emissions of parasite larvae in urine

RUQ right upper quadrant

Subject Index

MIX
Papier aus verantwortungsvollen Quellen
Paper from responsible sources
FSC® C105338

If you have any concerns about our products,
you can contact us on
ProductSafety@springernature.com

In case Publisher is established outside the EU,
the EU authorized representative is:
Springer Nature Customer Service Center GmbH
Europaplatz 3, 69115 Heidelberg, Germany

Printed by Libri Plureos GmbH
in Hamburg, Germany